PHYSIOTHERAPY in Community Health and Rehabilitation

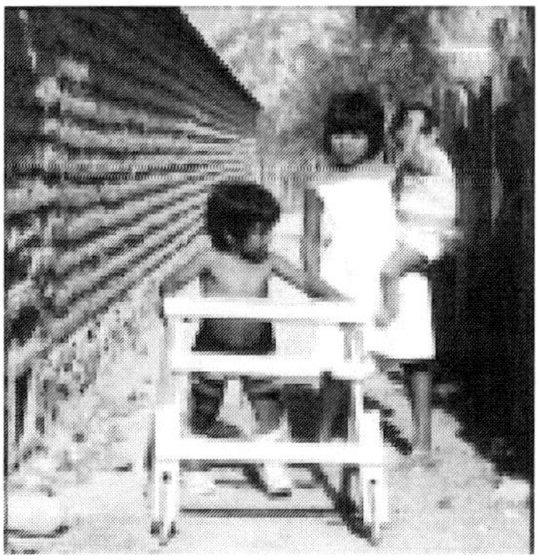

Waqar Naqvi

MPTH (Community Health and Rehabilitation)
Lecturer and *HOD*
Department of Physiotherapy
St Louis Higher institute of Biomedical Sciences
Bamenda, Cameroon, Africa

Foreword

Shalini J Sumbh

JAYPEE

JAYPEE BROTHERS MEDICAL PUBLISHERS
The Health Sciences Publisher
New Delhi | London

JAYPEE **Jaypee Brothers Medical Publishers (P) Ltd**

Headquarters
EMCA House
23/23-B, Ansari Road, Daryaganj
New Delhi 110 002, India
Landline: +91-11-23272143, +91-11-23272703
+91-11-23282021, +91-11-23245672
E-mail: jaypee@jaypeebrothers.com

Corporate Office
4838/24, Ansari Road, Daryaganj
New Delhi 110 002, India
Phone: +91-11-43574357
Fax: +91-11-43574314
E-mail: jaypee@jaypeebrothers.com

Overseas Office
J.P. Medical Ltd
83 Victoria Street, London
SW1H 0HW (UK)
Phone: +44 20 3170 8910
E-mail: info@jpmedpub.com

EU GPSR Authorised Representative
Logos Europe, 9 rue Nicolas Poussin
17000, La Rochelle, France
Phone: +33 (0) 6 67 93 73 78
E-mail: contact@logoseurope.eu

Website: www.jaypeebrothers.com
Website: www.jaypeedigital.com

Physiotherapy in Community Health and Rehabilitation

First Edition: **2011**

Reptint: **2026**

ISBN 978-93-5025-426-4

Typeset at JPBMP typesetting unit

Printed at: Samrat Offset Pvt. Ltd.

Dedicated to

My Mom and Dad.........

The Family is the country of the heart. There is an angel in the family who, by the mysterious influence of grace, of sweetness, and of love render the fulfilment of duties less wearisome, sorrows less bitter. The only pure joys unmixed with sadness which it is given to man to taste upon earth are, thanks to this angel, the joys of the Family.

***Thanks, Mom and Dad**........*

.......with love

This is for you

FOREWORD

It gives me an immense pleasure to write foreward to this book, because I have read it with great interest and I am convinced that supplies a long felt need. The scenario of Community health and Rehabilitation has changed considerably all over world; mainly because of need of the time. It is a purposeful attention paid to rehabilitation of geriatric, children, disabled, industries workers and national and international health care system. Physiotherapy plays an important and major role in this team work.

The author has covered all the areas related to Community health and Rehabilitation. It is up-to-date; and will be of great help to physiotherapy students.

Shalini J Sumbh
DPT, B.A, BSc (Physio) MPhT
Professor and Ex Principal, College of Physiotherapy PIMS Loni
Academic Council Member, Dean Faculty
Chair person Board of studies MUHS Nasik and PIMS Loni
Member Research and Ethical committee and Editorial board
PIMS Loni
Ahmednagar , Maharashtra, India

PREFACE

Physiotherapy in Community Health and Rehabilitation is combination of art and science in practical sense, serving for the improvement of Quality of life in Disabled people, Geriatrics, etc as well as a personality booster for the Physiotherapists; it is the combination of Physiotherapy with the social touch and technology making this field one of the Internationally renowned today and advanced, thus making the professions reaching from OPD to IPD and knocking door to door for serving the Humans society.

Physiotherapy in Community Health and Rehabilitation is one of the four important domains of syllabus of the final year graduation and we have all books of other specialty other than Physiotherapy community health. When, I was in graduation it was very difficult togather the notes from everywhere in the time of exam Preparation for the same subject, rest all subjects was very well-covered in lot of books, even today the students of final year are facing the same old difficulty for arranging the notes for subject, as none of the book covering the syllabus, all are scattered.......and difficult togather.

During my Postgraduation in Community Health and Rehabilitation from PIMS, Loni, I realized to start work on the book, covering maximum of final year syllabus of Physiotherapy in Community Health in one book, so I started arranging syllabus of PIMS, MUHS, RGHUS, Manipal, Jamia, etc. studied it thoroughly, and make a common conclusion of covering like—CBR, Geriatrics, Women's Health, Industrial therapy, Health care delivery system, Developmental disability and Disability evaluation, Orthotics and Prosthesis, Amputation, NGOs in a single book, so that it will be convenient for the students to study and read the subject that would reduce the time, energy and effort for searching notes elsewhere, I have tried my maximum level of effort and hard work for making this book.

The Chapter 1 covering "Introduction to Physiotherapy", a short review of literature of history of profession, when, how, where physiotherapy started and how we developed till here to be one of the demanding field in the field of medical sciences, Chapters 2 covering Indian Health care delivery system, PHC. Chapter 3 deals with Community based Rehabilitation, Models of Disability and Rehabilitation Team, Chapter 4 covering the Developmental Locomotor Disabilities like Polio, CP, Knee deformities, etc.

Chapter 5 dealing with physiological changes in Geriatrics, Theories of Aging, Osteoarthritis, specially Legal rights and Benefits for senior citizen etc., Chapter 6 covering the Amputation rehabilitation in the form of simple protocols that will be easy for student to read and understand.

The 7th Chapter deals with overview of Principles of Prosthetics and Orthosis with splints and ambulatory aids.

Chapter 8 includes the most important topic in Disability studies, i.e. disability evaluation and benefits to them according to India govt.

Chapter 9 signifies the importance of fitness in special populations like OA, DM, Asthma, CHD. Obesity, Osteoporosis, etc according to FITT program.

Chapter 10 has the topics including Ergonomics, Occupational hazards, Risk assessment, Health promotion, Work hardening and conditioning, etc.

Chapter 11 is the best chapter deals with NGOs, International bilateral Agencies like WHO, SIDA, etc and National Agencies like Spastic Society, the brief working and role of agencies in Health care.

Chapter 12, last chapter deals with various Internationally validated Questions like GFRS, PSMS, Clinical mobility index which are beneficial tools for the assessment need in Practical.

I have tried to present with you the recent knowledge in every part of the book, whether National Health policy from Govt. of India, or CBR from WHO, or Industrial Therapy from OSHA.

The book is designed for final year students of Physiotherapy but many topics are helpful for the Postgraduates which are covered in general Paper like Disability evaluation, Health promotion, CBR, Immunization program, National Health policy, Theories of Aging etc. This can be helpful for you also without searching elsewhere.

Suggestions and criticism are wellcome to upgrade this book, my knowledge, and the profession. As we are human beings there are chances of errors, so if even after many correction they exist. Kindly apologies and feel free to know me the same.

Waqar Naqvi
MPTH (Community Health and Rehabilitation)
Lecturer and HOD
Department of Physiotherapy
St Louis Higher institute of Biomedical Sciences
Bamenda, Cameroon, Africa
Ex Lecturer – Apollo College of Physiotherapy
Durg, Chattisgarh, India
Email – *vikkynaqvi@gmail.com*

ACKNOWLEDGEMENTS

I Came, I Saw and I Conquered........ Julius Caesar

First of all I would thank The Almighty God for creating me in this world and making me a proud son of my parents. I would like to thank Mohsin Naqvi, my father, Nighat Naqvi, my mother, Kashif and Kaif my two lovely brothers, and my Dadi for keeping belief on me and always praying for my best.

I am sincerely obliged to Navjyot S. Trivedi, my friend and dedicated professional in the field of physiotherapy for reviewing, correction and motivating me to complete the script for the book. I can credited him as second author of the book, it was impossible to deliver this book without him.

I cannot include the names of all those who have helped in so many ways, but the help of the following have been outstanding:

My teachers and motivators:

S.J Sumbh
Subhash Khatri
Prema Khatri
Suvarna Ganvir
Swati Meshram
Sucheta Golhar
Kashinath Sahoo

My friends and well-wishers:

Swapnil Ramteke
Varoon Jaiswal
Rahul Deshmukh
Prafull Patil
Peeyush Sinha
Rajkumar Jani
Kharsum Mohammed (Phillipines)
Amy Norona (Phillipines)
Nick Ngwanyam, my boss (Cameroon)

For this book I have borrowed information, ideas, illustrations, methods, and designs from many sources, published and unpublished. Often credit has been given, but not always. If you notice I have 'borrowed' from your material and neglected to give you credit, please accept our unspoken thanks and apologies.

For their excellent and dedicated work in preparing the manuscript for publication and making my dream project live, special thanks go to: JAYPEE Publication team.

I realized while working on this Dream Project. Dream is not we see in sleep, but thoughts which made us insomniac.

Waqar M. Naqvi

CONTENTS

One

Introduction to Physiotherapy

Physiotherapy is a health care profession concerned with human function and movement and maximizing potential:

- It uses physical approaches to promote, maintain and restore physical, psychological and social well-being, taking account of variations in health status.
- It is science-based, committed to extending, applying, evaluating and reviewing the evidence that underpins and informs its practice and delivery .
- The exercise of clinical judgments and informed interpretation is at its core.

Various modern approaches now exist in the field of Physiotherapy like different Manual Therapy techniques i.e. Maitland, Mulligan, Cyriax, Brunnstrom etc, and latest electronic physiotherapy equipments like Phyaction, EMG, as well as use of software like SPSS, Physio-office, E-pro, COES and so on.

Day by day new theories, new approaches, new researches, new thinking are developing in physiotherapy profession. Physiotherapy is heading towards becoming one of the dominant structures in the medical industry. And as described by D.W.L Parker an Orthopedics surgeon of Australia in 1960 as "A Physiotherapist will Move Mountains".

THE PAST OF OUR PROFESSION

The History of the practice of Physiotherapy is as old as the practice of medicine.

The word 'Massage' is derived through the Greek from an Arabic word Mass which means to press softly. Friction has been applied to the treatment of disease and injury of Limbs since the dawn of time.

Hippocrates, the father of Greek medicine wrote "the physician must understand many things and friction not the least of all. For friction can bind a joint that is too loose and loosen a joint that is too rigid. Friction warms the flesh, hardens it and makes it grow as it draws more nourishment through the vessels and increases its growth."

In 1894, Lucy Robinson, a trained masseuse and a mid-wife of the London Hospital and Roselind Paget, a trained nursing sister, also of London Hospital together with eight other enthusiasts, initiated their society of trained masseuses; their object was to hold exams and issue certificates.

Early in 1905, Miss L. Armstrong an English masseuse who was residing in New South Wales, Australia approached professor Anderson Stuart and convinced him about the merits of massage. Miss Armstrong possessed a great driving force and worked for the formation of The Australian Massage Association in 1905.

DEVELOPMENT ABROAD AND IN INDIA

- 1938 – First University level physiotherapy course established under University of Queensland, Australia.
- 1939 – Australian Massage Association renamed to Australian Physiotherapy Association.
- 1943 – Formation of Chartered Society of Physiotherapy United Kingdom.
- 1947 – 3 yrs training for Physiotherapy students was introduced in U.K.
- 1950 – First Degree in Physiotherapy offered under University of Queensland, Australia.
- 1951– World Confederation of Physiotherapists was inaugurated.
- 1953 – First Physiotherapy school in South-East Asia was started in collaboration with WHO at KEM Hospital, Mumbai with a strength of 10 students and were conferred with Diploma.

- 1955 – Indian Association of Physiotherapists formed.
- 1960 – Physio-Occupational therapy school started by Dr. Swaroop in Delhi.
- 1967/68 – Degree course in Physiotherapy started in Mumbai.
- 1979 – Masters of physiotherapy started in Mumbai.

USE OF ELECTROTHERAPY

It was Aeitus, a Greek Physician who had prescribed the shock of Torpedo, an electric field for the treatment of gout. It appeared to have been exploited, but in fact it was not in proper use until the middle of the 19th century, when Benjamin Franklin, Americas first scientist used Leydens jar in the treatment of paralysis and various Nervous disorders. The most of electrotherapy originates from the Roman and Greek era including Hydrotherapy, sunbath etc.

- 1646 – Sir Thomas Browne, Physician used the word for the first time.
- 1767 – The electric machine was first used for medical purpose in Middlesex Hospital, U.K.
- 1780 – Luigi Galvani, a professor of the Anatomy first observed the quick twitching of the muscle produced by the electricity in neuro-muscular preparation of the frog's leg.
- 1855 – G.B.A Duchenne described the application of faradic current for stimulation of muscles in the treatment of Muscle Atrophy.
- 1891 – Nicola Tesla of America observed the heating effect of High Frequency Current.
- 1908 – Nagel Schmidt in Berlin made experiment independently and named his method as 'Transthermy' Later changing it to "Diathermy."
- 1929 – Diathermy reached its greatest popularity when the King of England who had worsened on Ultraviolet treatment was improved by Diathermy.
- 1938 – Pierre Currie generated Ultrasound using the Quartz crystal.

USE OF TECHNOLOGY AND INFORMATION SYSTEMS

- Computer aided equipments
- Software
- Internet

Computer Aided Equipments

Computer aided equipment generously helped Physiotherapy in various aspects of evaluation, diagnosis, and management of various diseases. The commonly used Computer aided equipment are :

- EMG
- Gait analyzer
- Biomechanics expert
- Pulmonary function test
- Biofeedback etc.

Software

The Soul of the Computer, i.e. Software programs are becoming the need of physiotherapy profession starting from the patient's data entry to the statistics provider such as SPSS, INSTAT which takes less time to evaluate and interpret data and gives easy graphs and results. Various evaluation scales software are also available such as SF-36, VO2max calculator etc. Currently Software like Net-Physio, Physio-Office is being used for management of patients as well as staff, billing, attendance, evaluation etc.

Internet

This decade of extreme Internet use has provided an important source of up gradation of the knowledge, various websites provides Journals, Reviews, Articles related to physiotherapy, also there exists numerous digital libraries and databases that provide articles, and journals such as Cochrane library, Pubmed, Science-direct.

Different groups of physiotherapist are formed on various websites like Orkut, Hi5, etc. We can also find that there are well organized groups of Musculoskeletal physiotherapists, Neuro-physiotherapists, Manual therapists. The internet that has acted as a catalyst in the 'Development of Physiotherapy,' also communication played vital role in the development of Physiotherapy, and technology has filled all the communication gap via websites, posts, mails, SMSs, workshops, conference etc.

ROLE OF PHYSIOTHERAPIST IN VARIOUS SECTORS

Physiotherapists are spreading like a bright light in every part of medical profession where there is the need of Physiotherapy, Starting from the Massager to the Orthopedic Physiotherapist expanding to the Neurosciences, Cardio-Thoracic conditions, Geriatrics, Industrial Therapy, Women's Health and so on. Today the Chartered Society Of Physiotherapists, U.K. has formed 36 specialties of physiotherapy. Till date some of the recent advancement Physiotherapy in Oncology and Palliative Care, Reflexology, Animal Sciences, Mental Healthcare, Hemophilia.

"Physiotherapy does not add years to life, But adds Life to Years."

REFERENCE

1. D.Patel et al. Changing Concept in Physiotherapy, 1996, IAP.
2. Subhash Khatri. Basics of Electrotherapy. Jaypee Pub.
3. Parker D.W.L: The past and future of Physiotherapy, Aug, 1964, Australian Journal of Physiotherapy.
4. Wedlick L. Changing trends in Medical Electricity. 1964, Australian Journal of Physiotherapy.
5. May Frank. The changing face of physical medicine. 1954, Australian Journal of Physiotherapy.
6. And various resources on the internet.

Two

Indian Health Care Delivery System

Health is not valued till sickness comes. ***Dr. Thomas Fuller***

Health is the general condition of a person in all aspects. It is also a level of functional and/or metabolic efficiency of an organism, often implicitly *human*.

Health is defined as being *"A state of complete physical, mental, and social well-being and not merely the absence of disease or infirmity"*

Disease is defined as *"An abnormal condition of an organism that impairs bodily function associated with specific symptoms and sign"*.

Public health is "The science and art of preventing disease, prolonging life and promoting *health* through the organized efforts and informed choices of society, organizations, public and private, communities and individuals." It is concerned with threats to the overall health of a community based on *population health* analysis. The population in question can be as small as a handful of people or as large as all the inhabitants of several continents (for instance, in the case of a *pandemic*). Public health is typically divided into *epidemiology*, *biostatistics* and *health services*. *Environmental*, social, *behavioral*, and *occupational health* are also important subfields.

There are two distinct characteristics of public health:

1. It deals with preventive rather than curative aspects of health.
2. It deals with population level, rather than individual level health issues.

The focus of public health intervention is to prevent rather than treat a disease through *surveillance* of cases and the promotion of healthy behaviors. In addition to these activities, in many cases treating a disease may be vital to preventing it in others, such as during an outbreak of an *infectious disease*. *Hand washing*, *vaccination* programs and distribution of *condoms* are examples of public health measures.

The goal of public health is to improve lives through the prevention and treatment of disease. The United Nations and *World Health Organization* defines health as "a state of complete physical, mental and social well-being and not merely the absence of disease or infirmity."

Health care (often healthcare in British English), is the treatment and management of illnesses of the elderly, and the preservation of *health* through services offered by the *medical*, *dental*, complementary and *alternative medicine*, *pharmaceutical*, clinical sciences (*in vitro* diagnostics), *nursing*, and *allied health professions*. Health care embraces all the goods and services designed to promote health, including "preventive, *curative* and *palliative* interventions, whether directed to individuals or to populations". The definition of to recognize, tough to define."

The delivery of modern health care depends on an expanding group of trained *professionals* coming together as an *interdisciplinary team*.

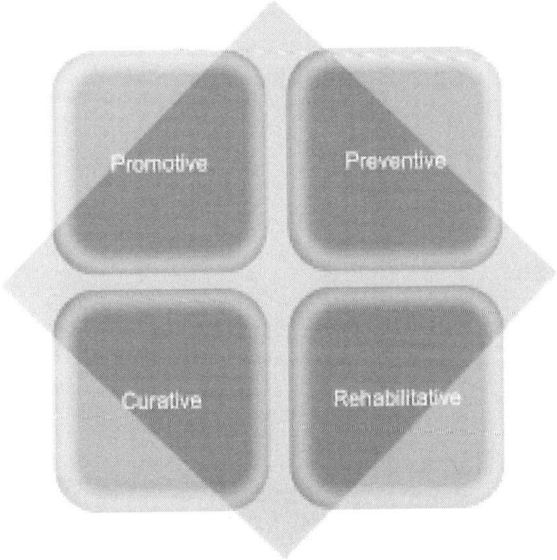

Fig. 2.1: Phases of Health Care

The health-care *industry* incorporates several sectors that are dedicated to providing services and products dedicated to improving the health of individuals. According to market classifications of industry such as the *Global Industry Classification Standard* and the *Industry Classification Benchmark* the health-care industry includes health care equipment and services and pharmaceuticals, biotechnology and life sciences. The particular sectors associated with these groups are: biotechnology, diagnostic substances, drug delivery, drug manufacturers, hospitals, medical equipment and instruments, diagnostic laboratories, nursing homes, providers of health care plans and home health care.

Evolution of the health system in India

- Phase 1 (1941 - 1983)
- Phase 2 (1983 - 2000)
- Phase 3 (Post 2000)

According to March 2008 statistics there are

- 146036 - Sub Centers
- 23458 - Primary Health Centers
- 4276 - Community Health centers

Public Health Care System in India

- National Level
- State Level
- District Level.

Rural Areas

- Community Health Center
- PHC
- Sub-Center

Community Health Center

- 80,000 – 1,20,000 population, Catchment- 4 PHCs
- Referral point for PHCs
- 30-bedded hospital located at the block headquarter

Secondary Level of Health Care

Specialist care:
- Medicine
- Surgery
- Obs and Gyn.
- Pediatrics
- Anesthesia
- Public health

Primary Health Care

- Maximum use of local resources, including traditional healers and trained community health workers
- Participation of the individual and the community
- Affordable and accessible care
- Integration of prevention, promotion, treatment and rehabilitation
- Coordination between the health care sector and other aspects of society, such as housing and education.

The *Declaration of Alma Ata (1978) states that Primary Health Care (PHC) is the key* to attaining health for all. It also states that PHC (Fig. 2.1) needs to address the main health problems in the community, providing promotive, preventive, curative and rehabilitative services.

"Primary health care is essential health care based on practical, scientifically sound and socially acceptable methods and technology made universally accessible to individuals and families in the community through their full participation and at a cost that the community and country can afford to maintain at every stage of their development in the spirit of self-reliance and self-determination.

It forms an integral part both of the country's health system, of which it is the central function and main focus, and of the overall social and economic development of the community. It is the first level of contact of individuals, the family and community with the national health system bringing health care as close as possible to where people live and work, and constitutes the first element of a continuing health care process.

Manpower at PHC

Medical Officer	1
Pharmacist	1
Nurse-midwife	1
Health workers (F)	1
Health Educator	1
Health Asstt. (Male and Female)	2
Clerks	2
Laboratory Technician	1
Driver	1
Class IV	4
Total	**15**

Role of PHC

- Maternal Child Health (MCH)
- 24 X 7 Delivery and New born care
- Adolescent Reproductive and Sexual Health (ARSH)
- Immunization
- National Health Programs
- Permanent FP methods-TT/ vasectomy/NSV
- Medically Terminated Pregnancy
- Common eye diseases and Refraction Services
- School Health
- Nutrition
- Selected surgeries.

Monitoring and Supervision

- MO to Sub-centres once a month
- Health Assistants (HA); Male and Lady Health Visitor (LHV) to Subcentres once a week
- Internal mechanism: Record maintenance, checking and supportive supervision
- External mechanism: Monitoring through the Village Health Committee
- Charter of patient's rights available at PHC
- RMRS.

Role of Physiotherapist

- Preventing disability and deformity
- Educating / training disabled people to move around
- Promoting self-care
- Educating, training and transferring skills to other staff.
- Consultancy, advice, support and supervision to other health care personnel
- Health promotion and disease prevention
- Curative and rehabilitation services
- Instigators of CBR services
- Team leaders and managers
- Providers of direct care
- Advocates for disabled people, local communities as well as the profession
- Advisers to governments, NGOs and local communities on establishing CBR programmes.

Manpower at Sub Centers

- Health Worker (F)
- Health Worker (M)
- Additional Health Worker (F)

Role of Subcenter

- All "Assured Services" (preventive, promotive, few curative and referral services and NHPs)
- Full immunization and Vitamin A prophylaxis
- Essential newborn care
- Antenatal, natal and postnatal care
- Prevention of malnutrition and common childhood diseases
- Family planning services
- Counseling
- Community needs assessment
- Minimum laboratory services
- Hemoglobin estimation
- Urine for albumin and sugar and
- Referral to PHC for blood grouping

- Malaria prophylaxis
- Provision of Janani Suraksha Yojana (JSY)
- Adolescent health care and school health services
- Appropriate and prompt referral services
- Providing treatment as per AYUSH according to local need
- Training of TBAs, ASHA/Community Health Volunteers
- Recording and reporting of vital events
- Syndromic surveillance to be done and reported to PHC every week
- Water Quality Monitoring and Disinfection of water sources.

The delivery of modern health care depends on an expanding group of trained *professionals* coming together as an *interdisciplinary team.*

REFERENCES

1. ^ *Princeton University.* (2007): Health profession. Retrieved June 17, 2007, from *Princeton University.*
2. United States Department of Labor. (February 27, 2007). Health Care Industry Information. Retrieved June 17, 2007, from *Employment and Training Administration (ETA) - U.S. Department of Labor.*
3. *Yahoo Industry Browser - Healthcare Sector - Industry List.*
4. *Welcome to the United Nations: It's Your World.*
5. *Albany Times-Union,* November, 12, 2009.
6. WHO: Joint paper on Community based Rehabilitation: Helsinki: 2003.
7. J. Kishore. Textbook of Social Medicine:2003
8. Tracy Bury, WCPT , PHC, CBR and Physical therapy, WCPT Briefing paper: 2005.
9. Maharashtra State Govt. Physiotherapy and Occupational therapy council Bill. 2007.
10. WHO: The UN rules on the Equalization of opportunities for PWD: 2001.
11. WHO reports : 1989, 1994, 1995a, 2001a, 2001b,2001c, 2001d, 2003
12. *WHO, int,* Preamble to the Constitution of the World Health Organization as adopted by the International Health Conference, New York, 19-22 June, 1946; signed on 22 July 1947 by the representatives of 61 States (Official Records of the World Health Organization, no. 2, p. 100); and entered into force on 7 April 1948.
13. *WHO.int* Constitution of the World Health Organization- *Basic Documents,* Forty-fifth edition, Supplement, October 2006.

14. Lalonde, Marc. *A New Perspective on the Health of Canadians.* Ottawa: Minister of Supply and Services; 1974.
15. *The UN World Water Development Report | Facts and Figures | Meeting basic needs.*
16. *Recreational Values of the Natural Environment in Relation to Neighborhood Satisfaction, Physical Activity, Obesity and Wellbeing.*
17. McEwen BS (2006). "Protective and damaging effects of stress mediators: central role of the brain". *Dialogues Clin Neurosci* **8** (4): 367–81. *PMID 17290796.*
18. Leavitt; World Health Organization and UNICEF 1978
19. Ministry of Health and family Welfare, Government of India, 1995.

Three

Principles in Rehabilitation

INTRODUCTION TO REHABILITATION

Definition

"The development of a person to the fullest physiological, social, vocational, avocational and educational potential consistent with his or her physiological or anatomic impairment and environmental limitations"

or

The process of restoration of skills by a person who has had an illness or injury so as to regain maximum self-sufficiency and function in a normal or as near normal manner as possible or the maintenance and restoration of physical and psychological health necessary for independent living and functional independence. Thus the restoration of someone to a useful place in society, transforming them from **disabled to differently abled.**

Rehabilitation of people with disabilities is a process aimed at enabling them to reach and maintain their optimal physical, sensory, intellectual, psychological and social functional levels. Rehabilitation provides disabled people with the tools they need to attain independence and self-determination.

Impairment (Flow chart 3.1)

- "Any loss or abnormality of psychological, physiological, or anatomical structure or function."

Flowchart 3.1:

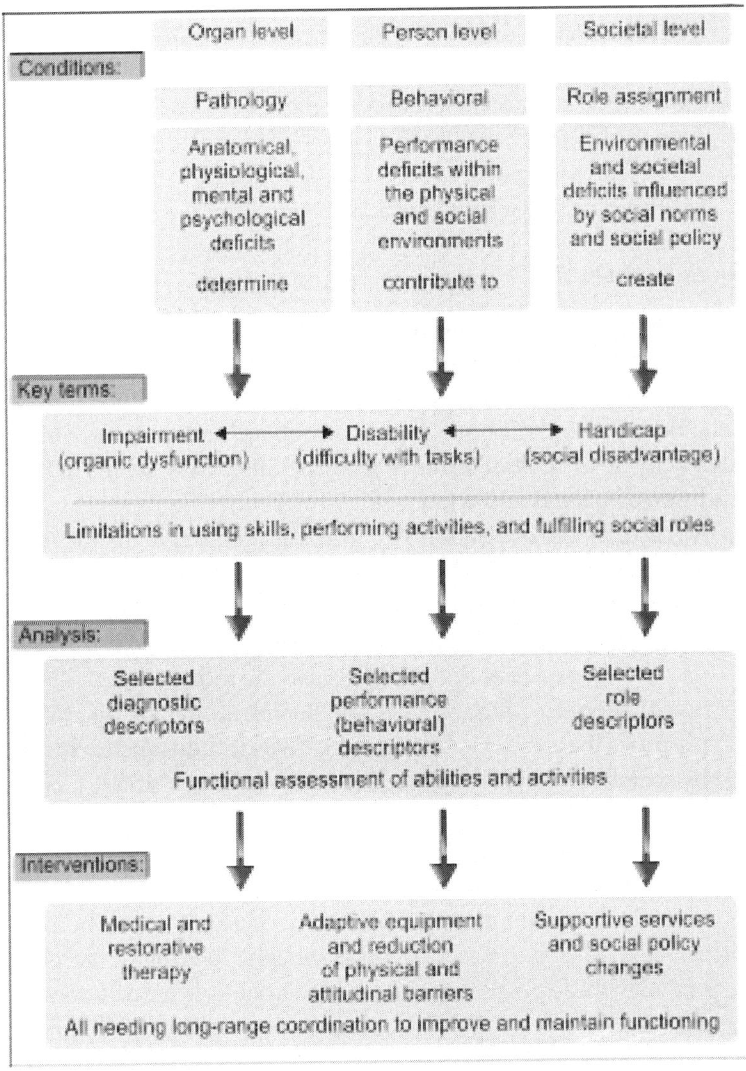

- Examples
  - Amputation
  - Fractured femur
  - Low back pain
  - Confusion.

Disability (Activity Limitation) (Flow chart 3.1)

- "Any restriction or lack, resulting from an impairment of ability to perform an activity in the manner or within the range considered normal for a human being."
- Examples:
  - Person with paraplegia is unable to walk
  - Pro-quarterback with broker finger dominant hand.

Models of Disability

The simplest, and maybe the initial, **definition of a disabled person** appears to be the following: "a person who in his/her society is regarded as disabled, because of a difference in appearance and/or behaviour". People "know" who is "disabled", and there are in all societies one or several terms to indicate this. There seems to be a tradition of what is and what is not "different."

- Medical model of disability - The **medical model of disability** is a model by which illness or *disability* is the result of a physical condition, is intrinsic to the individual (it is part of that individual's own body), may reduce the individual's *quality of life*, and causes clear disadvantages to the individual.
- Social Model of Disability - The **social model of disability** proposes that systemic barriers, negative attitudes and exclusion by society (purposely or inadvertently) are the ultimate factors defining who is disabled and who is not in a particular society. It recognizes that while some people have *physical*, sensory, intellectual, or *psychological* variations, which may sometimes cause individual functional limitation or *impairments*, these do not have to lead to *disability*, unless society fails to take account of and include people regardless of their individual differences.

The social model of disability often focuses on changes required in society. These might be in terms of:

- Attitudes, for example a more positive attitude towards certain mental traits or behaviors, or not underestimating the potential quality of life of those with potential impairments.
- Social support, for example helps dealing with the above barriers, resources, aids or *positive discrimination* to overcome them.

- Information, for example using suitable formats (e.g. *braille*) or levels (e.g. simplicity of language) or coverage (e.g. explaining issues others may take for granted)
- Physical structures, for example buildings with sloped access and elevators.

Handicap (Participation Restriction) (Flowchart 3.1)

- "A disadvantage for a given individual resulting from an impairment or a disability that limits or prevents the fulfillment of a role that is normal (depending on age, sex, social and cultural factors) for that individual."
- Examples:
  - Work environment not wheelchair accessible for person with paraplegia
    a. Impairment - *organ or tissue level*
    b. Disability - *whole person (functional) level*
    c. Handicap - *society level*

Goals of a Rehabilitation Program

- Reduction of disability
- Prevention of complications e.g., pressure sores
- Restoration of neuromuscular function - strength, ROM exercises, etc.

The Rehabilitation Team

A rehabilitation program is specifically designed for each individual depending on the injury, disorder, or illness. A multidisciplinary team approach for care and service is the basis of rehabilitation treatment. Multidisciplinary refers to the fact that many different disciplines work together towards a common goal.

The team is usually directed by a physiatrist, with other specialists playing important roles in the treatment and education process. Team members involved depend on many factors, including patient need, facility resources, and insurance coverage for services.

The major concern of the rehabilitation field is to improve the ability of the person to function optimally within the limitations placed upon them by a disease process for which there is no known cure. The emphasis is not on the full restoration to the premorbid level of function, but rather the optimization of the quality of life for those who may not be able to achieve full restoration. A team approach to chronic conditions is emphasized to coordinate care of the patients.

- Patient and Family:
  - The patient and family are considered the most important members of the rehabilitation team.
  - The multidisciplinary rehabilitation team may include, but is not limited to, the following team members are included:

The Rehabilitation Team can be Categorized Into

- Medical
  (Role – to limit Disability)
- Paramedical or Allied Health Professionals
  (Role – to reduce Handicap)
- Sociovocational

The Medical team Compromised of all Medical Specialties Such as

- Physiatrist – Team Leader
- Orthopedic surgeon
- General surgeon
- Physician
- Pediatrician
- Ophthalmologist
- Obstetrician and gynecologist
- Psychiatrist.

The Para - Medical Team Compromised of

- Physiotherapist
- Occupational therapist
- *Orthotist and Prosthetist*
- Speech-Language pathologist / Speech therapist
- Rehabilitation nurse

- Clinical psychologist
- Rehabilitation engineer
- Horticulture therapist
- Music therapist.

The Socio-Vocational Team Compromised of

- Social worker
- Health educator
- Mental health educator
- Rehabilitation counselor
- Vocational counselor
- NGOs
- Bank
- Special schools
- Special education teacher
- Community.

ROLES OF INDIVIDUAL

Physiatrist: Physical medicine and rehabilitation (PM&R) or Physiatry is a branch of *medicine* which aims to enhance and restore functional ability and quality of life to those with physical impairments or disabilities. A *physician* who has completed training in this field is referred to as a physiatrist.

Physiatrists are physicians who specialize in diagnosing problems in the musculoskeletal system and applying non-surgical solutions. The physiatrist manages, directs, and supervises a patient's rehabilitation program, assuring that the care, a patient receives is consistent with his or her diagnosis, functional limitations, and prognosis. The physiatrist also directs the interdisciplinary team towards facilitating treatment goals.

Physiotherapist: Physiotherapists evaluate and treat problems relating to mobility, strength, coordination, and endurance. They help patients to gain the highest level of functional independence within the limitations of their conditions. A physiotherapist will also instruct the patient and his or her family in activities and exercises to enhance recovery and decrease pain. The role of physiotherapist is to improve quality of life of the person. Members of the physiotherapy staff including rehabilitation assistants and technicians, all focus on the individual reaching their potential.

Once problem areas have been identified, a customized treatment program will be developed for that individual. The treatment plan will include short and long term goals designed to improve any of the following dependent upon the severity of the medical condition:

- Assessment of the patient's condition and its impact on everyday activities within the home and local community.
- Assessment, treatment and ongoing management of specific musculoskeletal (muscle and bone), respiratory (breathing) and neurological (brain and nerve) conditions.
- Recommendation and, wherever possible, provision of appropriate orthotics (surgical appliances - devices used to treat or support different parts of the body, e.g. collars, leg braces, shoe insoles), walking aids and minor equipment.
- Provision of individualized exercise programmes which patients can follow to improve their mobility, agility and strength in order to maintain independent living .
- Teaching family members and caregivers on how to assist the individual.
- Education of the individual, his/her family members or caregivers as to their disability.
- Recommendations for home and/or work modifications i.e ergonomics .
- Physiotherapy support for patients with long term and progressive conditions.
- Referral.

Occupational Therapist: Occupational therapists evaluate and treat physical and functional ability in daily activities. The occupational therapist can help improve the ability to perform everyday tasks, such as dressing, eating, personal hygiene, meal preparation, housekeeping, and community and prevocational skills. Members of the occupational therapy staff including rehabilitation assistants and technicians all focus on the individual reaching their potential. The evaluation assesses the individual's ability to complete everyday functional activities called activities of daily living ADLs consist of bathing, dressing, grooming, self-feeding, toileting, and homemaking skills. In addition to assessing these skills, occupational therapists also evaluate vision, balance, coordination, perceptual skills, and cognition.

For injured workers, occupational therapists can develop ergonomic assessments, assist in pre-employment screening, and creation of modified return to work jobs, work conditioning and transitioning programs. Once problem areas have been identified, the therapist will help the individual develop their abilities by focusing on a treatment plan designed to:

- Achieve maximum degree of independence in bathing, dressing, feeding and grooming
- Exercises to strengthen upper arms, hands and body positioning
- Determining the need for adaptive devices such as hand splints, use of grooming and other self care aids
- Homemaking skills based on individual's needs
- Money management based on individual's needs
- Cognitive skills and prevocational skills
- Driver training potential as indicated
- Job modifications.

Orthotists and Prosthetists

The prosthetist is the professional who designs and fabricates *prostheses* for individuals with partial or total absence of a limb.The orthotist provides care to individuals with disabling conditions of their limbs or spine by recommending, fitting, fabricating and maintaining orthopaedic braces that support or limit the movement of weakened joints or limbs.

The orthotist- prosthetist is a member of the rehabilitation team and enables people suffering from disabilities to live as normally as possible.

- Interpreting the surgeon's prescription by taking precise measurement, making traces from the patient's body and making plaster casts.
- Creating orthosis/prostheses that are both well-fitting and functional by examining the disability and modifying positive

plaster forms which will serve as models until both the patient and the orthotist-prosthetist are fully satisfied with the results.

- Welding, working with a variety of steels and undertaking minor fitting and turning, spray-painting, panel-beating and woodwork.
- Providing rehabilitative (prosthesis) and curative (orthotics) services to the public.
- Manufacturing surgical footwear for patients with deformities, such as club-feet.

Speech-Language Pathologist / Speech Therapist: A speech-language pathologist (speech therapist) evaluates and treats cognitive, communicative, and swallowing deficits that may interfere with the ability to speak, understand, read, write, focus, remember, or problem solve. Individual and group treatments will help to provide techniques to compensate for difficulties in these areas.

Rehabilitation Nurse: Nurses are an integral part of the entire rehabilitation team. A nurse who specializes in rehabilitative care and assists the patient in achieving maximum independence, especially in regards to medical care, prevention of complications, and patient and family education. They often help to facilitate the carry over of the rehabilitation program throughout the hospital stay. In addition to daily bedside care, rehabilitation nurses work on ensuring bowel and bladder continence, maintaining good skin care, ensuring healthy, nutritional intake, medication management and reinforcing carryover of learned skills. Education of the individual and family are vital to achieving a successful return back home.

Psychiatrist, Psychologist, or Neuropsychologist: A physician or counselor who conducts cognitive (thinking and learning) assessments of the patient and helps the patient and family adjust to the disability. Their role is to work with the individual, family and entire rehabilitation team to assist with adjustment difficulties and other psychological issues that can develop during the rehabilitation process. Counseling and support are essential for the individual and family during this time.

Rehabilitation engineering is the systematic application of *engineering sciences* to design, develop, adapt, test, evaluate, apply, and distribute technological solutions to problems confronted by individuals with disabilities. Functional areas addressed through rehabilitation engineering may include mobility, communications, hearing, vision, and cognition, and activities associated with employment, independent living, education, and integration into the community.

The rehabilitation process for *people with disabilities* often entails the design of assistive devices such as *walking aids* intended to promote inclusion of their users into the mainstream of society, commerce, and recreation.

Horticulture therapy included the following forms; imagining nature, viewing nature, visiting a hospital healing garden and, most important, actual gardening. It was expected to influence healing, alleviate stress, increase well-being and promote participation in social life and re-employment for people with mental or physical illness. The Horticultural therapy garden was described regarding the design of the outdoor environment, adaptations of garden tools, cultivation methods and plant material. This therapy programme for mediating mental healing, recreation, social interaction, sensory stimulation, cognitive re-organization and training of sensory motor function is outlined and pre-vocational skills and the teaching of ergonomical body positions are assessed.

Music therapist: The therapeutic effects of music are being recognized increasingly in the field of rehabilitation medicine. More music therapists are being employed in physical medicine and rehabilitation centers, with the goal of using music therapy services to assist in the physical recovery and health maintenance of clients. Inspite of the benefits of physical rehabilitation programs, client participation to their full potential is often not observed. Music encourages participation in exercises and activities. Music can ease the discomfort and difficulty associated with exercise and therapy activities, and ensure consistent participation. One of the goals of the music therapist is to provide a means for the client to express him/herself in a musical activity. Music therapy and rehabilitation medicine are starting to find a common niche in working together with clients who have various neurological, orthopaedic, and paediatric conditions. Therapeutic application of music in rehabilitation contributes to the quality of life of individuals with disabilities. Combined goals could include improving strength, range of motion, balance, communication, and cognition. Continued efforts in clinical practice and research will build on the information already available to further define possible applications of music therapy in rehabilitation, and its outcome and benefits.

Recreational therapists also referred to as *therapeutic recreation specialists;* provide treatment services and recreation activities for individuals with disabilities or illnesses. Using a variety of techniques, including arts and crafts, animals, sports, games, dance and movement, drama, music, and community outings, therapists improve and maintain the physical, mental, and emotional well-being of their clients. Therapists help individuals to reduce depression, stress, and anxiety; recover basic motor functioning and reasoning abilities; build confidence; and socialize effectively so that they can enjoy greater independence and reduce or eliminate the effects of their illness or disability. In addition, therapists help people with disabilities integrate into the community by teaching them how to use community resources and recreational activities. Recreational therapists are different from *recreation workers,* who organize recreational activities primarily for enjoyment.

Community based recreational therapists may work in park and recreation departments, special education programs for school districts, or assisted living, adult day care, and substance abuse rehabilitation centers. In these programs, therapists use interventions to develop specific skills, while providing opportunities for exercise, mental stimulation, creativity, and fun. Those few who work in schools help counselors, teachers, and parents address the special needs of students, including easing disabled student's transition into adult life.

Social Worker assist people by helping them cope with and solve issues in their everyday lives, such as family and personal problems and dealing with relationships. Some social workers help clients who face a disability, life-threatening disease, social problem, such as inadequate housing, unemployment, or substance abuse. Social workers also assist families that have serious domestic conflicts, sometimes involving child or spousal abuse. Additionally, they may conduct research, advocate for improved services, or become involved in planning or policy development. Many social workers specialize in serving a particular population or working in a specific setting.

The *medical social worker* is a liaison between the healthcare staff, the patient and family. Social worker record the patient's general background or psychosocial history, including information about the patient's pre-injury personality and lifestyle, emotional and financial resources, educational history, work and leisure interests, special relationships, and previous problems. The family can turn to social workers for advice, support, and counseling regarding treatment options and the various issues involved in the recovery process.

Health educators work to encourage healthy lifestyles and wellness through educating individuals and communities about behaviors that can prevent diseases, injuries, and other health problems.

Health educators attempt to prevent illnesses by informing and educating individuals and communities about health-related topics, such as proper nutrition, the importance of exercise, how to avoid sexually transmitted diseases, and the habits and behaviors necessary to avoid illness. They begin by assessing the needs of their audience, which includes determining the appropriate topics to cover. For example, they may hold programs on self-examination for breast cancer to women or may teach classes on the effects of being drinking to college students. Health educators must take the cultural norms of their audience into account. For example, programs targeted at the elderly need should be different from those aimed at a college-aged population.

Within medical care facilities, health educators tend to work one-on-one with patients and their families. In this setting, a health educator's goal is to educate individual patients on their diagnosis and how that may change or affect their lifestyle. To this end, they may explain the necessary procedures or surgeries as well as how patients will need to alter their lifestyles to manage their illness or return to full health. They may also direct patients to outside resources, such as support groups, home health agencies, or social services. Often, health educators work closely with physicians, nurses, and other staff to create educational programs or materials, such as brochures, Websites, and classes. In some cases, health educators train hospital staff about how to better interact with patients.

Mental health counselors work with individuals, families, and groups to address and treat mental and emotional disorders and to promote mental health. They are trained in a variety of therapeutic techniques used to address issues such as depression, anxiety, addiction and substance abuse, suicidal impulses, stress, trauma, low self-esteem, and grief. They also help with job and career concerns, educational decisions, mental and emotional health issues, and relationship problems. In addition, they may be involved in community outreach, advocacy, and mediation activities. Some specialize in delivering mental health services for the elderly. Mental health counselors often work closely with other mental health specialists, such as psychiatrists, psychologists, clinical social workers, psychiatric nurses, and school counselors.

Rehabilitation counselors help people deal with the personal, social, and vocational effects of disabilities. They counsel people with both physical and emotional disabilities resulting from birth defects, illness or disease, accidents, or other causes. They evaluate the strengths and limitations of individuals, provide personal and vocational counseling, offer case management support, and arrange for medical care, vocational training, and job placement. Rehabilitation counselors interview both individuals with disabilities and their families, evaluate school and medical reports, and confer with physicians, psychologists, employers, and physical, occupational, and speech therapists to determine the capabilities and skills of the individual. They develop individual rehabilitation programs by conferring with the client. These programs often include training to help individuals develop job skills, become employed, and provide opportunities for community integration. Rehabilitation counselors are trained to recognize and to help lessen environmental and attitudinal barriers. Such help may include providing education, and advocacy services to individuals to families, employers, and others in the community. Rehabilitation counselors work toward increasing the person's capacity to live independently by facilitating and coordinating with other service providers.

Special education teachers work with children and youths who have a variety of disabilities. A small number of special education teachers work with students with severe cognitive, emotional, or physical disabilities, primarily teaching them life skills and basic literacy. However, the majority of special education teachers work with children with mild to moderate disabilities, using or modifying the general education curriculum to meet the child's individual needs and providing required remedial instruction.

Special education teachers use various techniques to promote learning. Depending on the student, teaching methods can include intensive individualized instruction, problem-solving assignments, and small-group work. When students need special accommodations to learn the general curriculum or to take a test, special education teachers ensure that appropriate accommodations are provided, such as having material read orally or lengthening the time allowed to take the test.

Special education teachers help to develop an Individualized Education Program (IEP) for each student receiving special education. Special education teachers design and teach appropriate curricula, assign work geared toward each student's needs and abilities, and grade papers and homework assignments. They are involved in the student's behavioral, social, and academic development, helping them develop emotionally and interact effectively in social situations. Preparing special education students for daily life after graduational also is an important aspect of the job. Teachers provide students with career counseling or help them learn life skills, such as balancing a checkbook.

Technology is becoming increasingly important in special education. Teachers use specialized equipment such as computers with synthesized speech, interactive educational software programs, and audiotapes to assist children.

Vocational Counselor: The vocational rehabilitation counselor evaluates our vocational abilities and *employment* history. Vocational counselors can connect with career training or re-training and job placement services. They can recommend any adaptations and equipment that may be necessary for in a particular workplace, as well as related to your transportation to/from the workplace.

NGOs

NGOs supplement the efforts made by government. Local NGOs reach the grass-root level and provide relief to the people. The brief role of some NGOs is in 11th Chapter of the book.

APPROACHES OF REHABILITATION

These programmes use several different approaches, and should like to mention the main ones:

a. **Service projects:** personnel, equipment etc. are sent to a developing country for a limited time period. All services are provided by expatriates, and they return home without having trained the nationals.
b. **Development projects:** these aim at the transfer of knowledge and skills to a developing country. Nationals are trained by expatriates.

Development programmes may operate on several different levels. There are three main types:

a. **Institution-based:** professional services for people with disabilities are given in a center (boarding or day-care). Such centers are most often only set up to the capital or big cities.
b. **Outreach service programme:** the professional staff delivers services at home to the extent possible.
c. **Community-based programmes:** build on the idea of mobilizing community resources. The person with a disability is trained at home and in the community. A family member acts as the trainer, and a community worker as the local supervisor. Community workers are trained in rehabilitation tasks by an intermediate level supervisor, who in most cases is a professional. This programme needs the support of referral services.

The institution-based and the outreach service programmes require a lot of personnel and are costly to operate. It is unrealistic to assume that these approaches will contribute much to the reduction of the rehabilitation gap.

The community-based approach aims at a massive transfer of knowledge and skills to the person with disabilities, his or her family and the community. Such a transfer of skills and knowledge is a very clear characteristic also of modern rehabilitation programmes in the industrialized countries, where parents and other relatives are trained to become active partners in rehabilitation.

As we know there are various approaches of rehabilitation of persons with disabilities are being advocated both in theory and in practice. The two main approaches to rehabilitation are Community Based Rehabilitation (CBR) and Institutional Based Rehabilitation (IBR). (Table 3.1)

Table 3.1: Difference between CBR and IBR

	CBR	*IBR*
Cost of treatment	Cheaper	Costly
Accessibility of services	Accessible to all	Only few institutions are accessible to all
Extension of services	Can be done without of much cost	Not possible
Social rehabilitation	Possible	Not possible as patient is away from family
Psychological rehabilitation	Much Possible as they have support of family	Not much possible
Skilled personal care	Not given	Given
Application of advanced technique	Not possible	Possible
Quality of service	Not good	Good
Active participation	Possible	Not possible
Socio-Economic status	Considered	Not considered
Promotion of awareness	Yes	Not
Community interaction	Done	Not done
Evaluation	Difficult	Possible

Contd...

Contd...

	CBR	*IBR*
Goal of training	Interventions to prepare the re-entry of client to his home.	Interventions to discharge patient from hospital.
Location	Anywhere and community based	Cities and Institution based
Decision makers	PWD and their family	Service providers (one way traffic)
Service providers	CBR workers or semi professionals	Many Professionals
Action	Proactive	Usually responsive
Identification	Early	Delayed
Intervention	Early	Delayed
Follow-up	Guaranteed	Not guaranteed
Services	At door step Holistic	Far Medical
Complicated problems	Difficult	Easy to tackle

The distinctive features of CBR are that needs of persons with disabilities are met within their own environment, involving family members and community:

1. It refers to measures taken at community level to use and build on locally available resources of the community. These resources include the disabled persons, their families and others in the community
2. IBR on the other hand, is rehabilitation of persons with disabilities at or through institutions, often away from their homes. IBR generally leads to a transformation in social behaviour of persons with disabilities, making the process of their social integration difficult.

However, the quality of rehabilitation services provided through IBR tends to be better than through CBR, as services are provided by professionals and specialists, with the assistance of more sophisticated equipment and tools.

Many people need temporary assistance by special services that are often institution based. Among this group are people requiring corrective surgery, physical and occupational therapy, orthoses or prostheses. Therefore, for successful implementation of rehabilitation services, a close co-operation between these specialized services and CBR programs should be promoted.

Government of India set up Rehabilitation Council in 1986 as registered society. There after this was converted to a statutory body under the Rehabilitation council of India Act w.e.f.31 July, 1993. This is under the administrative control of Ministry of Social Justice and Empowerment. There are 31 PMR (Physical and Medical Rehabilitation) institutes, 9 of them are being upgraded. 11 District Rehabilitation Centers are functioning in 10 major states. Regional Rehabilitation Centers (RRC) are also functioning. The National Handicapped Finance and Development Corporation (NHFDC) has been incorporated by Ministry of Welfare, Government of India as a company not for profit. It extends loan to the persons with disability.

In recent years, community based rehabilitation has been advocated by various organisations and professionals. Their arguments are based on the greater effectiveness and low cost of the CBR approach. The CBR approach, according to them, enhances social integration of the persons with disabilities more easily, and keeps the social fibre largely undisturbed. The cost of rehabilitation is also lower as a majority of the resources used are local. However, despite the strong advocacy and emphatic world opinion in favour of CBR, efforts in India till now have been restricted to a few pockets, undertaken through a few NGOs, National Institutes and District Rehabilitation Centres. Even the organisations that implement the CBR approaches are doing it in a limited way, often in a small rural pocket in a town.

Although many definitions of CBR are given by different experts and people involved in various such programmes, however, in general, community based rehabilitation (CBR) and institution based rehabilitation (IBR) are clearly distinct from each other. It is also mentioned that through CBR, community takes part in activities to help provide rehabilitation services for the persons with disabilities at home. While usually through IBR, disabled people are abilitated at institutions, in a new strange environment, away from their homes and segregated from their communities. Thus CBR is considered a better way to rehabilitate disabled people in their own areas.

In some cultures, there can be such social barriers where CBR as a specific model is not allowed. Here, one of the solutions can be establishment of small scale, day-care rehabilitation units, supervised, run and managed purely by the local community, also involving persons with disabilities. Locally available, low-cost, appropriate technology and other resources can be widely utilized. For training personnel in such units, an appropriately planned resource centre is also needed.

2. COMMUNITY BASED REHABILITATION (CBR)

CBR is a strategy within general community development for the rehabilitation, equalization of opportunities and social inclusion of all people with disabilities.

CBR was designed as a model by which cost-effective community/home-based rehabilitation could be provided in developing countries. As defined it was not seen to equate to all rehabilitation that takes place outside an institutional setting, CBR, as internationally defined, is very much client-centric as opposed to profession centric.

In trying to clarify what CBR is and to draw a distinction with any care that takes place in a community environment there are a few key points.

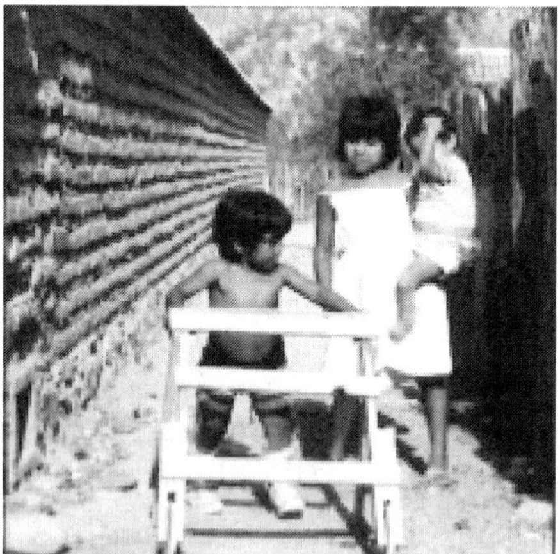

Fig. 1: Community based rehabilitation (Home made walker)

Flowchart 3.2: CBR is a strategy within general community development for the rehabilitation, equalization of opportunities and social inclusion of all people with disabilities.

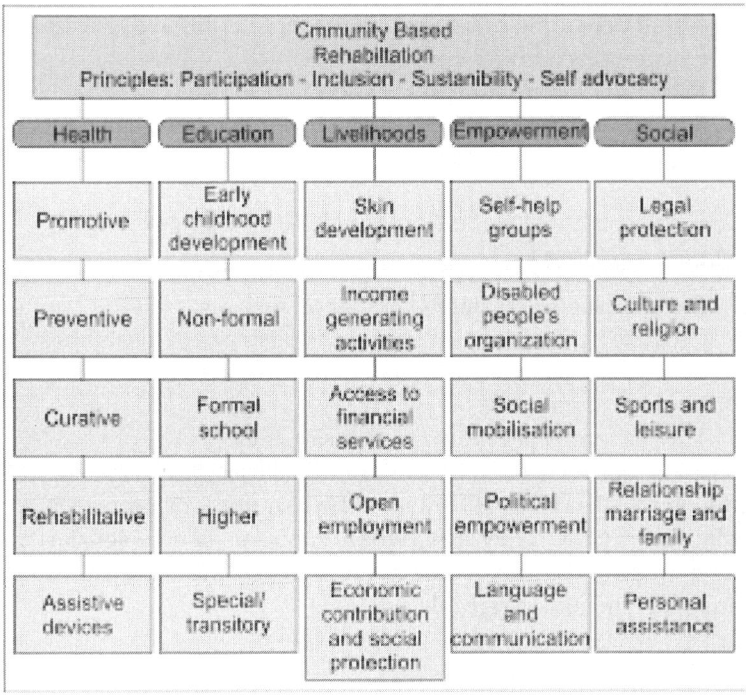

Conversely CBR Involves

- Partnerships with disabled people, adults and children, their families and carers.
- Capacity building of disabled people and their families, in the context of their community and culture.
- Holistic approach encompassing physical, social, employment, educational, economic and other needs.
- Promoting the social inclusion of disabled people in existing mainstream services.
- A system based in the community, using district and national level services for referral.

CBR is not

- An approach that only focuses on the physical or medical needs of a person.
- About delivering care to disabled people as passive recipients
- Only outreach from a centre.
- Rehabilitation training in isolation.
- An approach which is determined by the needs of an institution or groups of professionals.

CBR has been Described on the Basis of Component Features Such as

- Provision of functional rehabilitation services.
- Creating a positive attitude towards people with disabilities.
- The creation of micro and macro income-generation.
- Vocational training.
- The prevention of the causes of disabilities.

It has also been described on the basis of philosophical or ideological thinking. Helander (1999) has identified a number of key principles relating to CBR. They are; equality, social justice, solidarity, integration and dignity. These can be seen to relate to the principles embedded in human rights legislation.

2.1 Concept of CBR

CBR is a strategy within general community development for the rehabilitation, equalization of opportunities and social inclusion of all people with disabilities.

CBR is implemented through the combined efforts of people with disabilities themselves, their families, organizations and communities, and the relevant governmental and non-governmental health, education, vocational, social and other services.

2.2 Major Objectives

- To ensure that people with disabilities are able to maximize their physical and mental abilities, to access regular services and opportunities, and to become active contributors to the community and society at large.

- To activate communities to promote and protect the human rights of people with disabilities through changes within the community, for example, by removing barriers to participation.

2.3 Evolution of Concepts in CBR

Although its definition and major objectives have not changed, there has been an evolution of concepts within CBR and of stakeholder involvement. This evolution is around the concepts of disability and rehabilitation, the emphasis placed on human rights and action to address inequalities and alleviate poverty, and on the expanding role of DPOs.

2.3.1 Disability and Rehabilitation

Disability is no longer viewed as merely the result of impairment. The social model of disability has increased awareness that environmental barriers to participation are major causes of disability. No nation has eliminated all of the environmental barriers that contribute to disability.

Rehabilitation services should no longer be imposed without the consent and participation of people who are using the services. Rehabilitation is now viewed as a process in which people with disabilities or their advocates make decisions about what services they need to enhance participation. Professionals who provide rehabilitation services have the responsibility to provide relevant information to people with disabilities so that they can make informed decisions regarding what is appropriate for them.

2.3.2 Human Rights

CBR promotes the rights of people with disabilities to live as equal citizens within the community, to enjoy health and well being, to participate fully in educational, social, cultural, religious, economic and political activities. CBR emphasizes that girls and boys with disabilities have equal rights to schooling, and that women and men have equal rights to opportunities to participate in work and social activities.

2.3.3 Poverty

There is a strong correlation between disability and poverty. Poverty leads to increased disability, and disability in turn leads to increased poverty. Thus, a majority of people with disabilities live in poverty. Studies show that they have higher rates of unemployment compared to non-disabled people even in industrialized countries.

2.3.4 Inclusive Communities

The term 'Inclusive' is now commonly used with reference to educational provision that welcomes all children, including those with disabilities, to participate fully in regular community schools or centers of learning. The principle of 'Inclusion' is also being applied to policies and services in health, skills training and employment and to community life in general.

The concept of an inclusive community means that communities adapt their structures and procedures to facilitate the inclusion of people with disabilities, rather than expecting them to change to fit in with existing arrangements.

2.3.5 Role of Organizations of Persons with Disabilities (DPOs)

Today DPOs are prepared to take meaningful roles in the initiation, implementation and evaluation of CBR programmes. At the same time, they strive to reach more people with disabilities and to be more active in representing them. DPOs need to be recognized as a resource to strengthen CBR programmes.

3. INITIATORS OF CBR

Community action for CBR is often initiated by a stimulus from outside the community, most likely ministries or NGOs. Following initial discussions with representatives from outside the community, it is the community which decides whether CBR will become part of its ongoing community development activities. Various partners in the community, such as the community development committee, organizations of people with disabilities and other non-governmental organizations can provide leadership and take responsibility for the programme. Once a community chooses to initiate a CBR programme, the CBR programme management provides the necessary support, including training, access to referral services and the mobilization of resources.

4. ESSENTIAL ELEMENTS OF CBR

CBR requires community and DPOs involvement. But communities and DPOs cannot work alone to ensure equal opportunities for people with disabilities. National policies, a management structure, and the support of different government ministries, NGOs and other stakeholders (multi-sectoral collaboration) are also needed.

5. MULTI-SECTORAL SUPPORT FOR CBR

In CBR a multi-sectoral collaboration is essential to support the community, address the individual needs of people with disabilities, and strengthen the role of DPOs. In addition to collaboration between government ministries, collaboration is needed between these ministries, non-governmental organizations and the private sector. It is needed between the community and the referral services at local and intermediate levels, and also between the various referral services at local, intermediate and national levels.

Collaboration between national, intermediate and community levels within a sector can ensure that appropriate referral services are developed and delivered.

5.1 Supports from the Social Sector

Although the allocation of responsibility for social affairs varies from country to country, matters commonly addressed include disability pensions, technical aids and adaptations, housing, vocational training and employment, and co-ordination of referrals for individuals who require services from other sectors. If the social affairs ministry initiates CBR, social welfare officers, district collectors may be managers of the programme.

5.2 Supports from the Health Sector

The *Declaration of Alma Ata* (1978) states that Primary Health Care (PHC) is the key to attaining health for all. It also states that PHC needs to address the main health problems in the community, providing promotive, preventive, curative and rehabilitative services. The health care system is usually responsible for providing medical care and rehabilitation services, including assistive devices. Most basic rehabilitation activities can be carried out in the disabled person's own community using local resources.

5.3 Supports from the Educational Sector

Good co-operation between communities and the education sector is imperative if the goals of *Education for all* are to be met. The educational sector can make an important contribution to CBR by assisting community schools within the regular school system to become more inclusive. This involves, for instance, adapting the content of the curriculum and methods of teaching to meet the needs of all children rather than expecting them to adapt to a rigid curriculum. Schools may require assistance to change their methods of teaching in order to provide quality education for all children. Within the school system there are many people with knowledge and skills that could be shared with community schools. For example, there are schools that teach only child with special needs and the teachers from those schools can serve as resources to teachers in community schools. Schools that are already inclusive can help other schools learn how to respond to the needs of all learners, treat all children with respect, and be model schools.

5.4 Supports from the Employment and Labour Sector

Employment services organized by the sector help job seekers with disabilities to find employment opportunities in the open labour market. In addition, the civil service can set a good example by employing workers with disabilities.

5.5 Supports from NGOs

Most communities have a variety of non-governmental organizations (NGOs) and groups that can contribute to a CBR programme. These may include relief and development organizations, faith-based organizations, and service clubs as well as women's and youth groups. Some of these may provide services to people with disabilities, while others can make special efforts to include them in their activities.

5.6 Supports from the Media

Newspapers, radio, television and the internet can provide the public with information about disability issues, and also present a positive image of individuals with disabilities at school, work or in social settings.

5.7 Collaboration for Support to the Community

CBR will not work if the sectors mentioned above work in isolation. The following example illustrates the types of collaboration that can work well.

A CBR worker contacts a social welfare officer with information about an older child who has never been to school and who has difficulty with mobility and with learning. The officer and the CBR worker collaborate to encourage the family to contact the health services and the school. The health services assess the situation to see if something can be done to improve the child's mobility.

The teachers at the school assess the child's learning needs. If the child needs a wheelchair, for example, and there are no resources to pay for one, the social welfare officer requests assistance from other sectors, including NGOs.

Role of Physiotherapist in Community Based Rehabilitation

Physiotherapists undertake, or have the potential to undertake, a number of roles in primary health care and CBR dependent on local cultural and socioeconomic circumstances. These have been identified as:

- Preventing disability and deformity
- Educating/training disabled people to move around
- Promoting self-care
- Educating, training and transferring skills to other staff

- Consultancy, advice, support and supervision to other health care personnel
- Health promotion and disease prevention
- Curative and rehabilitation services
- Team leaders and managers
- Providers of direct care
- Advocates for disabled people, local communities as well as the profession
- Advisers to governments, NGOs and local communities on establishing CBR programmes

Physiotherapy in Institutions	Physiotherapy in CBR
• Direct service provision to the client	• Mainly indirect
• Predominantly 1:1 therapist: client ratio	• 1 therapist, to a given population
• Person receiving services usually addressed as patient	• Person receiving services addressed as client
• Rarely works in groups	• Often works in groups
• Allocates therapy time according to individual needs	• Allocates time based on the needs of the population
• Ideal to care for a few	• Good basic care to all
• Perceived higher professional status	• Perceived lower professional status
• Can focus on a strong biomedical model, although attitudes and approaches are changing	• Uses a strong social model • Teaches / trains local health workers and families to carry out day-to-day therapy acts as an expert resource

ROLE OF PHYSIOTHERAPY IN AIDS

The quality of life for people with human immunodeficiency virus (HIV) and acquired immune deficiency syndrome (AIDS) can be improved and expanded through physiotherapy intervention. With more than 13 million people throughout the world infected with HIV, it is imperative that rehabilitation professionals be prepared to access and utilize all possible modes of effective treatment.

People with AIDS have needs that may involve the services of virtually every member of the rehabilitation team. The physiotherapist is an important member of this multidisciplinary team, whose services include those that address the psychological, spiritual, vocational, and physical health of the individual. An understanding of the role of physiotherapist can facilitate the rehabilitation specialist's ability to make the best use of these professionals.

While AIDS is still regarded as a terminal illness, survival rates have increased to the point where rehabilitation is a predictable and necessary part of the person's plan of care. Rehabilitation needs are usually the result of disabilities caused as a primary or secondary result of the HIV infection or disabilities or injuries that result from etiologies unrelated to HIV. In either case, physiotherapy intervention may be divided into four major categories of goal-based activities. These are:

- Management of Pain
- Maintenance of Strength and Endurance
- Independence in Self-Care
- Education.

Management of Pain

Pain experienced by people with AIDS may come from any number of sources, ranging from those seen across the population in general to those more specifically associated with the sequelae of severe immune deficiencies. The key factor in pain as it relates to the role of the physiotherapist is its effect on function. Pain may be the primary cause of a reduction in function. This can lead to a rapid loss of independence and increased reliance on caregivers. The physiotherapist may use a combination of modalities and techniques for reducing pain. These include Ultrasound, Transcutaneous nerve stimulation (TENS), Laser, and counter-irritation. Manual therapy may be particularly successful in virus related myelitis. Reports of success in using techniques called myofacial release and craniosacral therapy also have been published.

Maintenance of Strength and Endurance

Since one of the hallmarks of AIDS is that it is a multisystem disease with a characteristically uneven clinical course, the maintenance of strength and endurance is critically important. In all cases, an individualized exercise program is designed after careful and thorough physiotherapy assessment.

The intensity of exercises designed for the AIDS client range from light resistive exercises—similar to those used for chronically ill persons—to assistive exercises, which are effective when strength to complete the appropriate motion on an independent basis is lacking. Whenever possible, the individual should be encouraged to participate in physical activities to his level of tolerance. Galantino and Pizzi (1991) report that they have found no data that support very aggressive exercise protocols. In fact, exercises that take the client to a point of fatigue may have negative consequences, including an increased feeling of a lack of control as well as general exhaustion. Based on the present body of literature, exercises should be limited to comfortable ranges that avoid fatigue (Spence, Galantino, Mossberg, & Zimmerman, 1990).

Self-Care

Self-care includes those activities relating to dressing, washing, feeding, taking medications, wound dressing, and exercise that are routinely employed by the client (Galantino, 1992; Spence, Galantino, Mossberg, and Zimmerman, 1990; Levinson & O' Connell, 1991). Of particular importance to the physiotherapist is the individual's ability to apply any necessary splints, braces, or other assistive devices necessary for maintaining function and independence. Techniques of energy conservation are also taught to enable the chronically ill person to achieve the maximum amount of self-care with the least amount of unnecessary effort.

Education

Education for the caregiver as well as the person with AIDS is of critical importance. In addition to developing, evaluating, and modifying the plan of care for the patient, the physiotherapist must be knowledgeable of and able to teach infection control to the client. Both the client and the caregiver must be carefully educated in methods to ensure that the activities of daily living are accomplished and that quality of life is maximized.

As the disease progresses, caregivers will become a more important part of the client's world. If they are to be effective, caregivers must be taught safe transfers from bed to chair as well as other important activities of daily living. Education to protect the health and safety of the caregiver is as important as that which pertains only to the individual with AIDS.

In all cases, AIDS education must include an in-depth coverage of universal precautions as defined by the Centers for Disease Control. Although sexual abstinence is the only real safe practice, those who remain sexually active should be educated in the safest procedures.

In summary, the physiotherapist's role in the treatment of AIDS related symptoms is an important one, and may include methods to reduce pain, increase strength and endurance, and maintain independence through self-care activities. Education that addresses all aspects of the client's life serves as the framework upon which safe, rational decisions can be made. AIDS is progressively becoming treatable. Effective and efficient treatment modalities can be selected only when the rehabilitation professional understands the scope of possibilities. Including the physiotherapist in this process can greatly augment the productivity and quality of life for people with AIDS.

REFERENCES

1. Helander E. Prejudice and Dignity - An Introduction to Community-Based Rehabilitation, New York; UNDP, 1999.
2. Helander E. Guest Editorial: 25 Years of Community-Based Rehabilitation. *Asia Pacific Disability Rehabilitation Journal*, 2000;*11(1)*: 4-9.
3. Helander E, Mendes P, Nelson G, Goerdt A, (1989). *Training in the Community for People with Disabilities.* Geneva, Switzerland: World Health Organization.
4. Henley E, Twible R. The value of physiotherapy and occupational therapy in community based rehabilitation. *Friday Meeting Transactions: Associate publication of Asia Pacific Disability Rehabilitation Journal* **1** (1), (1999).

5. International Labour Organization, United Nations Educational Scientific and Cultural Organization, United Nations Children's Fund, World Health Organization, (2002). *Community based rehabilitation (CBR) for and with people with disabilities. Draft Joint Position Paper. [now under revision]*. Geneva, Switzerland. International Labour Organization, United Nations Educational Scientific and Cultural Organization.
6. World Health Organization (1994). *Community-Based Rehabilitation for and with people with disabilities. Joint Position Pape,* Geneva, Switzerland.
7. Kaur R (2002). *The Physiotherapist in the Community.* The 8th General Assembly of Asian Confederation for Physical Therapy, Bangkok, Thailand.
8. Kay E, Kilonzo C, Harris M. Improving Rehabilitation Services in Developing Nations: The proposed role of physiotherapists. *Physiotherapy,*1994; 80(2): 77-82.
9. O. Toole B. Community-Based Rehabilitation Programmes. *Prospects,* 1995; **XXV**(2): 311-324.
10. United Nations (1994). *The Standard Rules on the Equalization of Opportunities for Persons with Disabilities.* New York; United Nations.
11. United Nations Economic and Social Commission for Asia and the Pacific (1997). *Understanding.*
12. *Community Based Rehabilitation.* UNESCAP, *www.unescap.org/decade/cbr.htm.*
13. World Health Organization (2001b). *The International Classification of Functioning, Disability and Health – ICF.* Geneva, Switzerland, World Health Organization.
14. World Health Organization (2001c). *Rethinking Care From the Perspective of Disabled People. Conference Report and Recommendations.* Geneva, Switzerland: World Health Organization, Disability and Rehabilitation Team.
15. World Health Organization (2001d). *The UN Standard Rules on the Equalization of Opportunities for Persons with Disabilities: government responses to the implementation of the Rules on medical care, rehabilitation, support services and personnel training I. Summary.* Geneva, Switzerland: World Health Organization.
16. World Health Organization (2002). *Innovative Care for Chronic Conditions Building Blocks for Action.* Geneva, Switzerland, World Health Organization.
17. World Health Organization (2003). *Review of CBR. International Consultation on Reviewing CBR 25- 28 May 2003, Helsinki, Finland.* AIFO,
18. World Health Organization, International Disability Consortium. (1996) *Guidelines for Conducting, Monitoring and Self-Assessment of Community Based Rehabilitation Programmes, Using Evaluation Information to Improve Programmes.* Geneva, Switzerland, World Health Organization.

19. World Health Organization, Swedish Organizations of Disabled Persons International Aid Association (2002). *Community Based Rehabilitation as we have experienced it..... voices of persons with disabilities.* Geneva, Switzerland: World Health Organization.
20. World Health Organization, UNICEF, (1978). *Report of the International Conference on Primary Health Care, Alma-Ata USSR, 6-12 September 1978. Jointly sponsored by the World Health Organization and the United Nations Children's Fund.* Geneva: World Health Organization.
Aids Watch (1992). PT Bulletin, 7 (32).
21. Centers for Disease Control. Revised classification system for HIV infection and expanded surveilance case definition for AIDS among adolescents and adults. Morbity and Mortality Weekly Report, 1992; 41, 1-13.
22. Galantino, M.L. (1992). Clinical assessment and treatment of HIV: Rehabilitation of a chronic illness. Thorofare, NJ: Slack.
23. Galantino, M.L., and Pizzi. M. Occupational and physical therapy for persons with HIV disease and their caregivers. Journal of Home Health Care Practitioners, 1991; 3 (3), 46-57.
24. Goodman, C.C (1990). Differential diagnosis in physical therapy: Musculoskeletal and systemic conditions. Philadelphia; W.B. Saunders.
25. Levinson, S.E, and O'Connell, P.G. Rehabilitation dimensions of AIDS: a review. Arch of Physical Rehabilitation, 1991; 72, 690-696.
26. O-Dell, M.W, and Dillon, M.E. Rehabilitation in adults with human immunodeficiency virus-related diseases. American Journal of Physical Medicine and Rehabilitation, 1992; 71 (3), 183-188.
27. Pamarola-Sune, T. Navia, B.A. Cordon Cardo, C. Cho E.S. and Price R.W. HIV antigen in the brains of patients with the AIDS dementia complex. Annals of Neurology, 1986; 21 (5), 490-496.
28. Spence, D.W, Galantino M.L, Mossberg K.A, and Zimmerman, S.O. Progressive resistance exercise: effect on muscle function and anthropometry of a select AIDS population. Archives of Physical Medicine and Rehabilitation, 1990; 71,644-648.
29. Wells P.E, Frampton V, and Bowsher D (1988). Pain management in physical therapy. Norwalk, CT; Appleton and Lange.

Four

Developmental Disabilities

Developmental disability is a term that refers to a permanent cognitive and/or physical impairment that usually occurs in the early years of life but can occur anytime before the age of 18 years. It usually results in significantly reduced capacity in three or more major life activities, such as communication, learning, mobility, living independently, decision making or self care, and the need for support, whether or not of an ongoing nature.

The term is used to refer to a range of conditions including intellectual disability, cerebral palsy, autistic spectrum disorder, spina bifida, cystic fibrosis, learning disability, muscular dystrophy and epilepsy. It is recognised that many people with a developmental disability may experience a number of impairments.

Developmental disabilities are usually classified as severe, profound, moderate or mild, as assessed by the individual's need for supports, which may be lifelong (Table 4.1).

Table 4.1: Crowe classification

Class	*Description*	*Dislocation*
Crowe I	Femur and acetabulum show minimal abnormal development	Less than 50% dislocation
Crowe II	The acetabulum shows abnormal development	50% to 75% dislocation
Crowe III	The acetabulum is developed without a roof. A false acetabulum develops opposite the dislocated femur head position. The joint is fully dislocated	75% to 100% dislocation

Contd...

Contd...

Class	Description	Dislocation
Crowe IV	The acetabulum is insufficiently developed. Since the femur is positioned high up on the pelvis this class is also known as "high hip dislocation".	100% dislocation

Causes of Developmental Disabilities

There are many social, environmental and physical causes of developmental disabilities, although for some a definitive cause may never be determined. Common factors causing developmental disabilities include:

- Brain injury or infection before, during or after birth.
- Growth or nutrition problems.
- Abnormalities of chromosomes and genes.
- Birth long before the expected birth date - also called Extreme prematurity.
- Poor diet and health care.
- Drug misuse during pregnancy, including alcohol intake and smoking.

DEVELOPMENTAL DYSPLASIA OF THE HIP

Developmental dysplasia of the hip (DDH) - Hip dysplasia, developmental dysplasia of the hip (DDH) or congenital dysplasia of the hip (CDH) is a congenital or acquired deformation or misalignment of the hip joint (see Fig 4.1).

Hip dysplasia can range from barely detectable to severely malformed/dislocated. The congenital form, teratologic or non-reducible dislocation occurs as part of more complex conditions.

The condition can be bilateral or unilateral:

- If both hip joints are affected one speaks of "bilateral" dysplasia. In this case some diagnostic indicators like asymmetric folds and leg-length inequality do not apply.
- In unilateral dysplasia only one joint shows deformity, the contralateral side may show resulting effects. In the majority of unilateral cases the left hip has the dysplasia.

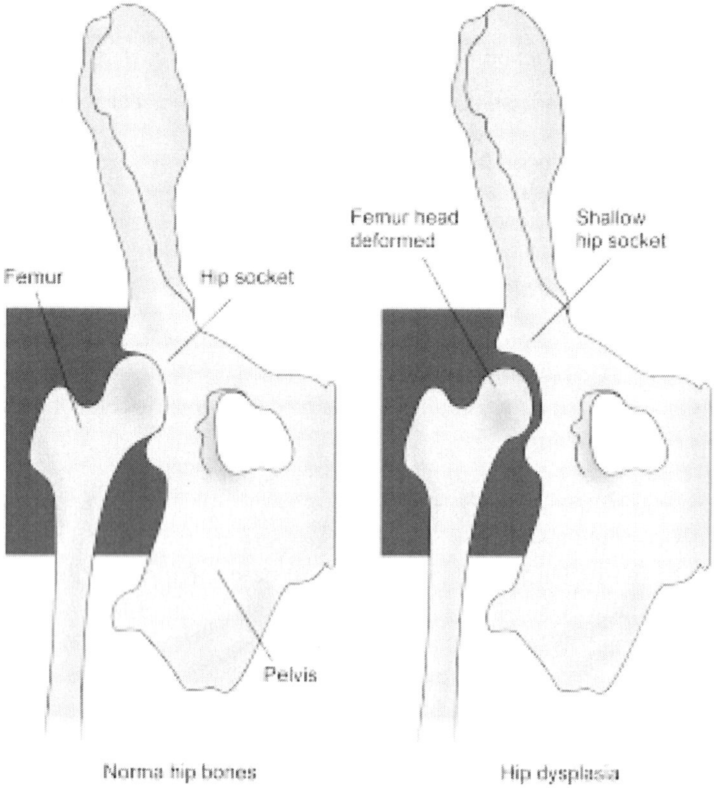

Fig. 4.1: Changes in DDH

If the joint is fully dislocated a false acetabulum often forms (often higher up on the pelvis) opposite the dislocated femoral head position.

In actetabular dysplasia the acetabulum (socket) is too shallow or deformed. The center-edge angle is measured as described by Wiberg . In coxa vara the femur head grows at too narrow an angle to the shaft, in coxa valga the angle is too wide.

Incidence

An instability rate of 1:60 has been described, though this rate drops to 1:240 at one week. The condition occurs with higher frequency in females than in males.

Causes

Hip dysplasia is considered to be a multifactorial condition. That means that several factors are involved in causing the condition to manifest. Cause is unknown but common in breech position or large fetal size.

Congenital

Some studies suggest a hormonal link. Specifically the hormone relaxin has been indicated.

Acquired

As an acquired condition it has often been linked to traditions of swaddling infants or use of a cradle board which locks the hip joint in an "abducted" position for extended periods. Modern swaddling techniques allow some room for leg movement.

Further risk factors include breech birth and first borns. In breech position the femoral head tends to get pushed out of the socket. A narrow uterus also facilitates hip joint dislocation during fetal development and birth.

Diagnosis

Most countries have standard newborn exams that include a hip joint exam screening for early detection of hip dysplasia. It can often be detected by a "click" or more precisely "clunk" in the hip (although not all clicks indicate hip dysplasia). Two maneuvers commonly

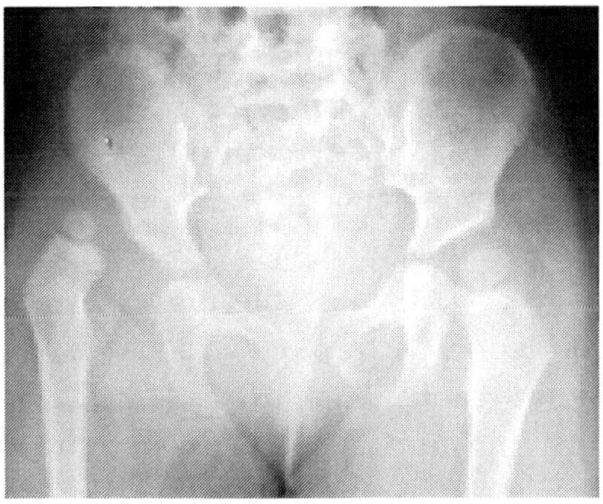

Fig. 4.2: Radiograph in DDH

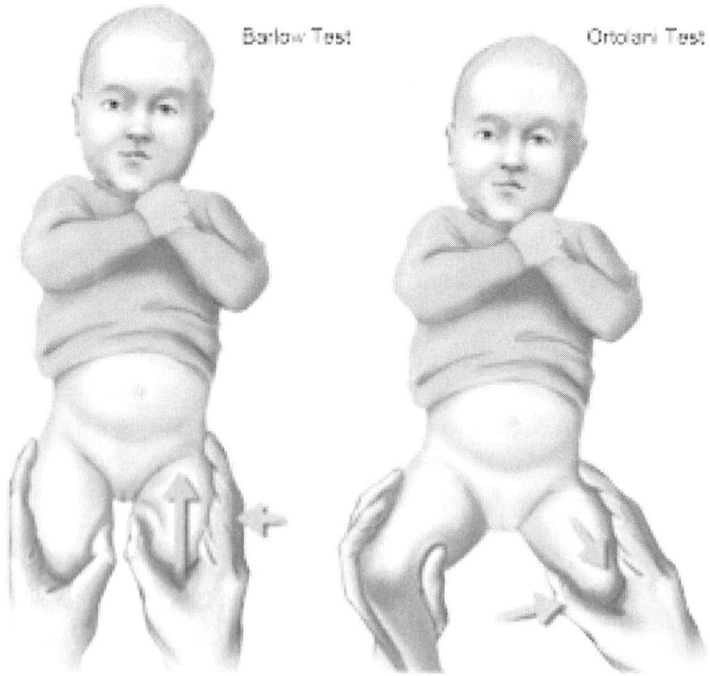

Fig. 4.3: Barlow test and Ortolani Test for DDH

employed for diagnosis in neonatal exams are the Ortolani maneuver and the Barlow maneuver (Fig 4.3)

Diagnostic Procedures may Include

- X-ray (Fig 4.2) - a diagnostic test which uses invisible electromagnetic energy beams to produce images of internal tissues, bones, and organs onto film.
- Ultrasound (also called sonography) - a diagnostic imaging technique which uses high-frequency sound waves and a computer to create images of blood vessels, tissues, and organs. Ultrasounds are used to view internal organs as they function, and to assess blood flow through various vessels.
- Computed tomography scan (also called a CT or CAT scan) - a diagnostic imaging procedure that uses a combination of x-rays and computer technology to produce cross-sectional images

(often called slices), both horizontally and vertically of the body. A CT scan shows detailed images of any part of the body, including the bones, muscles, fat, and organs. CT scans are more detailed than general x-rays.

- Magnetic resonance imaging (MRI) - a diagnostic procedure that uses a combination of large magnets, radiofrequencies, and a computer to produce detailed images of organs and structures within the body.

In X-ray imaging dislocation may be indicated if the Shenton's line (an arc drawn from the medial femoral neck through the superior margin of the obturator foramen) does not result in a smooth arc.

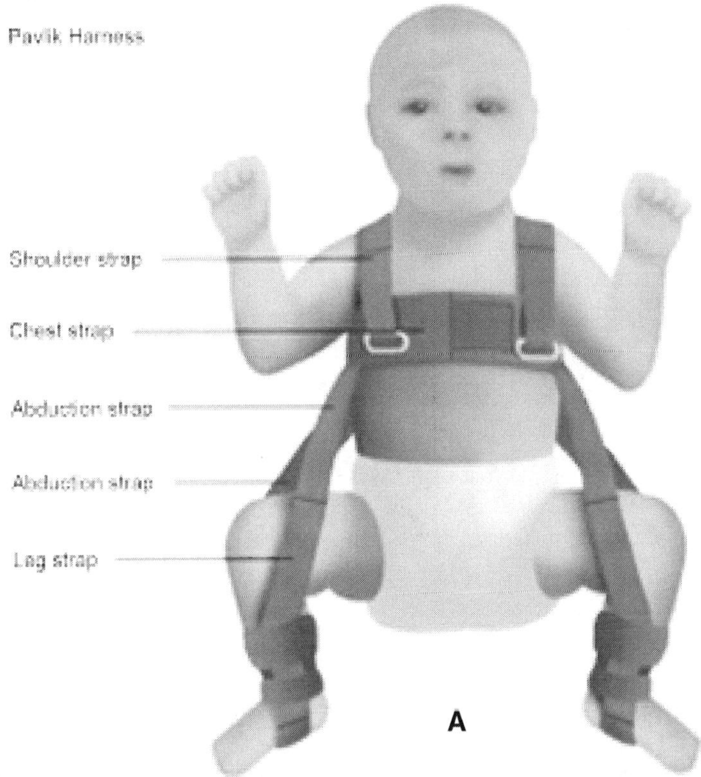

Fig. 4.4 A : showing A. Pavlik harness , B. Frejka splint , C. Hip spica cast

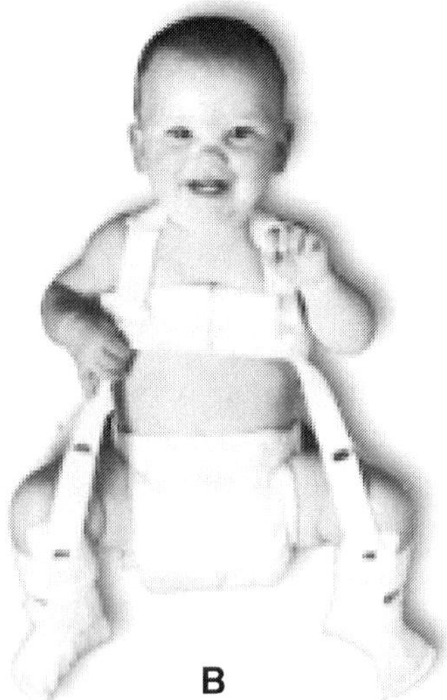

B

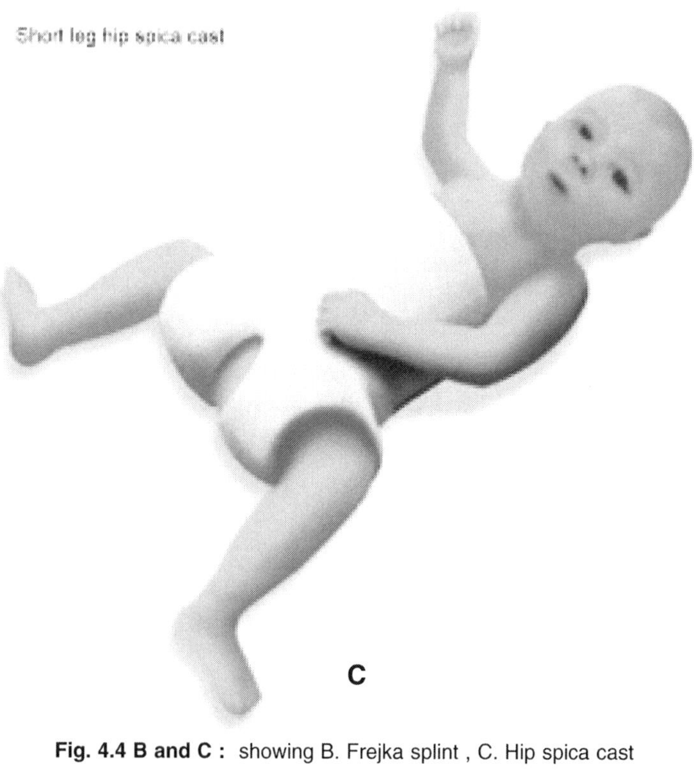

C

Fig. 4.4 B and C : showing B. Frejka splint , C. Hip spica cast

Management

Harnesses, Casts, and Traction

Early hip dysplasia can often be treated using a Pavlik harness (see Fig 4.4A) or the Frejka pillow/splint (see Fig 4.4B) in the first year of life with usually normal results.

Surgery

In older children the hip abductor and iliopsoas muscles have to be treated surgically because they adapt to the dislocated joint position (contracture). Braces and splints are often used following either of these methods to continue treatment.

Hip Replacement and Osteotomy

Hip dysplasia is often cited as causing osteoarthritis of the hip at a comparatively young age. Dislocated load bearing surfaces lead to increased and unusual wear. Subsequent treatment with total hip arthroplasty (hip replacement) is complicated by a need for revision surgery (replacing the artificial joint) due to skeletal changes as the body matures, loosening/wear or bone resorption.

Osteotomies are either used in conjunction with arthroplasty or by themselves to correct misalignment.

POLIOMYELITIS

Greek: Polio (gray) and Myelon (marrow)–Involvement of the Spinal Cord

- Classic manifestation: paralysis
- Other terminologies: poliomyelitis anterior acute, fatty atrophic paralysis of infancy, essential infantile paralysis, and Heine Medin disease.
  - Poliomyelitis is also known as infantile paralysis is, an infectious viral disease that affects the spinal cord or a part of the brain.
  - Poliomyelitis infection is caused by an enterovirus, which causes muscular paralysis. In some cases respiratory muscles are affected; in others limb muscles.

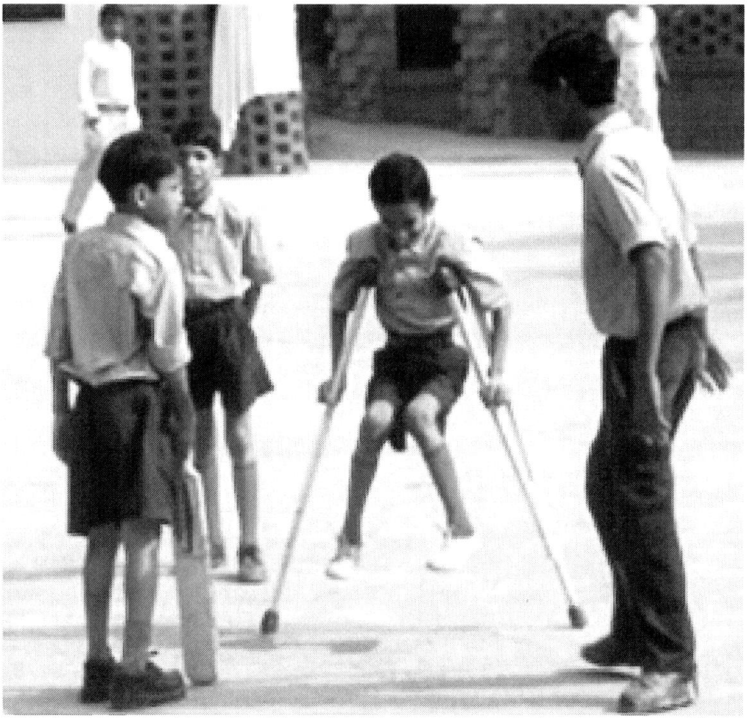

Fig. 4.5 : Poliomyelitis

Poliomyelitis is an acute viral infection caused by an RNA virus. It is primarily an infection of the human alimentary tract but the virus may infect the central nervous system, in a very small percentage (about 1 per cent) of cases resulting in varying degrees of paralysis, and possibly death (see Fig. 4.6).

Epidemiological Basis

- Poliomyelitis is eradicable because man is the only host.
- A long-term carrier state is not known to occur.
- The half-life of excreted virus in the sewage is about 48 hours, and spread can only occur during this period.

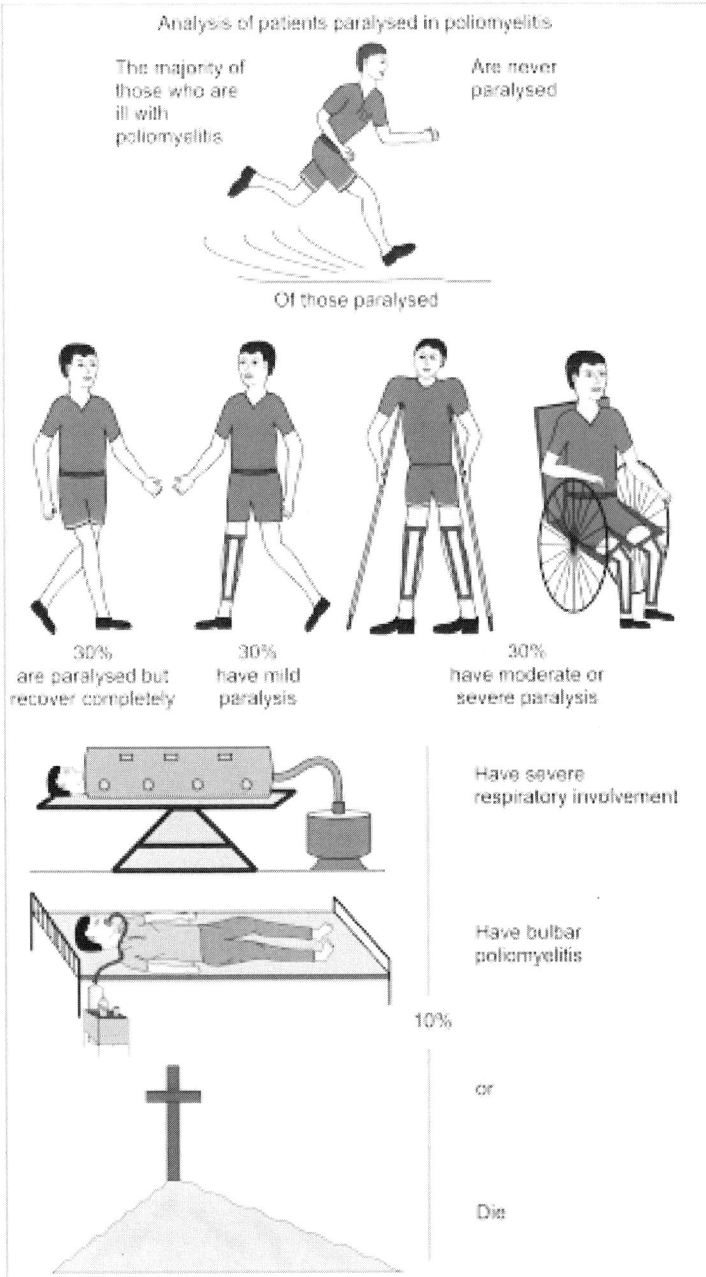

Fig. 4.6: Analysis of patients paralysed in poliomyelitis

Agent factors

- The causative agent is the poliovirus which has three serotypes 1,2 and 3. Most outbreaks of paralytic polio are due to type-1 virus.
- In a cold environment, it can live in water for 4 months and in faeces for 6 months, the virus may be rapidly inactivated by pasteurization, and a variety of physical and chemical agents.

Mode of Transmission

a. **Faecal-oral Route:**
   - The infection may spread directly through contaminated fingers where hygiene is poor, or indirectly through contaminated water, milk, foods, flies and articles of daily use.

b. **Droplet Infection:** This may occur in the acute phase of disease when the virus occurs in the throat.

Incubation Period

- Usually 7 to 14 days (range 3 to 35 days).

Early Symptoms of Polio

- These are similar to those of other viral infections, it includes; slight fever, headache dizziness, nervous irritability, and vomiting.
- Skin can become tender and sore.
- Stiffness and pain in the back and neck, and pain in the arms, legs, or abdomen.
- Muscles may be tender and spasmodic (subject to involuntary contractions).

Clinical Spectrum

a. Inapparent (Subclinical) Infection
b. Abortive Polio or Minor Illness
c. Non-paralytic Polio
d. Paralytic Polio

Paralytic Polio

- Occurs in less than one per cent of infections. The virus invades CNS and causes varying degrees of paralysis.
- The predominant sign is asymmetrical flaccid paralysis. A history of fever at the time of onset of paralysis is suggestive of polio.
- The other associated symptoms are malaise, anorexia, nausea, vomiting, headache, sore throat, constipation and abdominal pain.
- There might be signs of meningeal irritation, i.e., stiffness of neck and back muscles.
  - 2-5% of polioviral infection cases
  - Spinal cord anterior horn cells and other motor neurons: selectively susceptible
  - Incubation: 4-10 days, may extend to 4- 5 weeks
  - 1st symptoms: nonspecific fever and muscle weakness (?? >2-3 days).

Spinal Poliomyelitis

Affects LE > UE > Trunk

- Preceded by: ↑↑ muscle pain and spasm
- Paralysis: asymmetric, flaccid, patchy, proximal > distal ? may extent to other limbs after > 5-6 days
- Paralysis maximum in 48 hrs (some: > 1 wk)
- Paralysis progression: ↓↓ if the fever (-) in 48 hrs
- Reflexes ↓↓ (-) and bulbar involvement may follow
- Muscle atrophy: > 3 wks (max 12-15 wks ?permanent)
- Paresthesia: frequent without sensory disturbances.
- Rare accompanying conditions: trans. myelitis + paraparesis, urinary retention, sensory and autonomic disturbance.

Bulbar Poliomyelitis

A.K.A. brainstem poliomyelitis (10-15% of paralytic poliomyelitis cases)

- Isolated bulbar without limb weakness: more common in children (especially without history of tonsils and adenoids removal)
- Adult type: bulbospinal poliomyelitis

- Pain, nuchal rigidity and hypertonia: brainstem, spinal ganglia, and posterior column
- Cranial nerves: VII, IX, X, (rare: III) ? facial weakness, dysphagia, dysphonia, and oculomotor palsy (rare)
- Reticular formation: cardiorespiratory problems

Polioencephalitis

- Very rare and uncommonly occurs without paralysis
- Paralysis: may emerges 24-48 hrs > initial onset
- Clinical manifestations: tremulousness, obtundation, agitation, and autonomic dysfunction
- Autonomic: labile hypertension / hypotension, tachycardia, arrhythmias, and hyperhydrosis
- UMN signs: spasticity, hyperreflexia, and Babinski
- Other signs: muscle pains, muscle cramps, fasciculation, and radicular pain.

FUNCTIONAL ALTERATIONS

Activity
- Getting dressed
- Getting in and out of bed
- Feeding yourself
- Taking a bath or shower
- Using the miler
- Walking on level surfaces
- Climbing stairs
- Meeting physical demand of job, home, etc.

Change
- Less Walking
- Reduce social life
- More rest
- Reduced or stopped physical recreation
- Do less housework
- Employ household help
- Use more skills
- Get family to help more
- Plan more efficiently

- Moved house, modified house
- Less exercising
- Less standing
- Changed diet
- Other changes

Muscle Recovery (see Fig. 4.7)

- Muscle recovery: 6-9 month after onset (some >3 months)
- 50-70% of maximum capacities recover
- < 2 yrs: minimum improvement — slow progress
- >2 yrs: permanent

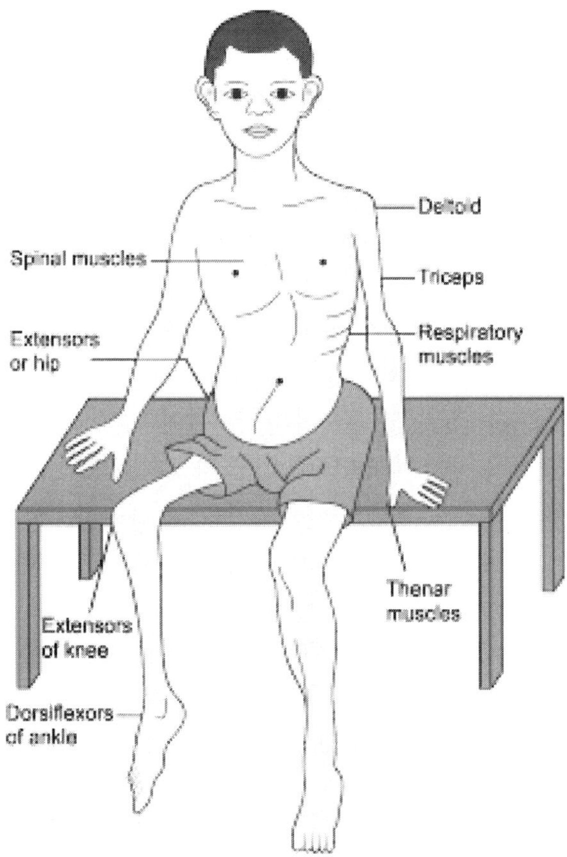

Fig. 4.7: Muscles commonly affected in poliomyelitis

- Severe cases: 50% functional strength and 20% complete recovery
- Children: progressive neurologic disorder
- Moderate cases: 90% recover
- Site of recovery: >> LE proximal muscles

Neuromusculoskeletal Function

Acute Flaccid Paralysis in polio: 3 phases ("triad two")
1st: Acute → subacute phase (1st 2 wks — 2 wks to 2 mo)
2nd : Convalescent phase (>2 mo - 2 yrs)
3rd : Chronic/Residual phase (> 2 yrs)
→ post polio condition → postpolio syndrome

- Paralysis in polio: UMN/LMN
- AFP: LMN type
- UMN type: rare
- UE paralysis: major predilection site → deltoids and triceps brachii— object manipulations may be normal
- Accompanying symptom of pain: devastating and may disturb other functions as well
- Pain: muscles, joints, and nerves (>> lower back)
- Hyperesthesia → pain ↑↑

  Children Physical Examination: transitional mobility activities and walking activity.
- Tests: standing on toes, standing on heels, squat-to-stand test, sit-to-stand test, jump in one leg, and walk test
- Infants PE: observe behavior on supine position
- Paralysis: frog-leg position (see Fig. 4.8)
- Other tests: sharp stimulus test and pendulum test

Musculoskeletal Complications

- Shortening and ↑↑ in diameter of the bone, due to:

  << Muscle pull, vascular supply disturbance + and nerve stimulation
- Bone will become << compact and may not able to support loading.

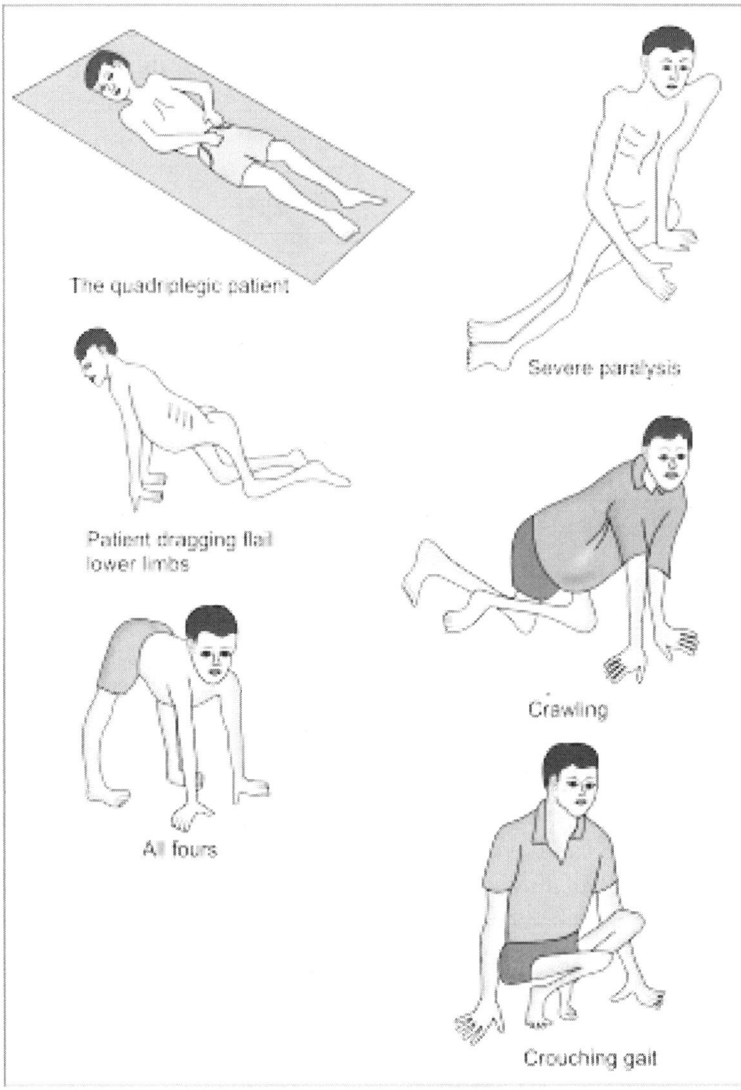

Fig. 4.8: The untreated poilio patient

Fractures May Easily Develop

- Bone-shortening in LE: result in LLD → disturb the posture balance on the vertebrae—deformity in vertebrae (scoliosis)

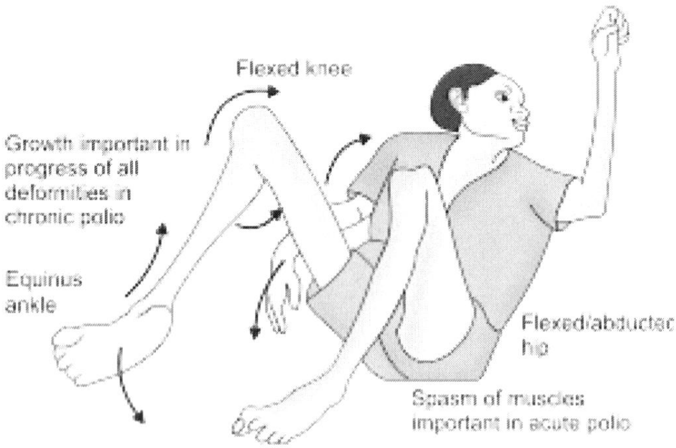

Fig. 4.9: Causion of Deformities (Imbalance of muscle)

Tripod Sign (see Fig. 4.10)

- The child finds difficulty in sitting and sits by supporting hands at the back and by partially flexing the hips and knees. Progression of the paralysis to reach its maximum in the majority of cases occurs in less than 4 days (may take 4-7 days).
- The paralysis is characterized as descending, i.e. starting at the hip and then moving down to the distal parts of the extremity.
- It is asymmetrical patchy paralysis; proximal muscle groups are more involved as compared to distal ones.

Cardiopulmonary Function

- Respiratory function (triple threat): weak respiratory muscles, poor cough efforts and risk of food aspiration
- Intercostal paralysis: AHC infection in thoracic region
- Diaphragm paralysis: AHC infection in the mid-cervical region
- Involvements in: dorsal nuclei of the Vagus and the medial reticular nuclei (vasomotor nuclei): pulmonary edema, CO2 retention, and papilledema

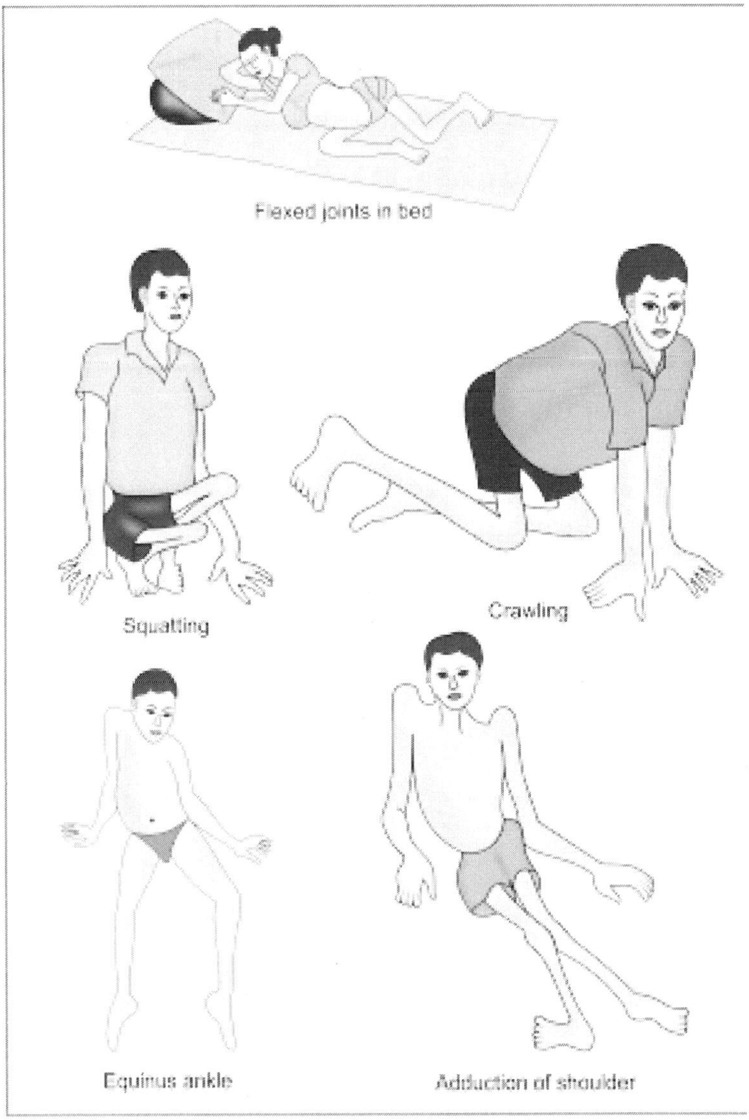

Fig. 4.10A: Causes of deformities

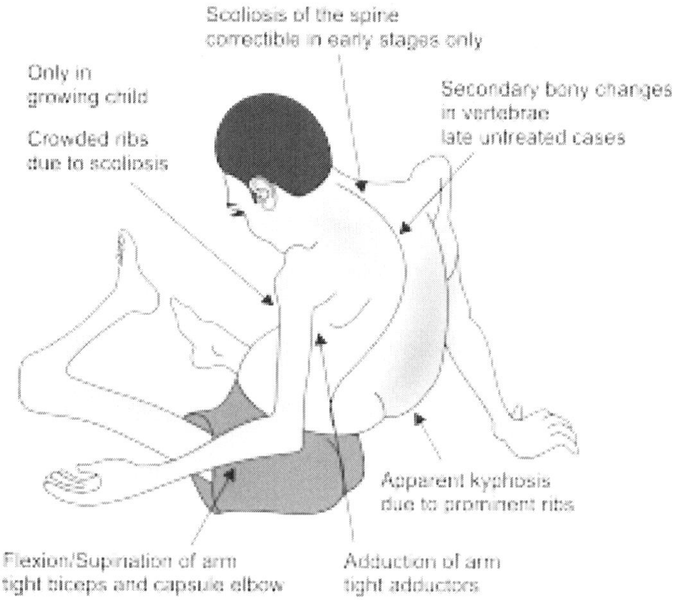

Fig. 4.10B: Maintenance and progression of contractures

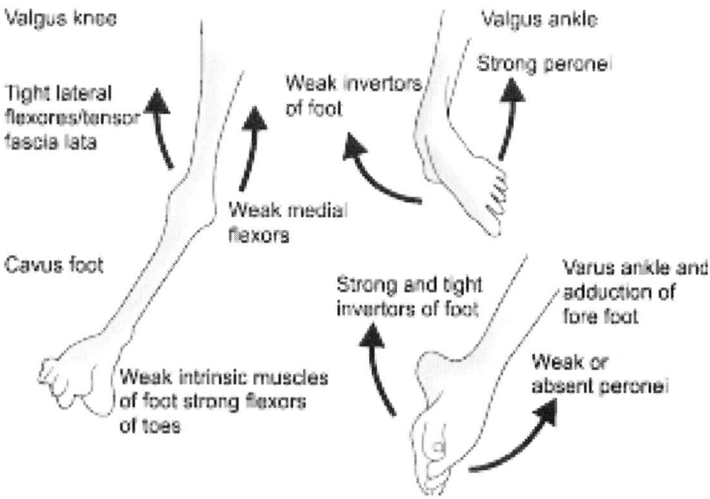

Fig. 4.11: Causation of Deformities (Imbalance of muscules)

- Involvement of nerve Vagu: dysphagia , (damaged innervation to the larynx ? potential airway obstruction (early tracheotomy)
- Paralysis of the larynx: saliva/mucus go down to the lower respiratory tract—pulmonary infection/edema
- Paralysis of the soft palate: speech disturbance
- Medullary/hypothalamus involvements: 2nd hypertension.

Behavioral Problems

- Tendencies in polio survivors: develop behavioral changes
- Type A personality: non-compliant to rehabilitation program, especially vocational
- Characteristic: hard-driving and excessive worker, pressured, easily angered, perfectionist, too sensitive to criticism and failure, hyperactive; have a chronic insecurity feeling, and low self-esteem.

GENERAL REHABILITATION MANAGEMENT IN POLIOMYELITIS

- Acute Phase
- Convalescent Phase
- Residual Phase

Acute Phase

- Physiatrist determines whether there are any bulbar involvements or not
- Respiratory assistance (life-saving intervention)
- Infants with respiratory failure : negative extra thoracic pressure ventilation (NEPV)
- Older children: intubation/intermittent positive pressure ventilation
- Bulbar involvement: inability of the patient to swallow ("drown" in his/her own secretions)
- Management: respiratory assistance and positioning technique.

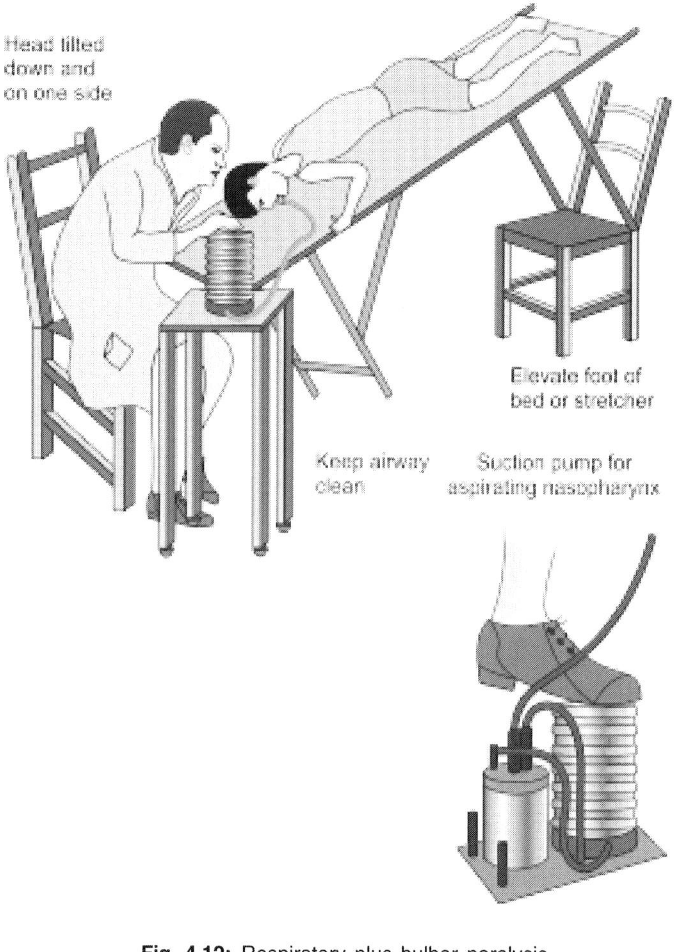

Fig. 4.12: Respiratory plus bulbar paralysis

Respiratory Assistance + Positioning Technique

- Bulbar palsy without respiratory failure: risk of aspiration (+) , owing to dysphagia
- Emergency management: posturing technique using a medially-angulated bed and pillows to support the center of the mattress
- Secretions will trickle down from the patient's mouth ? aspiration risk can be prevented (see Fig. 4.13C)

Other Rehabilitation Strategies

- Preventing complications secondary to prolonged bed rest/ immobilization (see 4.14 A and B)
- Pain management

Pain Management

Medications and supported by physical modalities:
- TENS
- Hot pack (Canny pack)
- Infrared therapy
- Electrical stimulation

EARLY MOBILIZATION

Goals of Early Mobilization

- Maintaining and exercising movement coordination
- preventing pressure ulcers
- prevention of deconditioning syndrome
  → (takes place after the febrile (-) and progression of paralysis ↓↓)
- Bed mobilization: rolling, side-lying, prone, sitting, or standing - using tilting table
  - Crawling activity: if possible
  - Abdominal breathing exercise and chest expansion exercise: as early as possible
  - Sitting balance exercise: if possible (preparation for ambulation).
- Instructions for patients and relatives (see Fig. 4.14A , B and C)

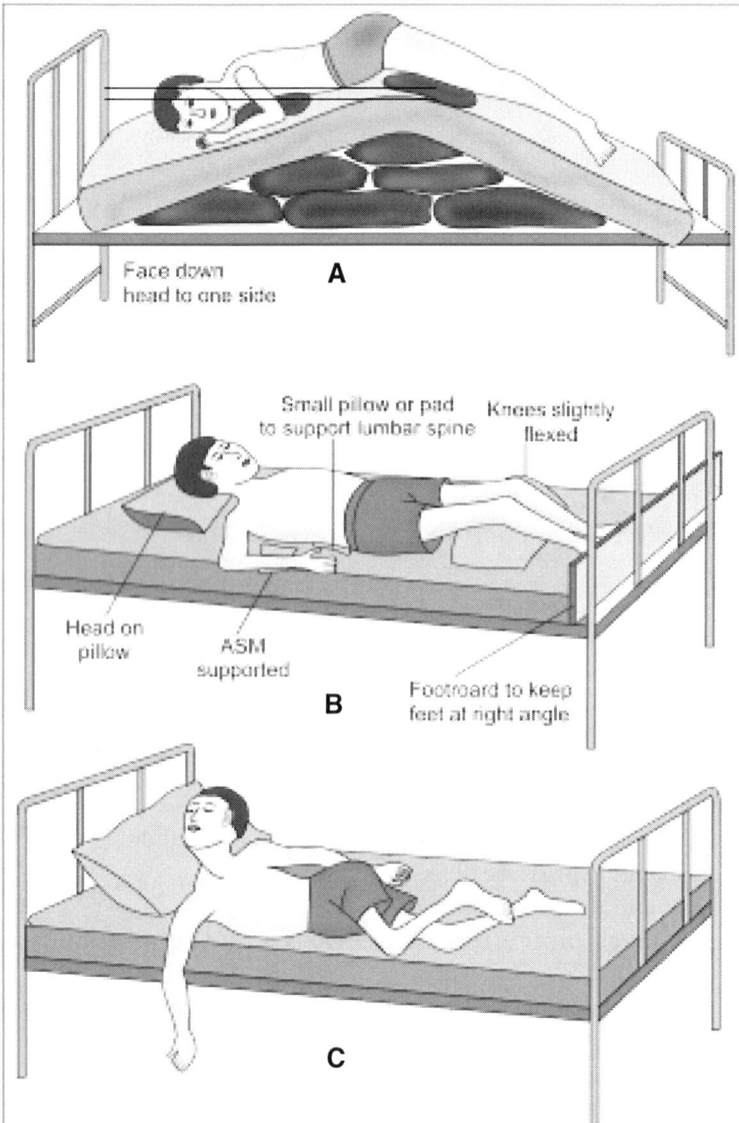

Fig. 4.13A, B and C: (A) Position of patient; (B) Nursing in acute poliomyelitis, Good mental and physical rest; (C)Treatment of patient with bulbar palsy alone

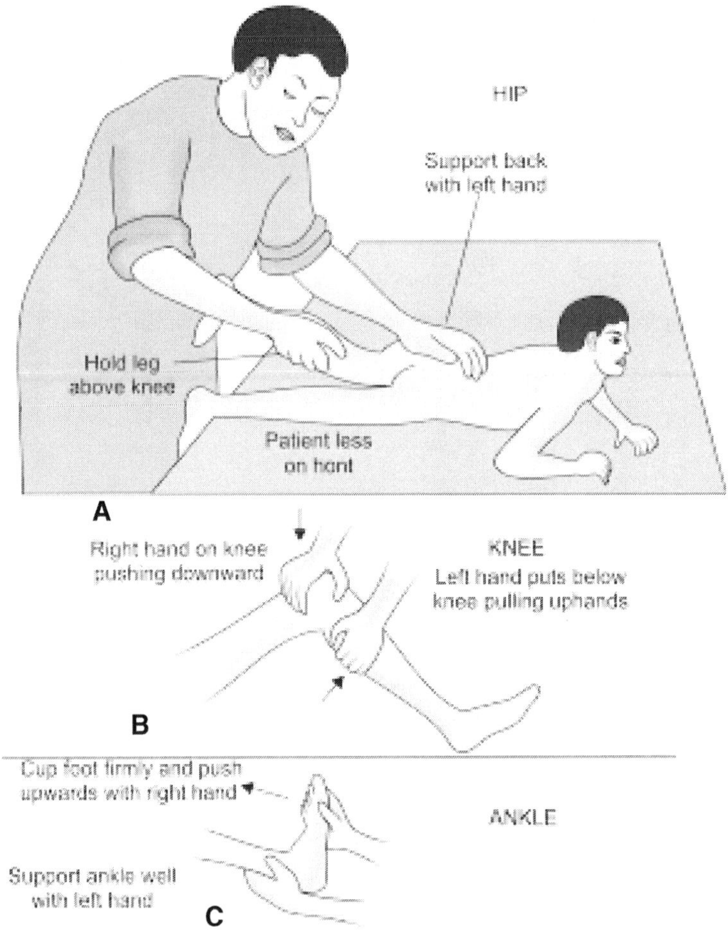

Fig. 4.14A, B and C: Stretching of tight muscles, A: Hip, B: Knee, C: Ankle

CONVALESCENT PHASE

- Mobilization (see Fig. 4.15)
- Hydrotherapy
- Muscle strengthening exercise (affected and unaffected limbs)

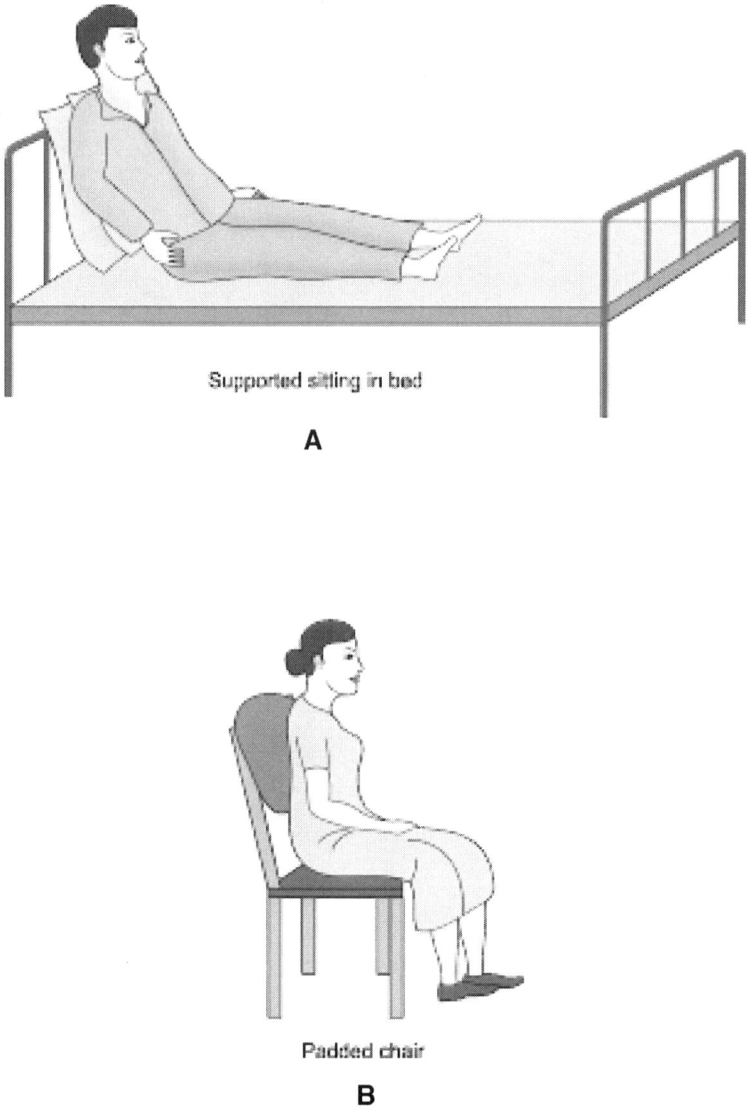

Fig. 4.15A and B: Mobilisation of the convalescent patient

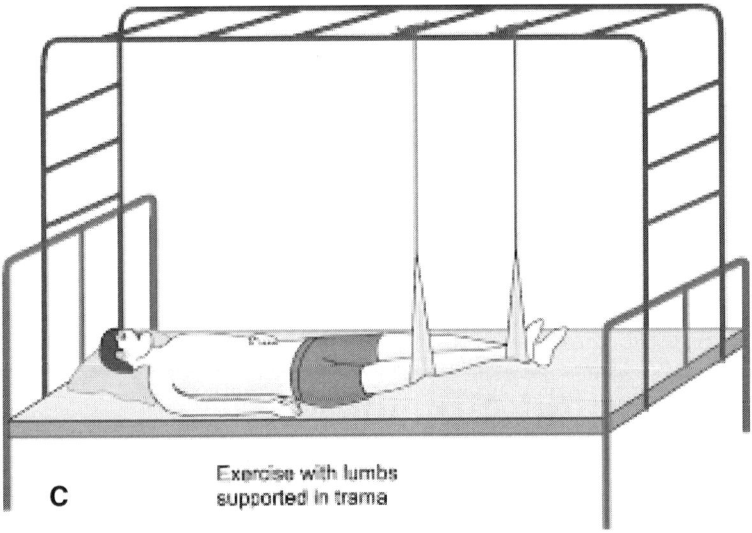

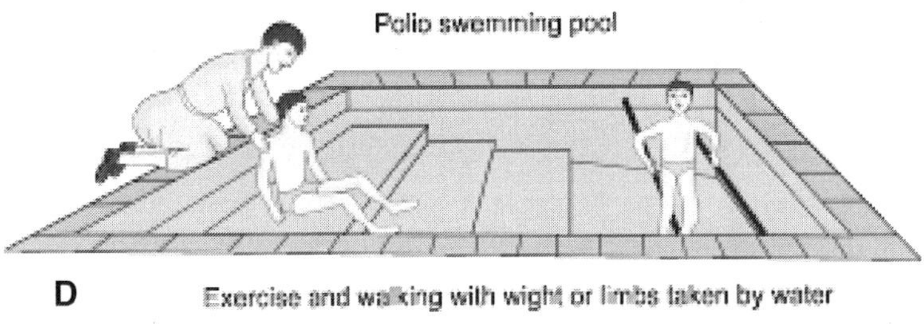

Fig. 4.15C and D: Mobilisation of the convalescent patient

- Standing and gait preparation
- Lower orthosis/spinal orthosis

LE orthosis

- HKAFO: MMT of hip extensors / flexors < 3
- KAFO: MMT of the knee < 3
- AFO: MMT of the ankle < 3
- FO: is indicated if there are ankle-foot deformities that require certain correction
- Spinal orthosis: scoliosis

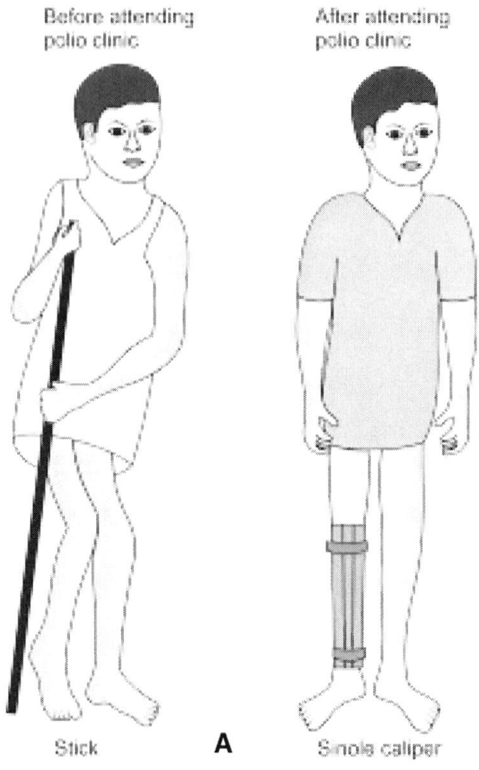

Fig. 4.16A: Supports in developing countries

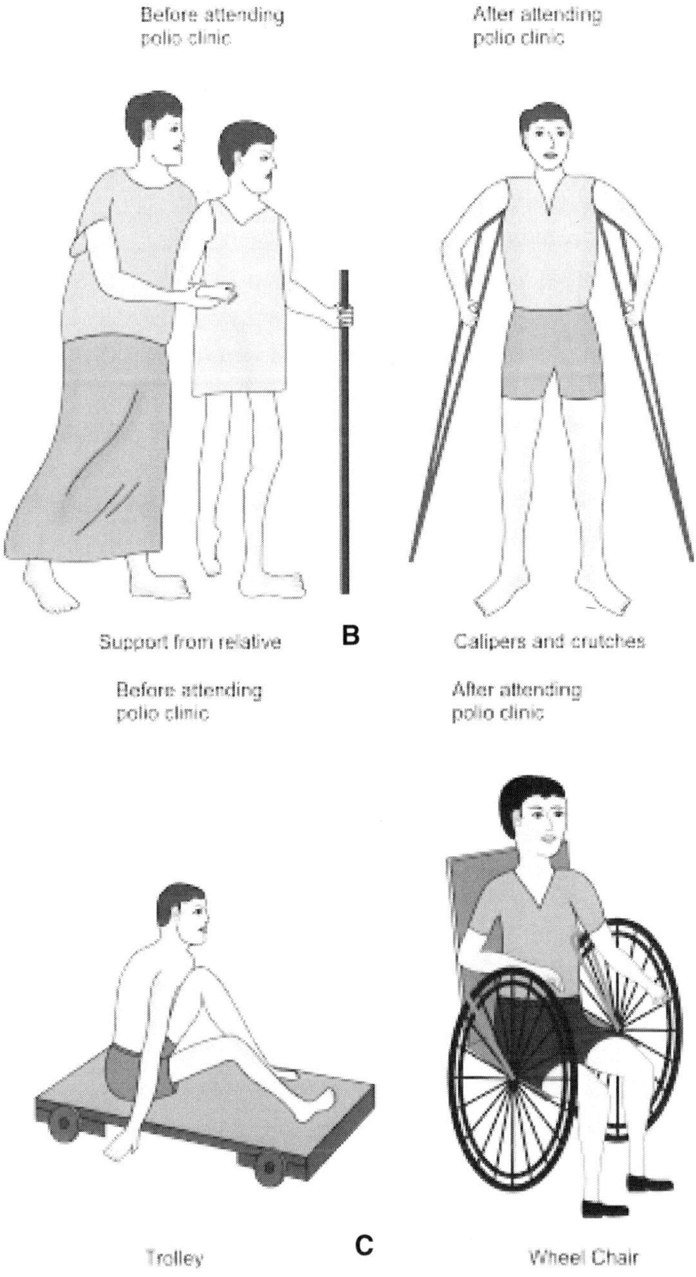

Fig. 4.16B and C: Supports in developing countries

SUPPORTS IN DEVELOPING COUNTRIES

RESIDUAL PHASE

Hallmark of rehabilitation: develop substitution pattern of the muscles (enabling patient to perform ADLs maximally)

- Orthosis: mandatory (exc. complete recovery)
- Operative management: sometimes necessary

Evaluation of the Patient

- 1st 2 months: every week (mo-1) and every 2 weeks (mo-2)
- > 2-6 months: evaluate every 2 months
- > 2 - 3 years: evaluate every 6 months

Management: (see 4.17, Fig. 4-18A and B)

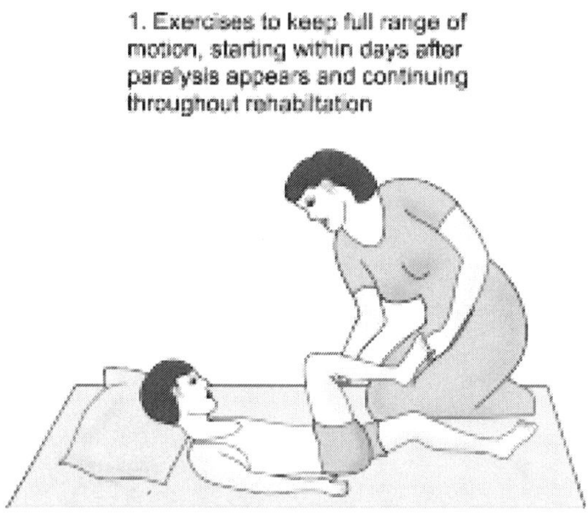

Fig. 4.17 (1): Corrective steps for residuel phase

2. Supported sitting in positions that help prevent contractures

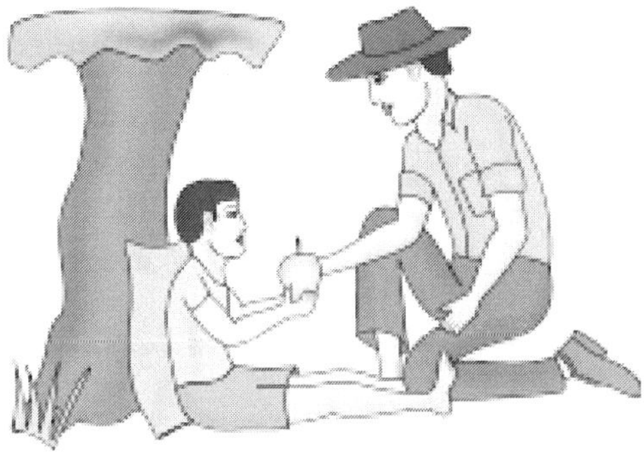

3. Active exercises with limbs supported, to gain strength and maintain full motion

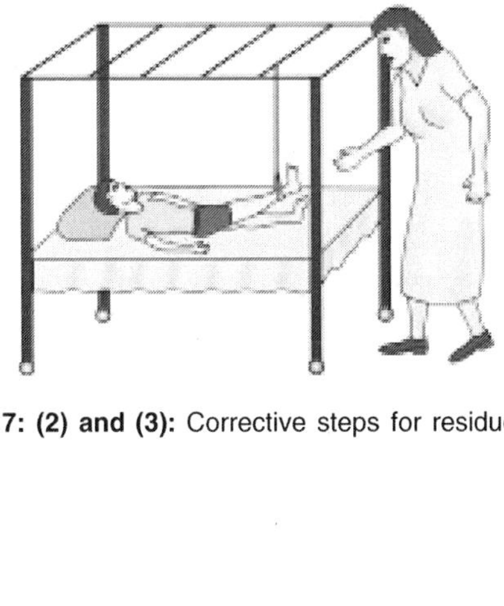

Fig. 4.17: (2) and (3): Corrective steps for residuel phase

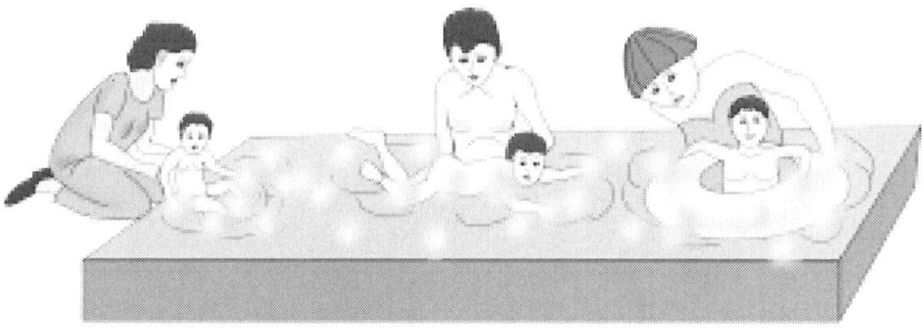

4. Exercise in water- walking, floating and swimming, with the weight of the limbs supported by the water

5. Wheelboard or wheelchair with supports to prevent or correct early contractures

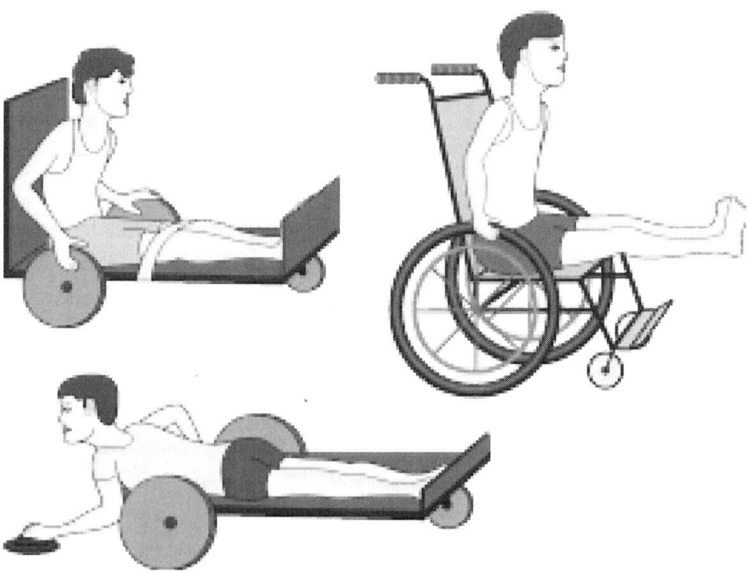

Fig. 4.17: (4) to (5): Corrective steps for residuel phase

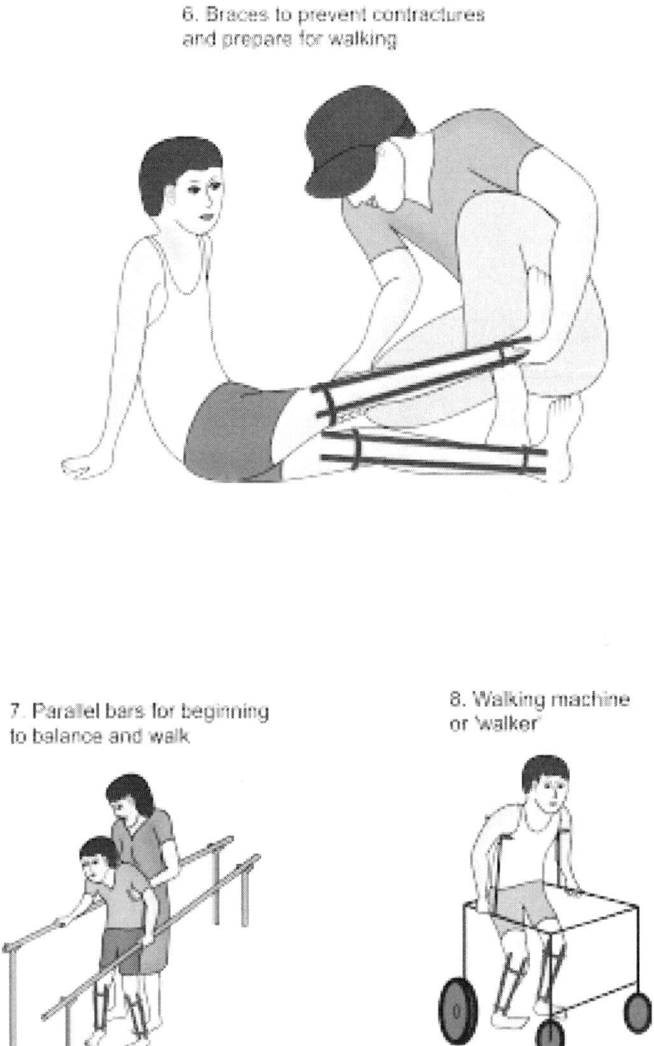

Fig. 4.17: 6 to 8: Corrective steps for residuel phase

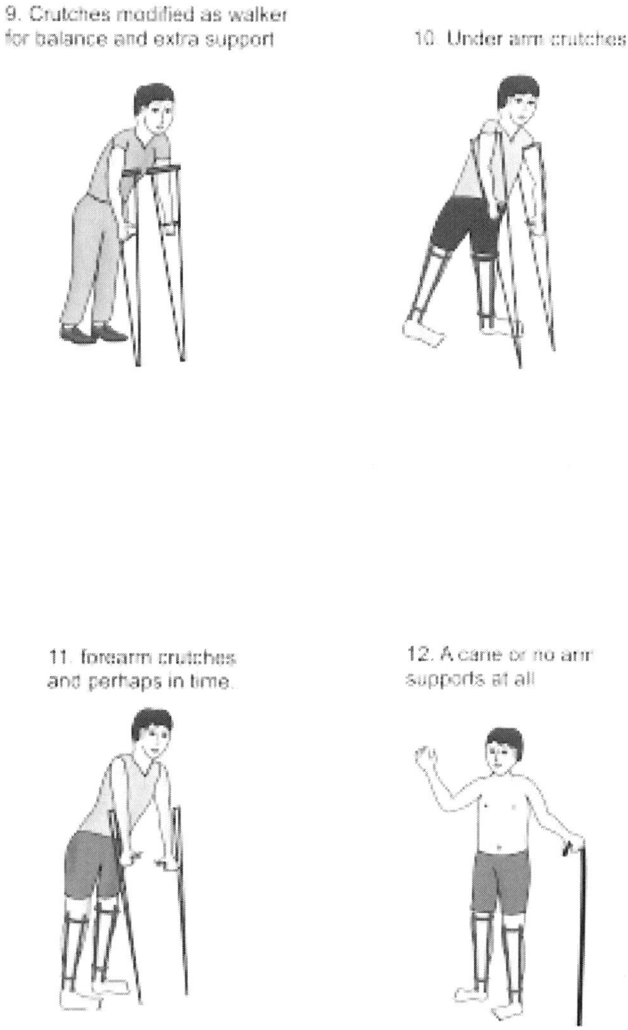

Figs 4.17: 9 to 12: Corrective steps for residuel phase

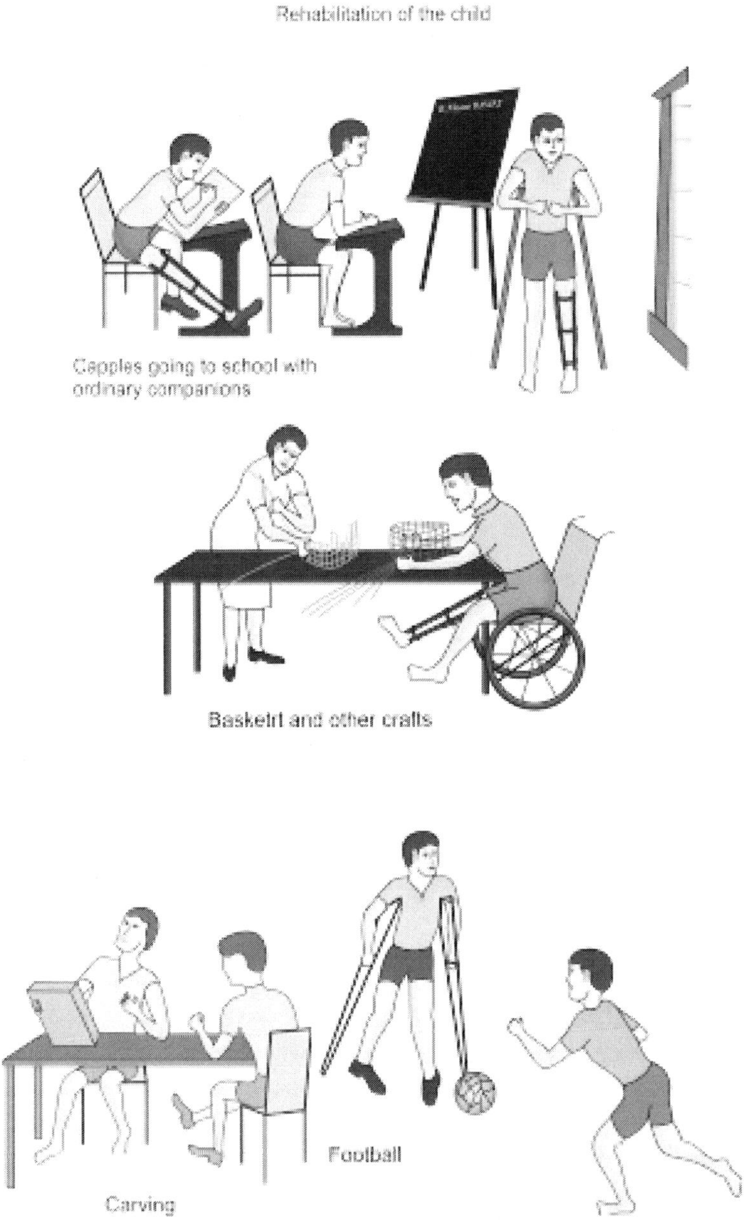

Fig. 4.18A: Rehabilitation of the child

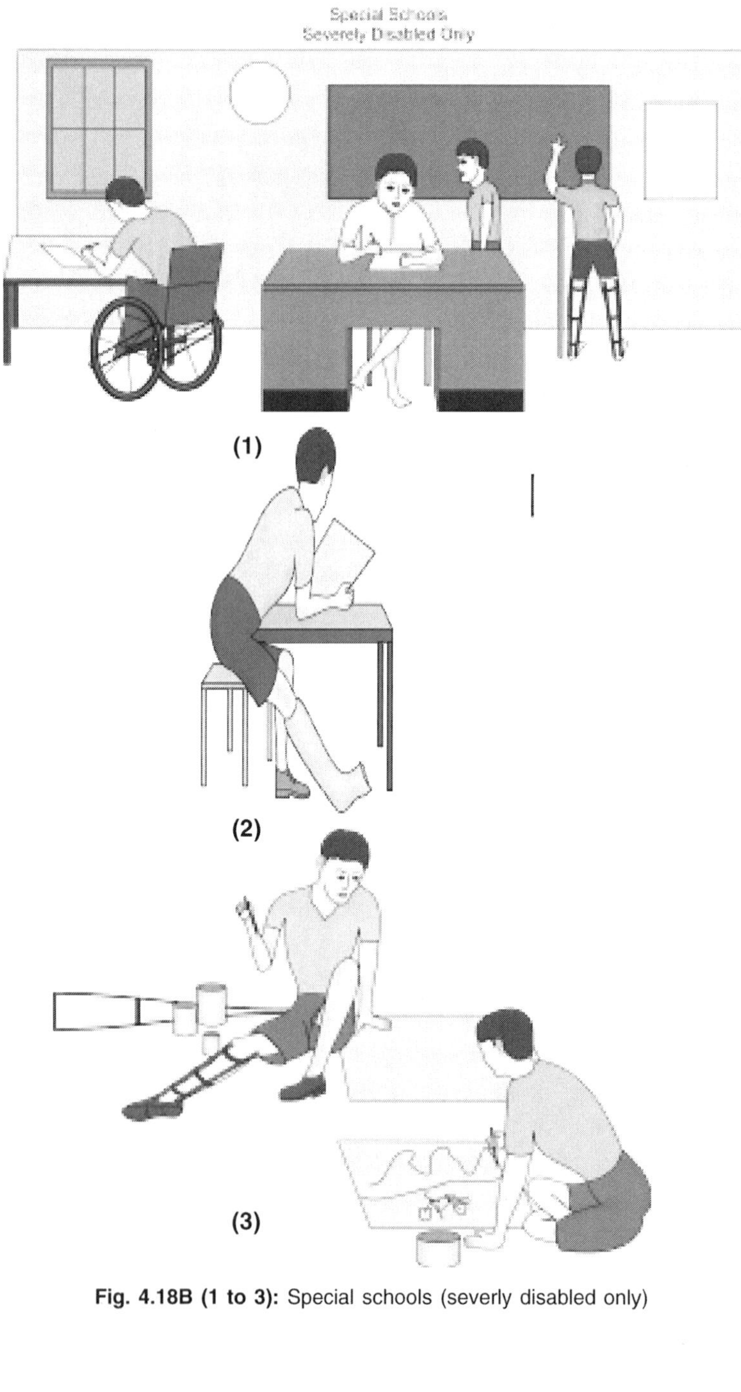

Fig. 4.18B (1 to 3): Special schools (severly disabled only)

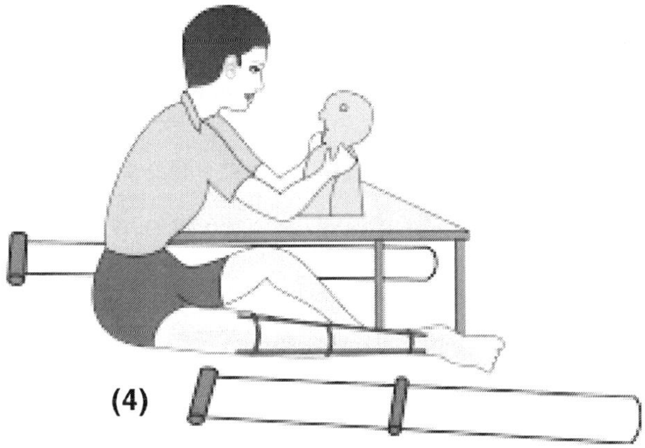

Fig. 4.18 (4): Special schools (severly disabled only)

POST-REHABILITATION MANAGEMENT

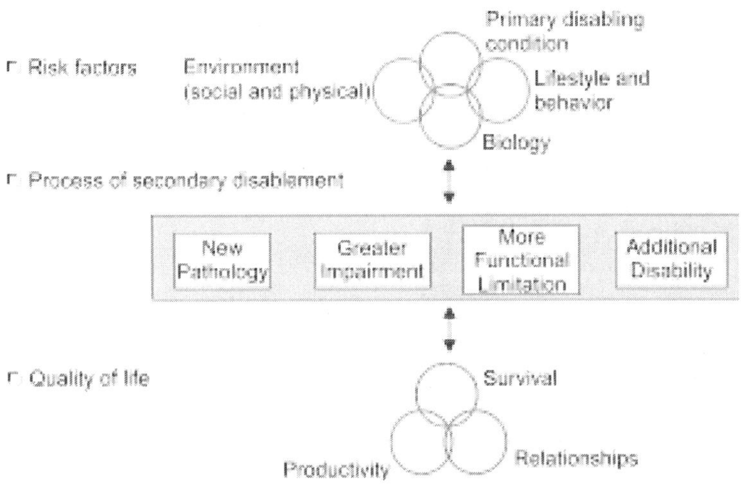

Fig. 4.19: Post Rehabilitation Management

AN APPROACH TO THE PATIENT WITH SUSPECTED POST POLIO SYNDROME

Prime Symptoms

Fatigue, Pain, and Weakness: Almost always present

- Fatigue (89%); pain in muscle/joint (86%); new weakness (83%) in previously symptomatic (69%) / asymptomatic (50%) muscles
- New Atrophy (28%) —Post Polio Muscular Atrophy (PPMA)
- ADL difficulties (78%) = functional loss
  ⇒ walking (64%); climbing stairs (61%); dressing (17%).

Additional Presenting Problems

- Pulmonary dysfunction
- Sleep Disorders
- Dysphagia
- Cold intolerance
- Degenerative arthritis
- Social and psychological problems.

Identify Areas of Dysfunction

- Hisory ⇒ identifying: fatigue, dysphagia, sleep disorders, and ADL alterations.
- Neurologic examination: atrophy/weakness, reflexes are not ↑↑
- Observe the "good" limb: (+) significant weakness without patient's awareness
- Leg muscles: use functional tests (MMT may not detect ↓↓ quadriceps strength to 30% of normal → although sufficient for routine ADLs)
  MMT: use mechanical advantage (e.g. Mm. triceps/quadriceps with the elbow/knee flexed > 900; m. psoas in supine position)
- General Physical examination and biomechanical examinaion: note obesity, joint deformity, overuses syndromes, and scoliosis
- EMG: document previous AHC disease (especially if previous polio is doubtful) and ruling out other neuromuscular pathologies/identifying subclinically involved muscles
- Lab: CK ↑ (may not correlate with progressive weakness).

REHABILITATION STRATEGIES

A. Management of PPS

1. Identification and treatment of other medical and neurological disorders which can mimic the symptoms of PPS
2. Management of weakness:
   - Strengthening exercises (isometric, isotonic, isokinetic)
   - Aerobic exercise
   - Stretching exercises (↓ / prevent contractures)
   - Avoidance of muscular overuse
   - Weight loss
   - Orthoses or other assistive devices.
3. Management of fatigue
   - Energy conservation techniques
   - Lifestyle changes
   - Pacing
   - Regular rest periods, naps during day
4. Management of pain.
   - Post-polio muscular pain, muscular cramps, muscular pain with activity
   - Activity reduction
   - Pacing (rest periods during activity)
   - Moist heat, ice, and stretching
   - Use of assistive devices
   - Life style modifications.

B. Fibromyalgia

- Medicines: Amitriptyline/cyclobenzaprine
- Aerobic exercise.

C. Joint and Soft Tissue Abnormalities

- Modification of extremity use
- Physiotherapy for use of physical modalities, strengthening, stretching.
- Orthoses/other assistive devices
- Medicins: NSAIDs, steroid injections/Surgery.

D. Treatment of other superimposed neurologic disorders (e.g. CTS, radiculopathy, spinal stenosis)

5. Pulmonary dysfunction
   - Preventive measures (pneumococcal vaccine, yearly influenza vaccine)
   - Ventilatory assistance (non-invasive methods preferred)
   - Identification and treatment of sleep apnea
   - Glossopharyngeal breathing.
6. Dysphagia
   - Changing or restricting diet
   - Use of special breathing techniques
   - Use of special swallowing techniques
   - Monitoring fatigue, and taking larger meals earlier, and smaller meals later
   - Avoiding eating when fatigued.
7. Psychosocial difficulties
   - Interdisciplinary approach
   - Post-polio support group
   - Evaluation and treatment by social workers, psychologists, psychiatrists.

Lifestyle Modifications

- The "sine qua non" of all attempts at successful management of PPS
- Patients: desperate, have a belief to overcome their disability through the "no pain, no gain" approach
- "No pain, no gain" approach: may be successful after the acute onset ⇒ now become self destructive
- Persistence in this approach: spiral of deteriorating function and ↓↓ self worth
- Understand the concept of "living with" PPS ↓↓
- Understanding the need for lifestyle modification: rarely achieved at 1st visit → must be reintroduced by an OT/PT and reinforced and monitored at subsequent physician visits

Increase Muscle Capacity

a. Achieving ↑↑ strength/endurance:
   - Strength: isometric exercise—select muscles carefully (some muscles will already be functioning at their maximum)
   - Exercise: may have a deleterious effect by forcing these muscles beyond their metabolic capacity and producing injury

b. Appropriate exercise: ↑↑ endurance, ↓↓ susceptibility to fatigue, ↓↓ long term deterioration:
   - Initial difficulties: occur in almost all patients (from overdoing)
   - May tend to associate fatiguing ADLs (challenge the weakest musculature and do not provide an effective aerobic training level) with exercise

   ⇒ can be an instructive opportunity for understanding the "lifestyle modification"

Goals in Aerobic Exercise

- Educate the patient to avoid potentially harmful exercise-induced fatigue
  ⇒ Strategy: establish the level of peak performance by patient history—start at 50% of peak performance and slowly ↑↑ performance as tolerated
- Select exercises which can create a training effective in the patient with weakened, atrophic musculature and overuse syndromes
  ⇒ Strategy: exercise intervals with intervening rests, just as is pacing of ADLs

c. Use of bracing, orthotics, or other aids which extend, amplify or substitute for muscles (to increase muscle capacity)

d. Pharmacologic treatment of fatigue: (↑↑ fatigue threshold) still observed and needs confirmation:
   - Amantadine
   - Deprenyl
   - Mestinon

Medications: just aid to give a running start for the rehabilitation process (patient should understand them as a non curative treatment)

Decrease Muscle Load to Less than Muscle Capacity

a. **Pacing of activity**
   - Implementation: patients must identify each of the ADL's length of time (before experiencing fatigue)
   - Break up activities into smaller modules of time (each with << duration (before fatigue occurs)
   - Concept of Pacing: Energy Budgeting—patient has a fixed energy expenditure (EE) for each day and should be spent on the highest priority of ADLs
   - Concept of exceeding use of this daily limit: acquire debt—correlates to metabolic injury of the motor unit (overuse).

b. Other means of decreasing muscle load:
   - Diet (for overweight >>)
   - Orthotics (improve mechanical efficiency)
   - Wheelchairs/scooters to save EE
   - Treatment of chronic overuse syndromes.

Treat Specific Complications

a. Attention to specific complications: e.g. dysphagia, pulmonary dysfunction and sleep disturbances
b. Functional consequences resulting from overuse syndromes (joint deformity)
   → Physiatry consultation/orthopedic intervention
   → Orthotic prescriptions (i.e., splints, braces, AFO's)
c. Somatization, depression, anxiety, and self worth problems: may occur as capacity ↓↓ (referral for counseling or polio support group)
d. Evaluate and/or modify work duties through referral to OT or vocational counselor.

Exercise in PPS Patients

- Include: isotonic, isokinetic and isometric strengthening exercise programs and aerobic exercise
- Average level of aerobic fitness in post-polio patients: 5.6 METS (similar to myocardial infarction patients)
- Aerobic exercise (UE + LE): bicycle ergometer or treadmill

- Bicycle ergometer: improved VO2 max, duration of exercise, watts attained during exercise, and maximum expired volume per unit time
- Treadmill training: improved economy or energy cost of walking (+ walking duration).

Exercise Prescription: Dependent on Several Factors

- Isometric: MMT < 3 or in muscles over a painful joint
- Isotonic: MMT > 3 and without a painful joint
- Aerobic exercise program: bicycle ergometer, walking, or swimming (should be an activity which the patient enjoys to increase compliance)
- Warm-up and cool-down period and stretching exercises should be included
- Early in the exercise program: monitored carefully (to ensure that the exercise prescription is being followed correctly and muscles and joints overuse is not occurring)
  - Encourage self-monitor.

Cardiovascular Exercise

The aims of aerobic exercise include:

- Improved heart function and efficiency—the average level of aerobic fitness in post-polio patient is 5 METS – similar to the fitness of patients following a myocardial infraction.
- Improved circulation.
- Improved respiratory function.
- Improved efficiency of working muscles; and
- Decreased blood pressure.

On the basis of scientific studies of the effects of aerobic exercise on post-polio subjects, the general features of aerobic exercise programs should be:

- Low intensity and non-fatiguing exercise
- Activities the patient enjoys–to improve compliance
- Low resistance activities that are least likely to fatigue compromised muscles. The activities may include walking cycling on a level surface, swimming and hydrotherapy.

Gentle stretching of tight muscle in the post-polio patient may:

- Improve posture
- Relieve muscle tension and cramping
- Reduce the risk of musculotendinous and joint range of motion.
- Prevent irrersible contractures, and
- Increase general flexibility before strengthening exercise.

It must be noted that reduced flexibility is not necessarily detrimental. Tightness of certain structure may help to provide stability and improve function. Therefore, stretching is not always appropriate.

Hydrotherapy

Hydrotherapy is often the exrcise method of choice for post-polio patients. When hydrotherapy is used in combination with other physiotherapy techniques. It has been found to improve muscle strength, range of movement, balance, coordination and endurance.

Hydrotherapy is particularly beneficial to the post-polio population because:

- The scope of water activities can benefit post-polio patiens with all levels of ability
- Exercising in water is a very pleasant and encouraging way to exercise particularly for non-mobile patients.
- Warm water promotes muscle relaxation and improved circulation.
- It allows particular movements to be either assisted, supported or resisted by the buoyancy of water.
- It reduce weight bearing and can decrease mechanical stress on limbs, depending on the level of immersion.

Prevention

- Immunization is the sole effective means of preventing poliomyelitis.
- Both killed (Salk) and live attenuated (Sabin) vaccines are available and both are safe and effective when used correctly.
- It is essential to immunize all infants by 6 months of age to protect them against polio.

Types of Vaccines

- Two types of vaccines are used throughout the world; they are :

1. Inactivated (Salk) polio vaccine (IPV)
2. Oral (Sabin) polio vaccine (OPV).

National Immunisation Schedule (see Table 4.2)

Table 4.2: National Immunisation Schedule

Sn.	*Age*	*Disease*	*Vaccination*
1.	At Birth	Hepatitis B	Hep B Vaccine -i
2.	At Birth	Polio	Oral Pv 0 Dose
3.	Birth To 6 Weeks	Tuberculosis	BCG
4.	4 -6 Weeks	Hepatitis B	Hep B Vaccine -ii
5.	6 Weeks	Diphtheria pertusis tetanus Polio	DPT-I OPV -I
6.	10 Weeks	Diphtheria Pertusis Tetanus Polio Hepatitis B	DPT-II OPV-II HEP B Vaccine III
7.	14 Weeks	Diphtheria Pertusis Tetanus Polio	DPT-III OPV- III HEP B Vaccine IV
8.	24 Weeks	Hepatitis B	HEP B Vaccine III
9.	9 -12 Months	Polio Measles	OPV-IV Measles
10.	15-18 Months	Mumps Measeles Rubella	MMR
11.	18 Months	Diphtheria Pertusis Tetanus Polio	DPT -Booster I OPV -V
12.	24 Months	Typhoid	Typhoid

Contd...

Contd...

Sn.	*Age*	*Disease*	*Vaccination*
13	4-5 Year	Diphtheria Pertusis Tetanus Polio	DPT Booster - II OPV -VI

RICKETS

Rickets is the softening and weakening of bones in children, usually because of an extreme and prolonged vitamin D deficiency. Vitamin D is essential in promoting absorption of calcium and phosphorus from the gastrointestinal tract, which your child needs to build strong bones. A deficiency of vitamin D makes it difficult to maintain proper calcium and phosphorus levels in bones. If a vitamin D or calcium deficiency causes rickets, adding vitamin D or calcium to the diet generally corrects any resulting bone problems for your child. Rickets due to a genetic condition may require additional medications or other treatment. Some skeletal deformities caused by rickets may need corrective surgery.

Symptoms

Vitamin D deficiency begins slowly before physical signs and symptoms of rickets appear. When rickets signs and symptoms develop, they may include:

- Skeletal deformities: These include bowed legs, abnormal curvature of the spine, pelvic deformities, and breastbone projection in the chest.
- Fragile bones: Children with rickets are more prone to bone fractures.
- Impaired growth: Delayed growth in height or limbs may be a result of rickets.
- Dental problems: These include defects in tooth structure, increased chance of cavities, poor enamel and delayed formation of teeth.
- Bone pain: This includes dull, aching pain or tenderness in the spine, pelvis and legs.
- Muscle weakness: Decreased muscle tone may make movement uncomfortable.

Causes

Vitamin D acts as a hormone to regulate calcium and phosphorus levels in bones. Due to Vitamin D deficiency it causes decreased absorption of calcium and phosphorus properly. The body senses the imbalance of calcium and phosphorus in bloodstream, it reacts by taking calcium and phosphorus from bones to raise blood levels to where they need to be. This softens or weakens the bone structure, which can result in skeletal deformities, such as bowlegs or improper curvature of the spine. Osteomalacia is the adult version of rickets. Vitamin D is adsorbed from two sources:

- Sunlight: Skin produces vitamin D when it is exposed to sunlight.
- Food: The intestines absorb vitamin D that's found naturally in the foods , or added to it during processing, or from supplements or multivitamins.

Rickets can also be caused by conditions that impair vitamin D absorption, such as the surgical removal of all or part of the stomach (gastrectomy) and celiac disease, in which the small intestine doesn't absorb certain nutrients from food. Additionally, conditions that impair the absorption of any fat soluble vitamin, which includes A, D, E and K, increases the risk of rickets. Other causes of rickets include:

Hereditary rickets (X-linked hypophosphatemia), an inherited form of rickets caused by the inability of the kidneys to retain phosphorus, or a complication of renal tubular acidosis, a condition in which your kidneys are unable to excrete acids into urine. Lack of exposure to sunlight, which stimulates the body to make vitamin D.

Risk factors

Children 3 to 36 months old are most at risk of rickets because they are growing rapidly and vitamin D, calcium and phosphorus play a major role in the growth process. Other risk factors for rickets include:

- Lack of vitamin D: Breast-fed infants who don't receive supplemental vitamin D are at increased risk of developing rickets because although vitamin D does cross from mother to baby in the breast milk, it's not enough to prevent a deficiency. While exposure to sunlight could produce the necessary amounts of vitamin D, sunburn and skin cancer are real dangers. Sunscreens,

which are used to protect against these dangers, can decrease vitamin D production by blocking the sun's ultraviolet rays.
- Lack of calcium and phosphorus: Children who don't get enough calcium and phosphorus in their diets are at increased risk of rickets.

Complications

While easily treated once it is diagnosed, rickets has a severe list of complications if left untreated. Untreated vitamin D deficiency rickets may lead to:
- Delays in child's motor skills development, failure to grow and develop normally
- Skeletal deformities
- Chronic growth problems that can result in short stature
- Seizures
- Dental defects.

Tests and Diagnosis

- Physical examination
- Blood tests
- X-rays
- Medical history.

Treatments and Drugs

The aim of treatment for rickets is to solve the underlying disorder. If deficiencies in vitamin D, calcium or phosphorus are at fault–replacing vitamin D and those minerals generally eliminates the signs and symptoms of rickets, such as bone tenderness and muscle weakness. Improvement generally occurs within three months. Vitamin D supplement to increase your intake of vitamin D-fortified foods, including fortified breakfast cereal, orange juice, fish and processed milk. Getting a sufficient intake of calcium is crucial to maintaining healthy bones. Appropriate level of calcium intake depending on your age and whether you have absorption problems. The combination of increased vitamin D intake with calcium may be enough to eliminate the effects of rickets entirely. Treating complications for some cases of bowlegs or spinal deformities, Special bracing to position child's body appropriately as the bones grow. More severe skeletal deformities may require surgery.

Prevention

Although most adolescents and adults receive much of their necessary vitamin D from exposure to sunlight, infants and young children need to avoid direct sun entirely or be especially careful by always wearing sunscreen. Vitamin D supplements in light of these factors, and because human milk contains only a small amount of vitamin D, all breastfed infants receive 400 international units (IU) of oral vitamin D daily beginning during the first two months of life and continuing until the daily consumption of vitamin D-fortified formula or milk is two to three glasses, or 500 milliliters (mL).

CONGENITAL TALIPES EQUINOVARUS (ALSO KNOWN AS)

Clubfoot (See Fig. 4.20A and B) is a condition in which one or both feet are twisted into an abnormal position at birth. The condition is also known as talipes.

It is a general term used to describe a range of unusual positions of the foot. This is present at birth and affects the foot and/or ankle. There is no known cause for clubfoot, and it is twice as common in male children as it is in female children. Most type of clubfoot is present at birth which can happen in one foot or in both feet. In almost half of affected infants, both feet are involved. Although clubfoot is painless in a baby, treatment should begin immediately. Clubfoot can cause significantly problems as the child grows, but with early treatment most children born with clubfoot are able to lead a normal life

Giles Smith syndrome, Talipes equinovarus; Talipes (Also known as)

Incidences

The frequency of congenital clubfoot is approximately 1 per 1,240 live births. In children there is a subtle imbalance in muscle forces in the lower leg resulting in the foot deformity. Often, the foot is 'kidney-

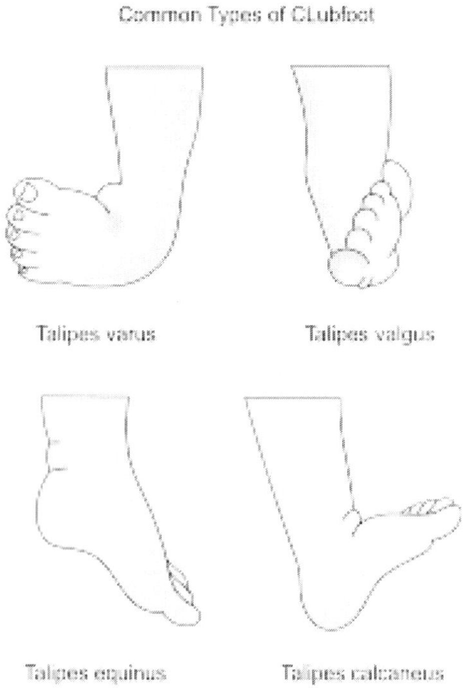

Fig. 4.20A: Common type of Clubfoot

shaped". About 50% of the time, both feet are affected with clubfoot. In USA, there are 1-2 cases for every 1000 live births. The ratio of males to females with clubfoot is 2.5 : 1.

Risk/Predisposing Factors

Risk Factors may Include

- Family history of clubfoot
- Position of the baby in the uterus
- Increased occurrences in those children with neuromuscular disorders, such as cerebral palsy (CP) and spina bifida
- Oligohydramnios (decreased amount of amniotic fluid surrounding the fetus in the uterus) during pregnancy.

Manifestation

Although there is no known cause of congenital clubfoot, some doctors believe the use of drugs or alcohol during pregnancy or the presence of other diseases can cause it. In some cases, clubfoot is just the result of the position of the baby while it is developing in the mother's womb.

Clubfoot is painless in a baby, but it can eventually cause discomfort and become a noticeable disability. Left untreated, clubfoot does not straighten itself out. The foot will remain twisted out of shaped, and the affected leg may be shorter and smaller than the other. These symptoms become more obvious and more of a problem as the child grows.

- Fixed plantar flexion (equinus) of the ankle, characterized by the drawn up position of the heel and inability to bring the foot to a plantigrade (flat) standing position. This is caused by a tight Achilles tendon.
- Adduction (varus), or turning in of the heel or hindfoot.
- Adduction (turning under), of the forefoot and midfoot giving the foot a kidney-shaped appearance.
- Abnormal (slightly smaller) size of foot and calf muscles.
- The heel cord (Achilles tendon) is tight causing the heel to be drawn up towards the leg.

Type/Stage/Classification

There are two categories of clubfoot/talipes equinovarus(TEV).

- Structural TEV is caused by: genetic factors, such as Edwards syndrome—a genetic defect with three copies of chromosome 18. Growth arrests at roughly 9 weeks and compartment syndrome of the affected limb also causes Structural TEV. Genetic influences increase dramatically with family history.
- Postural TEV could be caused by external influences in the final trimester such as intrauterine compression from oligohydramnios or from amniotic band syndrome. However, this is countered by findings that TEV does not occur more frequently than usual when the intrauterine space is restricted.

Pathophysiology (Fig. 20.B)

Theories of the pathogenesis of clubfeet are as follows:

- Arrest of fetal development in the fibular stage
- Defective cartilaginous anlage of the talus
- Neurogenic factors: Histochemical abnormalities have been found in posteromedial and peroneal muscle groups of patients with clubfeet. This is postulated to be due to innervation changes

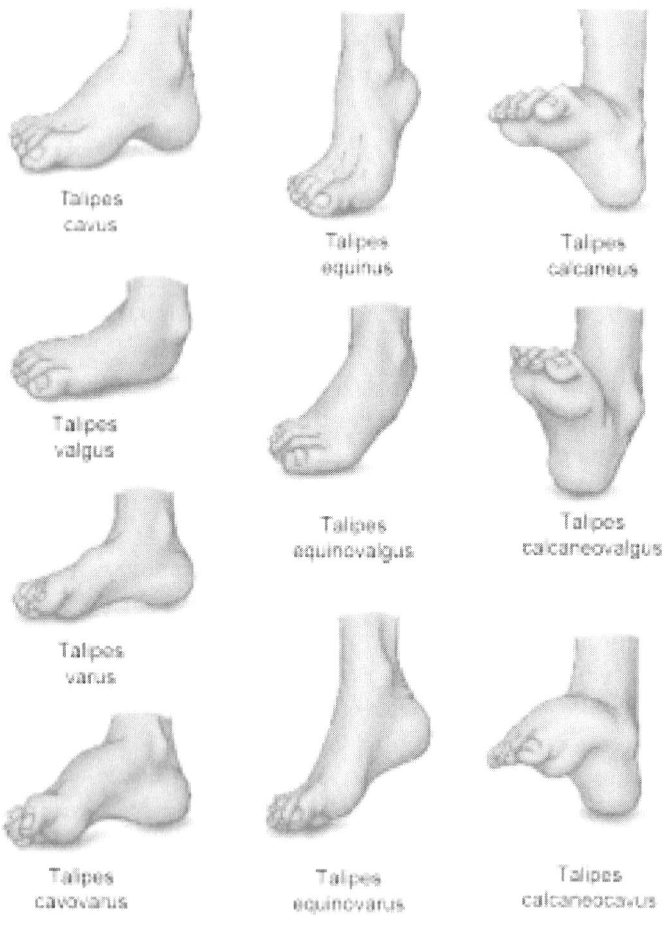

Fig. 4.20B: Other types foot

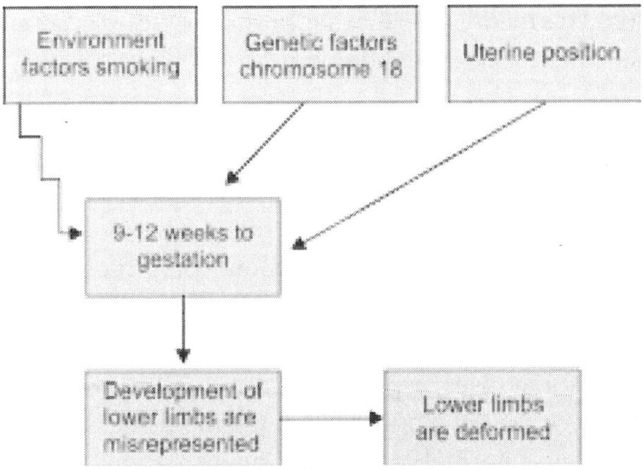

Fig. 4.21: Pathology

in intrauterine life secondary to a neurologic event, such as a stroke leading to mild hemiparesis or paraparesis. This is further supported by a 35% incidence of varus and equinovarus deformity in spinabifida.

- Retracting fibrosis (or myofibrosis) secondary to increased fibrous tissue in muscles and ligaments: In fetal and cadaveric studies, Ponseti also found the collagen in all of the ligamentous and tendinous structures (except the Achilles tendon), and it was very loosely crimped and could be stretched. The Achilles tendon, on the other hand, was made up of tightly crimped collagen and was resistant to stretching. Zimny et al found myoblasts in medial fascia on electron microscopy and postulated that they cause medial contracture.[1,2,9]
- Anomalous tendon insertions: Inclan proposed that anomalous tendon insertions result in clubfeet.[10] However, other studies have not supported this. It is more likely that the distorted clubfoot anatomy can make it appear that tendon insertions are anomalous.
- Seasonal variations: Robertson noted seasonal variations to be a factor in his epidemiologic studies in developing countries. This coincided with a similar variation in the incidence of poliomyelitis in the children in the community. Clubfoot was therefore proposed to be a sequela of a prenatal polio like con-

dition. This theory is further supported by motor neuron changes in the anterior horn in the spinal cord of these babies.

VIII. Diagnostic Studies

- Physical examination.
- Ultrasound: Ultrasound done while a fetus is developing can sometimes detect clubfoot. It is more common for your health professional to diagnose the condition after the infant is born, though, based on the appearance and mobility of the feet and legs. In some cases, especially if the clubfoot is due just to the position of the developing baby, the foot is flexible and can be moved into a normal or nearly normal position.
- X-ray
  - A diagnostic test which uses invisible electromagnetic energy beams to produce images of internal tissues, bones, and organs onto film.
- Computed tomography scan (also called a CT or CAT scan.) - a diagnostic imaging procedure that uses a combination of x-rays and computer technology to produce cross-sectional images (often called "slices"), both horizontally and vertically, of the body. A CT scan shows detailed images of any part of the body, including the bones, muscles, fat, and organs. CT scans are more detailed than general x-rays.

Management

Medical Intervention

There are two well-known non-surgical methods to treat talipes:

a. The Ponseti Method

A special splint called the Denis-Browne splint is put in place. This splint is made of two high-top, open-toed shoes connected by a bar, which is adjusted according to the correct position of the feet. The splint is worn full-time for two to three months and then only at night for the next two to four years.

Developed by Dr. Ignacio Ponseti of Iowa, the Ponseti method begins with a series of gentle manipulations and toe-to-thigh cast placements for the first five to seven weeks. The heel-cord is cut to complete the correction of the foot before the last cast is applied. Then, the last cast is placed for three weeks, by which time the heel-cord has healed properly.

b. French Method

This treatment requires daily one-hour therapy with a qualified physiotherapist. It consists of gentle stretching of the feet, followed by taping to maintain their improved position. At night, the taped feet are connected with a machine that allows for a continuous passive motion to maximize stretching. For two hours every day, the tape is removed to air the skin. Physiotherapy sessions continue daily for as long as three months, and taping is discontinued once the child begins walking.

In stretching and casting therapy the doctor changes the cast multiple times over a few weeks, gradually stretching tendons until the foot is in the correct position of external rotation. The heel cord is released (percutaneous tenotomy) and another cast is put on, which is removed after three weeks. To avoid relapse a corrective brace is worn for a gradually reducing time until it is only at night up to four years of age.

Surgical Intervention

The operative procedure includes:

- Z-lengthening of the heel cord with release of the medial fibers distally
- Capsulorrhaphy of the tibiotalar and fibulotalar joints complete
- Capsulorrhaphy of the deltoid ligament and plantar calcaneonavicular ligament maintaining a small tongue of capsule attached to the tibia
- Capsulorrhaphy of the talonavicular ligaments
- Capsulorrhaphy of the anterior tibiotalar ligament from medial to lateral malleolus (The talocalcaneal ligament and the posterior compartment for the foot should be avoided).

- The talus is then rotated laterally in the ankle mortise and the calcaneus with it. If derotation is not complete and if the scaphoid does not glide readily to the lateral side, a second incision is made laterally, opening the calcaneocuboid joint and the cuboid metatarsal joints. The sinus tarsi is entered and the lateral talonavicular and calcaneonavicular ligaments are released, as are the tibulotalar ligaments laterally.

This procedure usually allows full external rotation of the talus and the calcaneus as a unit and reestablishes the lateral border of the foot - the calcaneocuboid angle being changed from convex to neutral. The relationship between the talus and the calcaneus is reestablished and the foot is then lined up with the fibula and medial malleolus.

The anterior tibial tendon is detached from the first metatarsal on the medial side and transferred to the dorsum of the first metatarsal where it is reinserted into soft tissue and periosteum in the infant, or into a hole in the first cuneiform in the older patient.

All tendons that have been lengthened are resutured and none is resected. The posterior tibial tendon should be saved and every effort should be made to maintain its original action on the hindfoot. At this point in the operation, excessive correction or the creation of heel valgus is readily possible, particularly in the foot of a child under one year of age. Resuture of a portion of the deltoid ligament and the medial tendons will avoid excessive correction and allow active forces to be applied to the medial border of the foot as the child grows.

The tourniquet is released, the bleeding points are coagulated, and the skin is closed with absorbable suture. In the infant, fixation pins are usually unnecessary to maintain the relationship between the scaphoid and talus but may he required in the older child. Excessive abduction of the forefoot should be avoided and the relationship between the talus and the scaphoid, and the talus and ankle joint, should approach that seen in the physiologic position. If the skin is tight after closure, the foot should be inverted slightly and the tension taken off the skin.

Primary healing should be sought. Fluffed gauze and pads are applied, sheet cotton is used and split so that there is no pressure on the skin, and the cast is applied with the foot at right angles and in neutral position in relationship to the malleoli, with the knee at right angles. This cast is changed at 10 to 14 day's so that repositioning can be accomplished if there was tension on the skin initially. At this time the initial internal rotation of the foot and the apparent, but usually nonexistent, tibial torsion have been corrected. In over 90 percent of the clubfeet treated, the internally rotated position has been corrected by derotating the talus in the ankle mortise. In the author's opinion the ligamentous contracture, the position of the talus in the ankle mortise, and the relationship of the adjacent tarsal bones to the talus constitute the primary pathology in congenital talipes equino varus. If all aspects of the deformity are not corrected, then recurrent clubfoot is the rule.

Operative correction must be made from both the medial and lateral sides of the ankle joint and the midfoot in order to fully' correct the internal rotation of the talus and the medial positioning of the scaphoid, as well as the distortion of the calcaneocuboid joint. Any procedure that attempts to do this without correcting the talus may be successful only because the total deformity was very mild. Severe clubfeet will not be corrected permanently if the ankle joint is not released. Total subtalar release will not be successful in the severe foot and will result eventually in a distorted tibiotalar joint with a foot that is apparently corrected by external rotation but which eventually will either revert to varus or will be placed in a valgus position in overcorrection.

CEREBRAL PALSY

Cerebral palsy (**CP**) is an umbrella term encompassing a group of non-progressive, non-contagious motor conditions and is caused by damage to the brain at or around birth leading to physical disability in human development, chiefly in the spectrum of body movement. Though the condition is non-progressive but the clinical scenario alters during the development of nervous system. The prevalence is about 2 per 100 in school going kids.

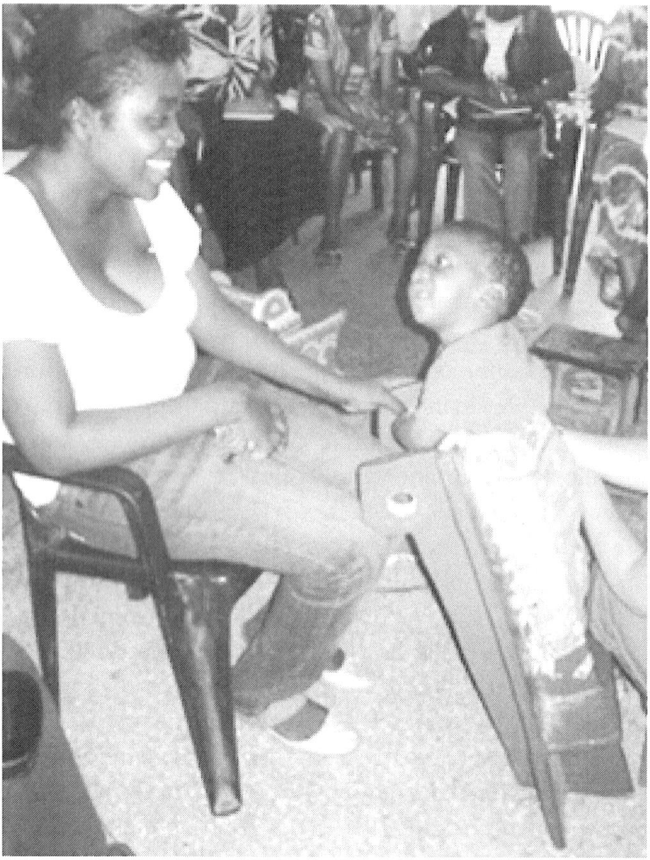

Fig. 4.23: Child with CP

CEREBRAL - PALSY

Cerebral refers to the cerebrum

which is the affected area of the brain (although the disorder most likely involves connections between the cortex and other parts of the brain such as the cerebellum)

Palsy refers to disorder of movement

CP is caused by damage to the motor control centers of the developing brain and can occur during pregnancy (about 75 percent), during *childbirth* (about 5 percent) or after birth (about 15 percent) up to about age three.

Cerebral palsy describes a group of permanent disorders of the development of movement and posture, causing activity limitation, that are attributed to nonprogressive disturbances that occurred in the developing fetal or infant brain. The motor disorders of cerebral palsy are often accompanied by disturbances of sensation, perception, cognition, communication, and behavior, by epilepsy, and by secondary musculoskeletal problems.

CP is divided into four major classifications to describe different movement impairments. These classifications also reflect the areas of the brain that are damaged.

Part Affected	*Diagnosis*
One side of the body	Hemiplegia
All four limbs(upper more than lower)	Quadriplegia
All four limbs(one side more than other)	Bilateral hemiplegia
Legs affected more than arms	Diplegia
One limb affected	Monoplegia

The four major classifications are:

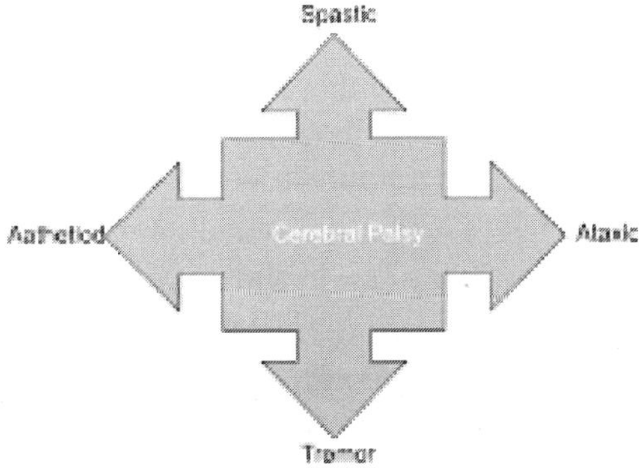

Fig. 4.24: Major classification of CP

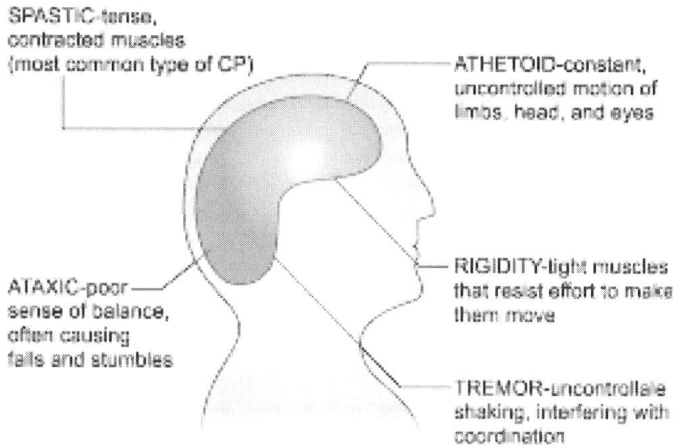

Fig. 4.25: Types of Cerebral Palsy

Spastic cerebral palsy is a disorder of increased tone characterized by increased resistance to stretch initially that in later stages may lessen and is manifested due to UMN, showing most common incidence, occurring in 70% to 80% of all cases. Moreover, spastic CP accompanies one of the other types in 30% of all cases. People with this type present with hypertonic and a neuromuscular condition stemming from damage to the corticospinal tract or the motor cortex that affects the nervous system's ability to receive gamma amino butyric acid in the area(s) affected by the disability.

CLINICAL PICTURE

- Increased initial tone.
- Exaggerated deep tendon reflexes and extensor response
- Abnormal positions (due to abnormal weakness of the antagonist)
- Contractures (due to deformity in joints)

Spastic CP is further classified by topography dependent on the region of the body affected; these include:

- *Spastic hemiplegia* (one side being affected).
  Generally, injury to muscle-nerves controlled by the brain's left side will cause a right body deficit, and vice versa. Typically, people that have spastic hemiplegia are the *most ambulatory*,

although they generally have dynamic equinus on the affected side and are primarily prescribed ankle-foot orthoses to prevent said equinus.

- *Spastic diplegia* (the lower extremities are affected with little to no upper-body spasticity).
  - The most common form is the spastic forms. Most people with spastic diplegia are fully ambulatory and have a scissors gait. Flexed knees and hips to varying degrees are common. Hip problems, dislocations, and in three-quarters of spastic diplegics, also strabismus (crossed eyes), can be present as well. In addition, these individuals are often nearsighted. The intelligence of a person with spastic diplegia is unaffected by the condition.
- *Spastic tetraplegia* (all four limbs affected equally).

  People with spastic quadriplegia are the least likely to be able to walk, or if they can, to want to walk, because their muscles are too tight and it is too much effort to do so. Some children with quadriplegia also have hemiparetic tremors, an uncontrollable shaking that affects the limbs on one side of the body and impairs normal movement.

Occasionally, terms such as monoplegia, paraplegia, triplegia, and pentaplegia may also be used to refer to specific manifestations of the spasticity.

- *Ataxic*

  Ataxia type symptoms can be caused by damage to the cerebellum or its pathways. The forms of ataxia are less common types of cerebral palsy, occurring in at most 10% of all cases and may be a part of dysmorphic syndrome or may be associated with intra-uterine infection. The most presenting features are hypotonia,disturbance of balance,inco-ordination,intention tremor,dysarthria and sometimes nystagmus. Mental handicap is most common. Motor skills such as writing, typing, or using scissors might be affected, as well as balance, especially while walking. It is common for individuals to have difficulty with visual and/or auditory processing.

- *Athetoid/dyskinetic*
  Athetoid or **Dyskinetic** is mixed muscle tone — People with athetoid CP have trouble holding themselves in an upright, steady position for sitting or walking, and often show involuntary motions. For some people with athetoid CP, it takes a lot of work and concentration to get their hand to a certain spot (like scratching their nose or reaching for a cup). Because of their mixed tone and trouble keeping a position, they may not be able to hold onto objects (such as a toothbrush or pencil). About one quarter of all people with CP have athetoid CP. The damage occurs to the extrapyramidal motor system and/or pyramidal tract and to the basal ganglia. It occurs in 10% to 20% percent of all cases.. In newborn infants, high bilirubin levels in the blood, if left untreated, can lead to brain damage in certain areas (kernicterus). This may also lead to athetoid cerebral palsy.
- *Hypotonic*
  People with hypotonic CP appear limp and can move only a little or can't move at all.

Incidence and Prevalence

In the industrialized world, the incidence of cerebral palsy is about 2 per 1000 live births. The incidence is higher in males than in females; the Surveillance of Cerebral Palsy in Europe (SCPE) reports an M: F ratio of 1.33:1. Variances in reported rates of incidence across different geographical areas in industrialized countries are thought to be caused primarily by discrepancies in the criteria used for inclusion and exclusion. When such discrepancies are taken into account in comparing two or more registers of patients with cerebral palsy (for example, the extent to which children with mild cerebral palsy are included), the incidence rates converge toward the average rate of 2:1000.

In the United States, approximately 10,000 infants and babies are diagnosed with CP each year, and 1200–1500 are diagnosed at preschool age.

Overall, advances in care of pregnant mothers and their babies have not resulted in a noticeable decrease in CP. This is generally attributed to medical advances in areas related to the care of premature babies (which results in a greater survival rate). Only the introduction of quality medical care to locations with less-than-adequate medical care has shown any decreases. The incidence of CP increases with premature or very low-weight babies regardless of the quality of care.

Apgar scores have sometimes been used as one factor to predict whether or not an individual will develop CP.

CAUSES OF CEREBRAL PALSY

Antenatal Causes

- Genetic causes: first and second degree consanguineous marriage
- Intrauterine viral infections by rubella and cytomegalovirus.
- Hypoglycemia (infant of a diabetic mother are more prone to CP)
- Trauma or infection to mother
- Malnourishment of foetus
- Exposure to X-rays
- Prolong use of steroids by mother

Neonatal Causes

- Premature babies are more prone to CP
- Occlusion in the mid carotid artery and mid cereberal artery during birth
- Trauma during delivery
- Neonatal meningitis
- Asphyxia

Postnatal Causes

- Jaundice
- Trauma due to disproportion, forcep delivery etc.
- Delayed cry
- Infection

CLINICAL MANIFESTATIONS

- Visual disturbances as cortical blindness and splint.
- Nerve deafness

- Disorders of speech articulation
- Epilepsy
- Mental handicap
- Emotional problems.

DIAGNOSIS

The diagnosis of cerebral palsy has historically rested on the patient's history and physical examination. Once diagnosed with cerebral palsy, further diagnostic tests are optional. The American Academy of Neurology published an article in 2004 reviewing the literature and evidence available on CT and MRI imaging. They suggested that neuroimaging with CT or MRI is warranted when the etiology of a patient's cerebral palsy has not been established - an MRI is preferred over CT due to diagnostic yield and safety. When abnormal, the neuroimaging study can suggest the timing of the initial damage.

MANAGEMENT OF CP

Medical Management

- *Diazepam*- helpful in relaxing a baby.
- *Balcofen*-used for antispasticity.

PHYSIOTHERAPY MANAGEMENT

PRINCIPLES OF MANAGEMENT

- A Physiotherapist or other health care provider should be consulted before initiating an exercise program, particularly if you have health problems or are taking medication for a chronic health problem
  - Careful assessment should be carried out.
  - Incorporation of early treatment.
- The assistance of a professional knowledgeable in exercise principles and techniques is often useful to achieve the goals.
- An exercise program should be individualized to meet the goals and potential of each person and the recording of the child should be ongoing rather than isolated process.

- An exercise program can be carried out at home, in a general facility, or in a specialized facility. Special arrangements for accessibility, equipment, or assistance hold importance.
- Realistic performance goals need to be set at the beginning while the reassessment of the goals should be carried out ones in six months in order to check the level of recovery
- Exercise should be engaged in regularly; at least 3-5 times a week.
- The duration of each exercise session needs a periodic assessment. In general, 20-30 minutes per session is the minimum goal. However, during the first few weeks, several short sessions (e.g.: 5-10 minutes) per day can be better than a longer period.
- Exercise should aim at strengthening weak muscles and stretching tight muscles.
- It is particularly important to increase the duration, intensity, and frequency of the exercise activity gradually. At initiation, duration should be increased progressively rather intensity.
- Physical activity and exercise need not be overly strenuous to achieve health benefits. A moderate level will accomplish the same purpose. Muscle soreness may accompany early progress.
- Exercise with a partner for both social and safety benefits.
  For people with severe contractures or weakness, extra caution is advised to minimize muscle strain as end range work would lead to microtraumas.
  - Maximization of sensory motor experiences
  - Modification of abnormal tone by facilitation of functional patterns.
  - The therapist should try to use adequate afferent stimuli
  - Prevention of secondary impairments as contractures and deformity.
  - Achievement of functional independence with or without assistance
- Light headedness, chest pain, difficulty breathing, excessive fatigue, nausea, moderate to severe joint or muscle pain are red flag signs and are an indication to danger. Stop exercising! Discontinue the exercise program and seek a physician or other health care provider's advice before starting again.

COUNSELING

Early counseling of the parents should be done.

LIFTING THE CHILD

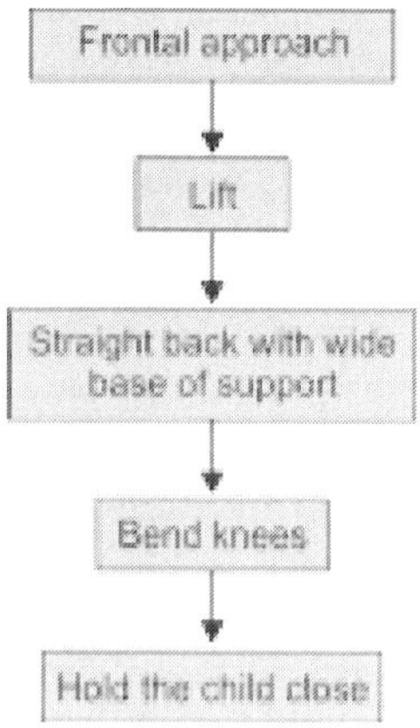

- **Positioning**
  Variety of positions should be encountered everyday

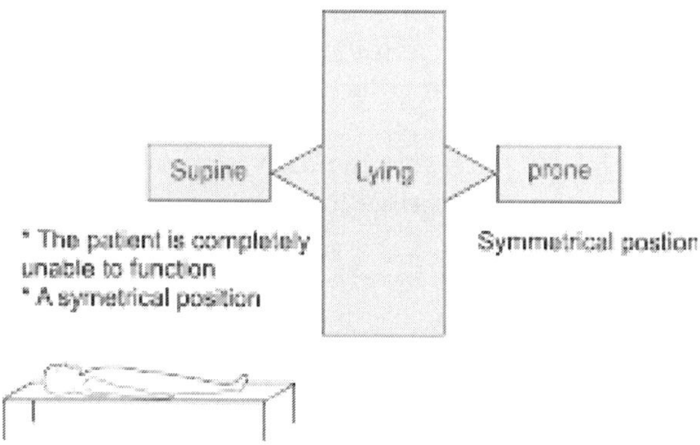

Fig. 4.26: Positioning

- **Lying**
- **Sitting**
  In a long sitting position a normal baby learns to establish a base of support while a CP child flexes his trunk over his legs and then brings the trunk more upright

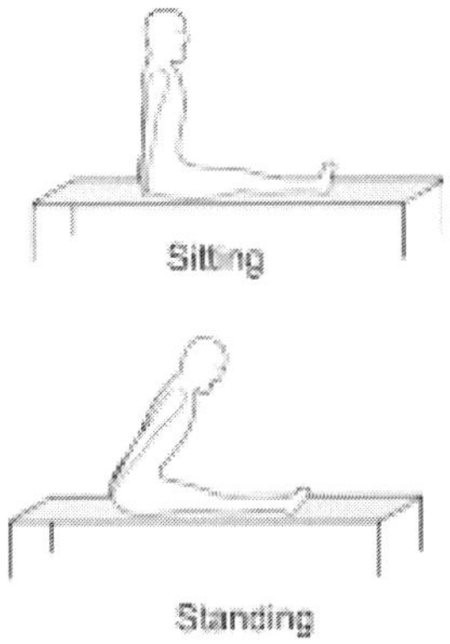

Fig. 4.27: Sitting and Standing

STANDING

- Prevention of flexion deformity
- Social benefits as no inferiority is witnessed
- Development of weight bearing surfaces
- Sensory feedback

Exercise Principles and Guidelines for Persons with Cerebral Palsy

Health and well being arc thc result of many factors:

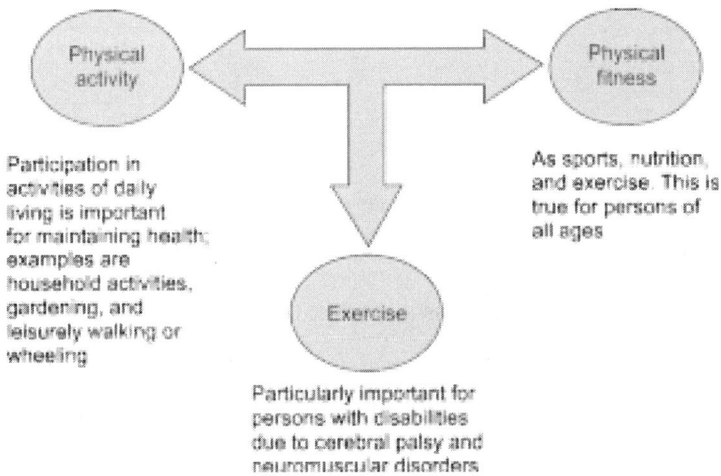

Fig. 4.28: Factors affecting health

Benefits of Exercise

- Increases participation in individual and community activities
- Improves the sense of well being and reduces anxiety
- Increases and maintains heart and lung efficiency
- Increases and maintains strength, flexibility, mobility and coordination
- Improves and maintains bone structure and strength
- Assists in weight control
- Reduces risks of several chronic diseases (e.g.: high blood pressure, osteoporosis)

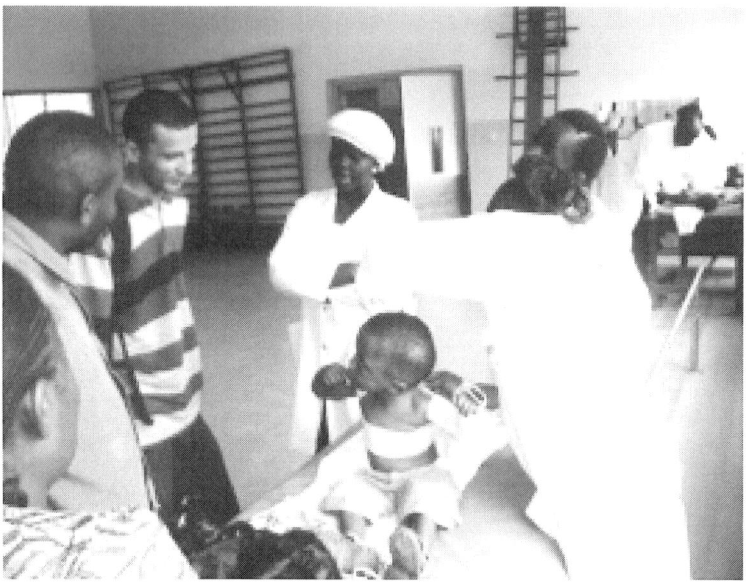

Fig. 4.29: Physiotherapy management in CP

Health and Safety

Certain health and safety issues must be sustained in all exercise activities.

- Plenty of water should be taken, during, and after exercise however the exact amount will depend upon a number of factors including temperature, humidity, and length of the workout.

- Clothing and footwear appropriate for each specific exercise program should be worn at all times. Apparel that could cause an accident and/or injury should be avoided (e.g.: loose slacks or pants that could get caught in the chain of a bicycle). Head gear and knee and elbow pads may be needed in some activities.
- Extra precautions should be taken for strenuous outdoor activity during times of extreme heat or cold. The amount of time exercising often must be adjusted for extremes of heat, cold and high humidity. The length and intensity of the workout should decrease as the temperature and humidity increase.
- If exercising outdoors, care should be taken to wear the appropriate clothing depending upon the weather. Clothing should be layered so that items can be removed or replaced if the participant becomes too warm or too cold.
- If exercising outdoors at night or in poor visibility, use brightly colored clothing and/or reflectors on shoes, bicycles or wheelchairs.
- Medications can alter the body's response to an exercise program. Individuals should be familiar with how their medication affects their participation in an exercise program or they need to consult their physician or health care provider about this.
- Weight bearing and joint flexing exercises must be done with caution by persons with significant contractures and/or loss of bone density.

Components of an Exercise Session

An exercise session should always include:

- A warm-up period of 5-10 minutes:
    a. 2-5 minutes to warm-up the muscles and joints to be exercised by gentle activity such as slow walking/slow wheeling.
    b. 2-5 minutes of stretching that includes the muscles and joints of primary concern.
- A specific exercise activity such as aerobic exercise, resistance exercise, swimming, aquatics, cycling, etc. for at least 20-30 minutes.

- A cool-down period of 5 minutes or longer; continues until you feel cooled-down and your pulse rate has returned to near the resting level.
  a. 3-5 minutes of slow walking or slow wheeling.
  b. 2-5 minutes of stretching that includes the muscles and joints of primary concern.

EXERCISE SUGESSTIONS

Arm Cycling	* improves heart and lung efficiency * improves muscle strength and endurance * improves flexibility and range	• bicycling is done with arms instead of legs. * ergometer or arm driven cycles are taken into consideration. * wearing a helmet is recommended during outdoor cycling.
Chair Aerobics	* improves heart and lung efficiency * improves muscle strength and endurance	* A combination of upper body and stretching techniques are used to facilitate cardiovascular endurance. * usually preformed in seated position with music.
Dancing	* improves heart and lung efficiency. * improves flexibility and range. * improves bone structure and strength.	* an exercise done to the music so that the tempo of the music determines the speed of the exercise. * predetermination of specific heart rate zone. * monitoring of body alignment, breathing intensity and range. * special care must be taken regarding bone density loss and unsignificant contractures.

Contd...

Contd...

Exercise Bands	* improves muscle strength and endurance. * improves bone structure and strength.	* wide elastic bands are used for resistance training and stretching. * these are latex bands with various size and resistance * one end is attached to a stationary object while the other is used for strengthening * Precaution should be taken that the band is not to be removed in stretched position.
Jogging	* improves muscle strength and endurance. * improves bone structure and strength. * improves heart and lung efficiency	* It is the act of fast walking and running at a steady pace. * it can be done in place,trademill,on track or outdoors. * proper fitted exercise shoes is recommended. * initially muscle soreness may occur but however if there are any flags hoisting for joint dysfunction then lower type of exercises as walking, swimming are to be taken into consideration. * special care must be taken regarding bone density loss and unsignificant contractures

Contd...

Contd...

Leg Cycling	* improves heart and lung efficiency * improves muscle strength and endurance * improves flexibility and range	* an activity on a mobile vehicle or stationary equipment. * use of helmet is recommended.
Rowing	* improves heart and lung efficiency * improves muscle strength and endurance * improves flexibility and range	* total body exercise in a seated position using stationary equipment. * involves repetitive pulling of both arms against resistance with the bending and straightening and bending of leg.
Start Climbing	* improves heart and lung efficiency * improves muscle strength and endurance. * improves bone structure and strength	* Action of walking up stairs. * mid upper leg muscle soreness and joint soreness initially.
Swimming	* improves heart and lung efficiency * improves muscle strength and endurance * improves flexibility and range	* act of moving progressively in water by the forceful use of arms and legs. * ideal temperature is 75'F-85'F. * wear goggles in chlorinated pools. * don't swim alone.
Walking	* improves heart and lung efficiency * improves bone structure and strength.	* act of advancing by foot. * convenient, can be done with or without assistance anywhere. * special care must be taken regarding bone density loss and usingnificant contractures.

Contd...

Contd...

		* Joint pain is a warning sign of too much impact.
Water Exercise	* improves heart and lung efficiency * improves bone structure and strength. * improves flexibility and range	* Exhibits features as swimming. * gradually increase the strength and duration.
Weight Training	* improves bone structure and strength. * improves muscle strength and endurance	* use of free weight and exercise machines either outdoor or indoor. * weak muscles can be made stronger by resistance of weight. * level of resistance and the number of repitions varies according to the goals. * lifting of free heavy weight is prohibited.
Wheeling	* improves heart and lung efficiency * improves muscle strength and endurance	* propulsion of wheel chair by arms or legs through extended distance. * can be done with a conventional wheelchair or a sports wheelchair. * if moving out care should be taken regareding traffic.
Yoga and Thi Chi	* improves flexibility and range * improves bone structure and strength	* physical form of yoga involving breathing and stretching. * dance like movements linked in smooth flowing sequence. * non binding comfortable clothing should be worn.

Specific Goals

- To Increase and Maintain Heart and Lung Efficiency
- To Improve Flexibility and Range of Motion
- To Strengthen Muscles and Increase Endurance
- To Improve and Maintain Bone Structure and Strength

To Increase and Maintain Heart and Lung Efficiency

- Often referred to as aerobic exercises. These exercises can also contribute to weight control.
- Characterized by increasing your heart rate to a moderate level above the resting level for a sustained period of time during moderate to vigorous activity.
- Start the program with 5 minutes of exercise, gradually increasing the length of exercise as tolerated to 20-60 minutes.
- Best if done at least 3 times a week; can be done daily.
- Cautions: It is important to choose exercises that minimize stress on joints and muscles, particularly in already overstressed areas.

To Improve Flexibility and Range of Motion

- Persons with cerebral palsy are at risk of having muscle tightness that limits motion at joints; loss of functional mobility can be associated with pain.
- Focus on muscles that are causing the most problems with mobility in activities of daily living.
- Stretch the muscle slowly to the point of tension, but not pain.
- Hold each stretch for 10-60 seconds; do it 2-3 times.
- Stretch the muscle to improve both flexibility and range of motion several times daily.

To Strengthen Muscles and Increase Endurance

- Higher weight, not repetition, increases strength. Moderate weight and more repetition increases endurance. You can exercise one muscle or joint at a time or several muscles. Focus on a balanced program with emphasis on those muscles that will help you in everyday activities.

- Following a strength training exercise for a particular muscle group, a one day rest period is necessary before repeating the exercise for that muscle group.
- Expect mild temporary soreness for up to 48 hours at the beginning of the program and as you increase the intensity.
- Initiate the program for each muscle group by performing 10 comfortable movements against a resistance over time. Gradually increase the load and decrease the number of repetitions. Two sets of each of the movements can be performed in a beginning program.
- If muscles fatigue after 2-4 repetitions, the load is too high. If you can perform 12-15 repetitions, the load is too low. Aim for 10 repetitions.
- Muscle strengthening exercises are most effective when they are focused primarily on the muscle group opposite the tight muscle group. For example, if the muscles that bend the elbow are tight, stretch and strengthen the muscles that straighten the elbow.
- It is particularly important to have a period of warm up and stretching before and after strength training exercises to prevent muscle strain.

Precautions

Loads should not be at a maximum. Weights should not be allowed to dangle on the limb. Free weights (e.g. bar bells) should be used with caution by persons with athetosis (involuntary body movement). Weights are not advisable for persons who cannot control the weights. If using free weights, it is recommended to have a partner or spotter. Do not hold your breath during the resistance phase. If there is significant muscle or joint pain or swelling for more than 48 hours, seek consultation.

To Improve and Maintain Bone Structure and Strength

- Persons with cerebral palsy and neuromuscular disabilities are at risk of being inactive or immobile.
- Inactivity or immobility decreases bone density and strength (e.g.: osteoporosis).

- Weight bearing in conjunction with movement of the body and limbs, and muscle exercises are believed to prevent loss of bone structure and strength.
- If you have been inactive, start at a level that is comfortable for you. Increase the effort and duration gradually

Exercise Concerns

- **Age:** Exercise is not reserved for any age group. At all ages, exercise can strengthen bone, enhance mobility, build strength and improve coordination.
- **Trauma:** An appropriate exercise program does not aggravate conditions that accompany cerebral palsy or neuromuscular disorders.
- **Fatigue:** Exercise does utilize energy; however, by exercising regularly, people build stamina that makes it easier to meet daily demands.
- **Falls:** Exercise does not cause falls or injuries; if done properly exercise improves balance, mobility, strength and coordination that protect against injury in activities of daily living.

GENU VARUM

Genu Varum (Fig. 4.30) (also called bow-leggedness or bandiness), is a deformity marked by medial angulation of the leg in relation to the thigh, an outward bowing of the legs, giving the appearance of a bow. It is also known as bandy-leg, bowleg, and tibia vara. Usually there is an outward curvature of both femur and tibia. "Genu varum" is distinguished from Blount's disease because it involves both the femur and the tibia, while Blount's disease affects only the tibia with no femur involvement.

Children until the age of 3 to 4 have a degree of Genu Varum. The child sits with the soles of the feet facing one another; the tibia and femur are curved outwards; and, if the limbs are extended, although the ankles are in contact, there is a distinct space between the knee-joints. During the first year of life a gradual change takes place. The knee-joints approach one another; the femur slopes downward and inward towards the knee joints; the tibia becomes straight; and the sole of the foot faces almost directly downwards.

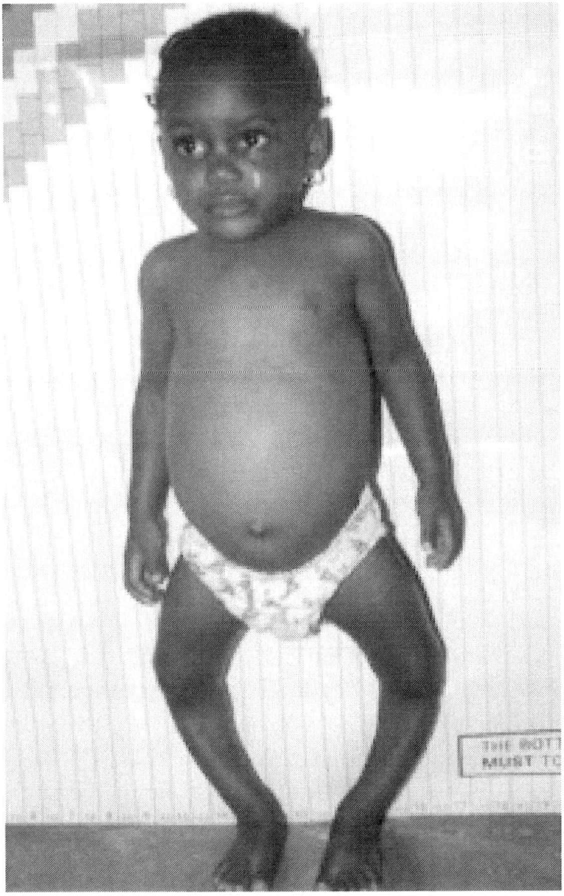

Fig. 4.30: Genu Varum

While these changes are occurring, the bones, which at first consist principally of cartilage are gradually becoming ossified. By the time a normal child begins to walk the lower limbs are prepared, both by their general direction and by the rigidity of the bones which form them, to support the weight of the body.

Causes

If a child is sickly, either with rickets or suffering from any ailment that prevents the due ossification of the bones, or is improperly fed, the bowed condition may remain persistent. Thus the chief cause of this deformity is rickets. Skeletal problems, infection, and tumors can also affect the growth of the leg, sometimes giving rise to a one-sided bow-leggedness. The remaining causes are occupational, especially among jockeys, and from physical trauma, the condition being very likely to supervene after accidents involving the condyles of the femur.

Expectations

In most cases persisting after childhood, there is little or no effect on the ability to walk. Due to uneven stress and wear on the knees, however, even milder manifestations can see an accelerated onset of arthritis. Those with bowlegs and a genetic predisposition for developing arthritis will likely start having arthritic symptoms around age 30.

Treatment

Generally, no treatment is required for idiopathic presentation as it is a normal anatomical variant in young children. Treatment is indicated when it persists beyond 3 and half years old, Unilateral presentation, or progressive worsening of the curvature. When caused by rickets, the most important thing is to treat the constitutional disease, at the same time instructing the mother never to place the child on its feet. In many cases this is quite sufficient in itself to effect a cure, but matters can be hastened somewhat by applying splints. When the deformity arises in older patients, either from trauma or occupation, the only treatment is surgery.

GENU VALGUM (SEE FIG. 4.31)

Genu Valgum, commonly called "knock-knees", is a condition where the knees angle in and touch one another when the legs are straightened. Females have a wider pelvis than men and a relatively shorter length of the thigh bone, and as a result, have a greater static genu valgum than men. Individuals with severe valgus deformities are typically unable to touch their feet together while simultaneously straightening the legs. The term originates from the Latin genu,

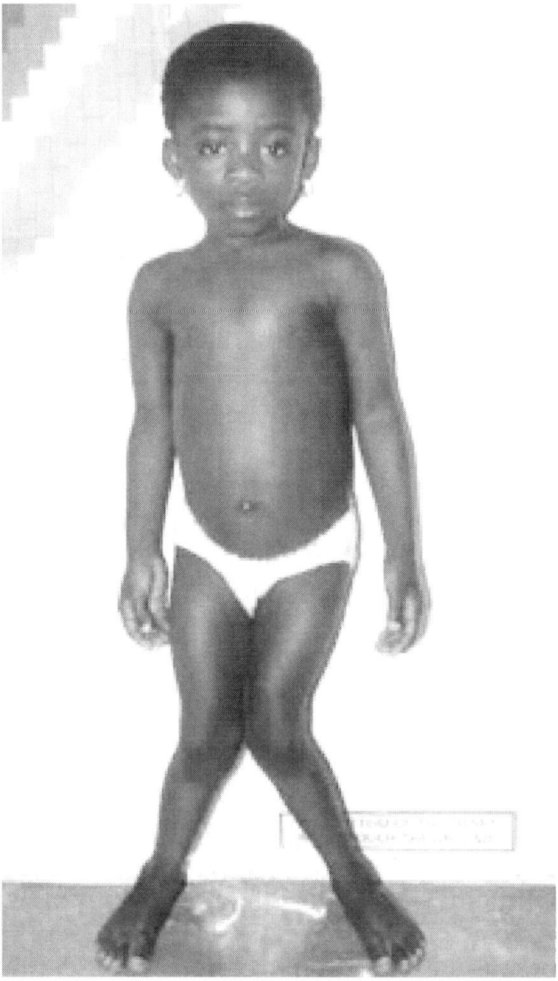

Fig. 4.31: Genu Valgun

"knee", and valgus, "bent inward". For a discussion of the etymology of valgus, see the entry under varus.

Mild genu valgum can be seen in children from ages 2 to 5, and is often corrected naturally as children grow. However, the condition may continue or worsen with age, particularly when it is the result of a disease, such as rickets or obesity. Idiopathic is the term used to describe genu valgum that is congenital or has no known cause.

Other systemic conditions may be associated, such as Schnyder Central Corneal Dystrophy, an autosomal dominant condition frequently reported with hyperlipidemia.

Diagnostic test

The Q angle which is formed by a line drawn from the anterosuperior iliac spine through the center of the patella and a line drawn from the center of the patella to the center of the tibial tubercle should be measured next. In women, the Q angle should be less than 22 degrees with the knee in extension and less than 9 degrees with the knee in 90 degrees of flexion. In men, the Q angle should be less than 18 degrees with the knee in extension and less than 8 degrees with the knee in 90 degrees of flexion.

Treatment

Generally, there is no known cure for knock knees post-childhood. Contrary to common belief, no amount of orthotic treatment or bodybuilding exercise will straighten knock knees for adults. If the condition persists or worsens into late childhood and adulthood, a corrective osteotomy may be recommended to straighten the legs. This however is more of a cosmetic remedy, and may hamper athletic performance in the future.

Adults with uncorrected genu valgum are typically prone to injury and chronic knee problems such as chondromalacia and osteoarthritis. In some cases, total knee replacement (TKR) surgery may be required later in life to relieve pain and complications resulting from severe genu valgum.

Leg braces are also an alternative for the problem.

REFERENCES

DDH

1. Jacobsen S, Romer L, Soballe K. The other hip in unilateral hip dysplasia. Clin. Orthop. Relat. Res, 2006;446: 239-46, doi:10.1097/01.blo.0000201151.91206.50. PMID 16721954.
2. Wiberg G. Studies of acetabular and congenital subluxation of the hip joint with special reference to complication of osteoarthritis. Acta Chir Scand, 1939; 83(Suppl. 58)

3. Cilliers HJ, Beighton P. Beukes familial hip dysplasia: an autosomal dominant entity. Am. J. Med, Genet, 1990; 36 (4): 386-90. doi:10.1002/ajmg.1320360403. PMID 2389793.
4. http://www.onsmd.com/Jon-F-Crowe-MD
5. Crowe JF, Mani VJ, Ranawat CS (1979). "Total hip replacement in congenital dislocation and dysplasia of the hip". J Bone Joint Surg Am 61 (1): 15-23. PMID 365863.
6. Bialik V, Bialik GM, Blazer S, Sujov P, Wiener F, Berant M (1999). Developmental dysplasia of the hip: a new approach to incidence. Pediatrics; 103 (1): 93-9. doi:10.1542/peds.103.1.93. PMID 9917445.
7. Kokavec M, Bialik V. Developmental dysplasia of the hip. Prevention and real incidence. Bratisl Lek Listy, 2007; 108 (6): 251-4. PMID 17972535.
8. UNSW Embryology- Musculoskeletal System - Abnormalities.
9. Clinical Practice Guideline: Early Detection of Developmental Dysplasia of the Hip - Committee on Quality Improvement, Subcommittee on Developmental Dysplasia of the Hip 105 (4): 896 - AAP Policy
10. Lynn T Staheli. Fundamentals of Pediatric Orthopedics; p 13.
11. Forst J, Forst C, Forst R, Heller KD (1997). Pathogenetic relevance of the pregnancy hormone relaxin to inborn hip instability. Arch Orthop Trauma Surg 116 (4): 209-12. doi:10.1007/BF00393711. PMID9128773.

Poliomyelitis

1. Cohen JI. Chapter 175: Enteroviruses and Reoviruses. In Kasper DL, Braunwald E, Fauci AS, et al. (eds.). Harrison's Principles of Internal Medicine (16th ed.), McGraw-Hill Professional, 2004; pp. 1144. ISBN0071402357.
2. Chamberlin SL, Narins B (eds.): The Gale Encyclopedia of Neurological Disorders. Detroit: Thomson Gale, 2005; pp. 1859-70. ISBN 0-7876-9150-X.
3. Ryan KJ, Ray CG (eds.) : Enteroviruses". Sherris Medical Microbiology (4th ed.). McGraw Hill. 2004; pp. 535-7. ISBN 0-8385-8529-9.
4. Atkinson W, Hamborsky J, McIntyre L, Wolfe S (eds.): Poliomyelitis. Epidemiology and Prevention of Vaccine-Preventable Diseases (The Pink Book) (10th ed.): Washington DC: Public Health Foundation, 2007; pp. 101-14.
5. Paul JR. A History of Poliomyelitis. Yale studies in the history of science and medicine. New Haven, Conn: Yale University Press. 1971; pp. 16-18. ISBN 0-300-01324-8.
6. Trevelyan B, Smallman-Raynor M, Cliff A. The Spatial Dynamics of Poliomyelitis in the United States: From Epidemic Emergence to Vaccine-Induced Retreat, (2005); 1910-1971. Ann Assoc Am Geogr 95 (2): 269-93. doi:10.1111/j.1467-8306.2005.00460.x. PMID 16741562.

7. Aylward R. Eradicating polio: today's challenges and tomorrow's legacy. Ann Trop Med Parasitol, 2006; 100 (5-6): 401-13. doi:10.1179/136485906X97354. PMID 16899145.
8. Heymann D. Global polio eradication initiative. Bull. World Health Organ, 2006; 84 (8): 595. doi:10.2471/BLT.05.029512. PMID 16917643.
9. Falconer M, Bollenbach E. Late functional loss in nonparalytic polio. American journal of physical medicine and rehabilitation / Association of Academic Physiatrists, 2000; 79 (1): 19-23. doi:10.1097/00002060-200001000-00006. PMID 10678598.
10. Leboeuf C. The late effects of Polio: Information For Health Care Providers.. Commonwealth Department of Community Services and Health. 1992; ISBN 1-875412-05-0. Retrieved 2008-08-23.
11. Frauenthal HWA, Manning JVV. Manual of infantile paralysis, with modern methods of treatment.. Philadelphia Davis, 1914; pp. 79-101. OCLC 2078290.
12. Wood, Lawrence D. H, Hall, Jesse B, Schmidt, Gregory D. Principles of Critical Care (3rd ed.). McGraw-Hill Professional, 2005; pp. 870. ISBN 0-07-141640-4.
13. Katz, Samuel L. Gershon, Anne A., Krugman, Saul, Hotez, Peter J. Krugman's infectious diseases of children. St. Louis: Mosby, 2004; pp. 81-97. ISBN 0-323-01756-8.
14. Ohri, Linda K, Jonathan G. Marquess. Polio: Will We Soon Vanquish an Old Enemy?. Drug Benefit Trends, 1999;11 (6): 41-54. Retrieved 2008-08-23. (Available free on Medscape; registration required.)
15. Kew O, Sutter R, de Gourville E, Dowdle W, Pallansch M. Vaccine-derived polioviruses and the endgame strategy for global polio eradication. Annu Rev Microbiol, 2005; 59: 587-635.doi:10.1146/annurev.micro.58.030603.123625. PMID 16153180.
16. Parker SP (ed.): McGraw-Hill Concise Encyclopedia of Science and Technology. New York: McGraw-Hill, 1998; pp. 67. ISBN 0-07-052659-1.
17. Durstine JL, Moore GE (Eds):.ACSM's Exercise management for persons with chronic diseases and disabilities. Champaign, IL. Human Kinetics. 24. Borg G. (1970) Perceived exertion as an indicator of somatic stress. Scand. J. Rehabil. Med, 2003; 2(2):92-8. 25.
18. Borg K. Postpolio Fatigue, In: Silver, JK, Gawne AC. PostPolio Syndrome. Philadelphia: Hanley and Brews, 2004; pp77-86.
19. Horemans HL, Beelen A, Nollet F, Lankhorst GJ. Reproducibility of walking at self-preferred and maximal walking speed in patients with postpoliomyelitis syndrome. Arch. Phys. Med. Rehabil, 2004; 85(12):1929-1932.
20. 27. Clark, DR, Perry J, Lunsford TR. Case studies - Orthotic management of the adult post-polio patient. Orthotics and Prosthetics; (1986); 40(l):4350.

21. Hebert JS, Liggins AB. Gait evaluation of an automatic stance-control knee orthosis in a patient with post poliomyelitis. Arch. Phys. Med. Rehabil. 2005;86(8); 1676-80.

Cerebral Palsy

1. Cerebral Palsy. (National Center on Birth Defects and Developmental Disabilities, October 3, 2002; www.cdc.gov.
2. Cerebral palsy at Dorland's Medical Dictionary.
3. Beukelman, David R. Mirenda. Augmentative and Alternative Communication: Management of severe communication disorders in children and adults. Pat (2 ed.). Baltimore: Paul H Brookes Publishing Co, 1999; pp. 246-249.
4. Cerebral Palsy - Topic Overview. Retrieved 2008-02-06.
5. WebMD Medical Reference from Healthwise.
6. Anonymus. Definition and classification of cerebral palsy. Developmental medicine and child neurology, Feb 2007; 49(8): 8.
7. Economic costs associated with mental retardation, cerebral palsy, hearing loss, and vision impairment-United States. MMWR Morb. Mortal. Wkly. Rep, 2003; 53 (3): 57-9. 2004. PMID 14749614. Retrieved 2007-08-12.
8. Summary of The Epidemiology of cerebral palsy: incidence, impairments and risk factors." United Cerebral Palsy Research and Education Foundation (U.S.). Retrieved 5 July 2007.
9. Information: Scope. Retrieved 2007-12-08.
10. Groch, Judith. Medical News: Cerebral Palsy Rates Decline in Very Low Birthweight Children - in Neurology, General Neurology from MedPage Today". MedPage Today. Retrieved, January 5, 2007;12-08.
11. Birol Balaban, Evren Yasar, Ugur Dal, Kamil Yazicioglu, Haydar Mohur and Tunc Alp Kalyon The effect of hinged ankle-foot orthosis on gait and energy expenditure in spastic hemiplegic cerebral palsy. Disability and Rehabilitation, January 2007; 29(2): 139-144.
12. Athetoid/Dyskinetic Cerebral Palsy. Retrieved 2009-10-27.
13. Thames Valley Children's Centre - Cerebral Palsy - Causes and Prevalence. Retrieved 2007-06-11.
14. Johnson, Ann. Prevalence and characteristics of children with cerebral palsy in Europe. Developmental medicine and child neurology, 2002; 44 (9): 633- 0. doi:10.1017/S0012162201002675. PMID12227618.

Five

Principles in Geriatric Rehabilitation

Ageing or aging (see Fig. 5.1) is the accumulation of changes in an organism overtime or latter part of animate life.

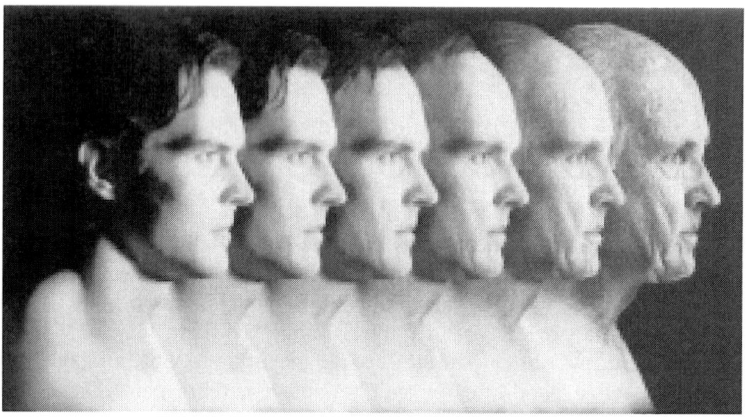

Fig. 5.1: Ageing

Ageing (see Fig. 5.2) in humans refers to a multidimensional process of physical, psychological, and social change. Some dimensions of ageing grow and expand over time, while others decline. Reaction time, for example, may slow with age, while knowledge of world events and wisdom may expand. Research shows that even late in life potential exists for physical, mental, and social growth and development. Ageing is an important part of all human societies reflecting the biological changes that occur as years goes on, but also reflecting cultural and societal conventions. Age is usually

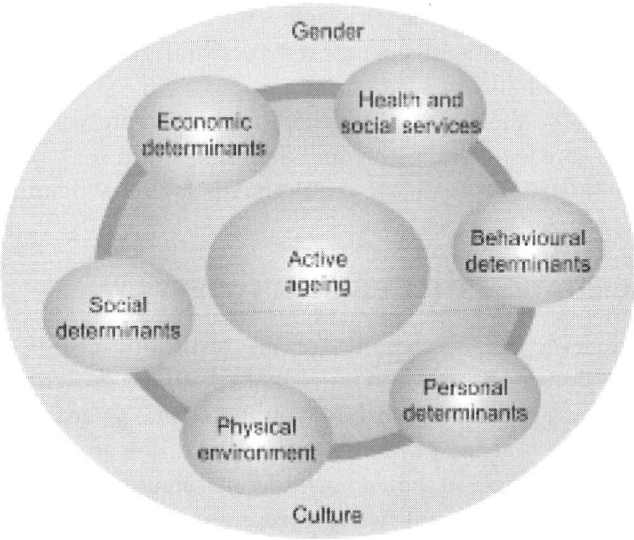

Fig. 5.2: Ageing

measured in full years and months for young children. A person's birthday is often an important event. Roughly 100,000 people worldwide die each day of age-related causes.

- Gerontology- The scientific study of the biological, psychological, and sociological phenomena associated with old age and aging.
- Geriatrics- treats the clinical problems of later life.
- Rehabilitation is a critical component of geriatric health care, because disabling conditions, which are common among older adults, profoundly affect their quality of life and are amenable to treatment. In older adults chronic disease almost always underlies disability; for example, stroke occurs most commonly in people with other vascular diseases, and hip fractures occur most commonly in people with osteoporosis and gait disorders. Worsening disability also occurs in progressive chronic diseases, such as osteoarthritis, Parkinson's disease, and amyotrophic lateral sclerosis, or in the context of deconditioning from inactivity during acute illness. In order to provide the best functional recovery possible, those providing geriatric rehabilitation must:

- Use systematic approaches to assess the causes of disability,
- Be familiar with the advantages and disadvantages of the various sites of rehabilitative care,
- Understand the role of multidisciplinary teams and care plans,
- Adapt care to other diseases and disabilities, and
- Be familiar with the basic requirements for rehabilitation of common geriatric conditions.

REHABILITATION STRATEGIES: AN OVERVIEW

The primary goals of rehabilitation are restitution of function, compensation or adaptation to functional losses, and prevention of secondary complications. Rehabilitation should maximize the older person's potential for participation in social, leisure, or work activities. Rehabilitation should not be defined simply as improving independence in ADLs but also as a program to prevent disability. A wide variety of strategies can be used to achieve these goals.

Restitution of physical function usually depends on therapeutic exercises (see Table 5.1 and 5.2) to improve flexibility, strength, motor control, and cardiovascular endurance. Although exercise has been shown to improve strength and motor control in well-defined populations of disabled older adults, there is still uncertainty about whether these gains translate into changes in mobility, activities of daily living, participation, or risk of falling.

Table 5.1: Benefits of Exercise in Older Adults

Cardiovascular	*Osteoporosis*	*Cancer*
Improves physiologic parameters (VO_2 max, cardiac output, decreased submaximal rate-pressure product) Improves blood pressure Decreases risk of coronary artery disease Improves congestive heart failure symptoms	Decreases bone density loss in postmenopausal women Decreases hip and vertebral fractures Decreases risk of falling **Osteoarthritis** Improves function	Potential decrease in risk of colon, breast, prostate, rectum Improves quality of life and decreases fatigue **Other** Decreases all-cause mortality Decreases all-cause morbidity

Contd...

Contd...

Cardiovascular	*Osteoporosis*	*Cancer*
and decreases hospitalization rate Improves lipid profile **Diabetes mellitus, type 2** Decreases incidence Improves glycemic control Decreases hemoglobin A_{1C} levels Improves insulin sensitivity	Decreases pain **Neuropsychologic health** Improves quality of sleep Improves cognitive function Decreases rates of depression, improves Beck depression scores. Improves short-term memory	Decreases risk of obesity Improves symptoms in peripheral vascular occlusive disease

Table 5.2: Common Barriers to Exercise in Older Adults

Barrier	*Approach*
Self-efficacy	Begin slowly with exercises that are easily accomplished; advance gradually; provide frequent encouragement.
Attitude	Promote positive personal benefits of exercise; identify enjoyable activities.
Discomfort	Vary intensity and range of exercise; employ cross-training; start slowly; avoid overdoing.
Disability	Specialized exercises; consider personal trainer or physical therapist.
Poor balance/ataxia	Assistive devices can increase safety as well as increase exercise intensity.
Fear of injury	Balance and strength training initially; use of appropriate clothing, equipment, and supervision; start slowly.
Habit	Incorporate into daily routine; repeat encouragement; promote active lifestyle.
Subjective norms	Identify and recruit influential others; education of patient and influential family/friends.
Fixed income	Walking and other simple exercises; use of household items; promote active lifestyle.
Environmental factors	Walk in the mall; use senior centers; promote active (e.g., inclement lifestyle, weather)
Cognitive decline	Incorporate into daily routine; keep exercises simple.
Illness/fatigue	Use a range of exercises/intensities that patients can match to their varying energy level.

Speech and language therapy can be used to treat aphasia in stroke patients, and cognitive rehabilitation can be used to improve their alertness and attention. As yet, however, there is no clear evidence that speech and language therapy or cognitive rehabilitation improves functional deficits.

Equipment such as mobility aides, orthotic and prosthetic devices and splints, and dressing and bathroom aids can augment or replace the function of impaired body parts and thereby reduce limitations in activities and participation.

Repeated practice of task-specific activities, such as bed mobility, transfers, and walking, can improve functional mobility. Upper-extremity function can also be improved with specific functional training activities, such as grasps, reaches, and fine manipulations. Balance training may reduce the risk of falls. Many older adults benefit from retraining in instrumental activities of daily living (IADLs), such as cooking, managing finances, or driving a car.

Contextual factors, both environmental and personal, need to be addressed in rehabilitation to minimize restrictions on the older person's activities and participation. Environmental modifications such as grab bars and raised toilet seats in the home or curb cutouts on public streets may be required to optimize the older person's independence in the home and the community.

A collaborative approach to goal setting, good patient and family education, and support groups may be used to address such personal factors as motivation. Each patient must be encouraged to accept responsibility for managing his or her condition and well-being.

ASSESSMENT AND REHABILITATION PLANNING

Comprehensive assessment of each elderly patient is necessary for appropriate clinical management and evaluation of outcomes. The treatment plan should be guided by the results of the assessment. The primary components of any assessment include patient demographics, social support, place of residence prior to illness, medical comorbidities, severity of current illness, and patient's prior functional status. Impairments such as deficits in range of motion and flexibility, strength, sensory functions, balance, cognition, and mood should always be assessed. The patient's functional status should be assessed with standardized measures of ADLs (eg, the Functional Independence Measure, the Barthel ADL Index), and of IADLs. The patient's participation or quality of life should also be assessed.

Assessment of the Geriatric Patient

Geriatric patients tend to have a lengthier past medical history than other patients due to their advanced age, medication use, and chronic illness. Due to physical impediments, such as hearing loss, visual impairment, or simple patient fatigue, the history taking process may take longer. When communicating with the geriatric patient, the physiotherapist should:

- Always identify yourself
- Speak at eye level to ensure that the patient can see you
- Locate a hearing aid, eyeglasses, or dentures (if needed)
- Speak slowly, distinctly, and respectfully
- Use the patient's surname, unless requested otherwise
- Listen closely
- Be patient
- Use gentleness
- Preserve dignity.

History Taking

When obtaining history from older age patients, it is noteworthy to examine the living conditions of the patient for:

- Alcohol or medication use (compliance, noncompliance, or abuse)
- Medications (current or expired, from one physician or multiple doctors)
- Health information
- Evidence of nutritional status
- Signs of adequate, personal hygiene
- Sometimes it helps to obtain additional history from caregivers (if any are available), due to an increased incidence of poor memory or dementia in some geriatric patients.

Note: Obtaining a current list of the patient's medications is important for the following reasons:

- It can be determined if the patient has multiple doctors prescribing conflicting medications.
- This information can assist the paramedic in making a working diagnosis.
- It can be determined if the patient is compliant with all of their medications.
- It can be determined if the patient is perhaps abusing their medication.

Physical Examination

While assessing and examining the geriatric patient, the paramedic should be considerate of the following:

- The patient may fatigue easily
- Geriatric patients commonly wear many layers of clothing for warmth, which may hamper the exam
- Respect the patient's need for privacy unless it interferes with patient care procedures
- Explain actions clearly, particularly if patient is visually or hearing impaired
- Be aware that patients may minimize or deny problems due to fear
- Try to differentiate between chronic and acute problems

THEORIES OF AGING

Senescence as the process of ageing is the steady deterioration of cell function following the period of development in youth.

- Cellular senescence- cells lose the ability to divide in response to DNA damage -cells either senesce, or self-destruct (apoptosis) if the damage is irreparable
- Organismal senescence is the aging of whole organisms.
- Species have different "rates of aging"- a mouse is elderly at 3 years; humans at 85 yrs
- Apart from species specific genetics, chance events determine the probability of death

The theories of ageing can be brodly classified in to Biological theories and Non-Biological theories

Biological Theories

At present, the biological basis of ageing is unknown. Most scientists agree that substantial variability exists in the rates of ageing across different species, and that this to a large extent is genetically based. Nevertheless, even in the relatively simple organisms, the mechanism of ageing remains to be elucidated. Because the lifespan of even the simple lab mouse is around 3 years, very few experiments directly test specific ageing theories (most of the evidence for the ones listed below is correlative).

Telomere Theory

Telomeres (structures at the ends of chromosomes) have experimentally been shown to shorten with each successive cell division. Shortened telomeres activate a mechanism that prevents further cell multiplication. This may be an important mechanism of ageing in tissues like bone marrow and the arterial lining where active cell division is necessary. Importantly though, mice lacking telomerase enzyme do not show a dramatically reduced lifespan, as the simplest version of this theory would predict.

Reproductive-Cell Cycle Theory

The idea that ageing is regulated by reproductive hormones that act in an antagonistic pleiotropic manner via cell cycle signaling, promoting growth and development early in life in order to achieve reproduction, but later in life, in a futile attempt to maintain reproduction, become dysregulated and drive senescence (dyosis).

Wear-and-Tear Theory

The very general idea that changes associated with ageing are the result of chance damage that accumulates over time. Proposed by Dr August Weismann (1982), the theory postulates that the daily grind of life, in particular abuse or overuse, literally wears the body out, leading to disease states. The degeneration of cartilage and eventual grinding of bone on bone is an example of the aging process on body joints, as wear and tear exceeds the body's ability to repair.

Waste Accumulation Theory

This theory proposes that, as we age, our cells accumulate waste products as a consequence of normal metabolic processes in the cells. It is believed that this build-up of toxic "sludge" eventually compromises normal cell functions. Lipofuscin pigments or liver spots, common on aging skin, are an example of this waste material. The brownish pigments consist of oxidized (rancid) fats that accumulate in the skin, as well as in the internal organs of our body, as we age.

Somatic Mutation Theory

The biological theory that ageing results from damage to the genetic integrity of the body's cells.

Faulty Reconstruction Theory

Throughout life the body is constantly re-building and repairing itself. The Faulty Reconstruction Theory argues that, as we age, the repair process begins to produce faulty reconstruction materials that compromise the repair job and weaken the cell - much like renovating a house with poor quality building supplies that diminish its final structure.

Immuno-suppression Theory

It is well known that the thymus gland, or gland of youth, which is located at the base of the throat, declines in size from infancy (250 gm) to adulthood (3 gm) the thymus is known to play a role in the auto-immune system, the body's primary defense against disease. Age-related reduction in the size of the thymus appears to correspond to a reduction in our immune systems, suggesting that the thymus may play a significant role in the aging process.

Errors and Repair Theory

According to this theory, the aging process is, in part, caused by damage to the genetic structure of the DNA, the genetic blueprint of our cells. Geneticist Bruce Ames of the University of California at Berkeley, states that, while the cell can repair over 99 percent of these point mutations, thousands of errors go un-repaired each day, leading to a life-long accumulation of molecular rubbish that, in turn, leads to errors in the manufacture of related proteins and helps accelerate the aging process.

Error Accumulation Theory

The idea that ageing results from chance events that escape proof reading mechanisms, which gradually damages the genetic code.

Accumulative-Waste Theory

The biological theory of ageing those points to a buildup of cells of waste products that presumably interferes with metabolism.

Autoimmune Theory

The idea that ageing results from an increase in autoantibodies that attack the body's tissues. A number of diseases associated with ageing, such as atrophic gastritis and Hashimoto's thyroiditis, are probably autoimmune in this way. While inflammation is very much evident in old mammals, even SCID mice in SPF colonies still senescence.

Ageing-Clock Theory

The theory that ageing results from a preprogrammed sequence, as in a clock, built into the operation of the nervous or endocrine system of the body. In rapidly dividing cells the shortening of the telomeres would provide just such a clock. This idea is in direct contradiction with the evolutionary based theory of ageing.

Molecular Cross-linkage Theory

Postulated back in 1942 by Johan Bjorksten, the theory advances the thought that molecular cross-linking between protein molecules, such as the collagen found in our skin, tendons and ligaments and the glycation (cross-linking) of other structural proteins and lipids (fats) with excess glucose, disrupts the functions of these molecules, leading to acceleration of the aging process. Glycation is one of the likely reasons that diabetics, who have chronically high levels of blood sugar (glucose), exhibit accelerated aging.

Mitochondrial Damage Theory

Mitochondria are minute organelles that are the respiratory centres within the cells of our body. Think of them as the "powerhouses of the cell," miniature blast furnaces where the foodstuffs of the cell are converted into useable energy to drive the cell's metabolic machinery. The Mitochondrial Damage Theory postulates that the oxidative processes occurring deep within the mitochondrial membranes eventually damage the organelle, leading to a loss of function. Once mitochondria are lost to the cell, they cannot be replaced, leading to a gradual but inexorable loss of energy and function in cells over time.

Reliability Theory of Ageing and Longevity

A general theory about systems failure. It allows researchers to predict the age-related failure kinetics for a system of given architecture (reliability structure) and given reliability of its components. Reliability theory predicts that even those systems that are entirely composed of non-ageing elements (with a constant failure rate) will nevertheless deteriorate (fail more often) with age, if these systems are redundant in irreplaceable elements. Ageing, therefore, is a direct consequence of systems redundancy. Reliability theory also predicts the late-life mortality deceleration with subsequent levelling-off, as well as the late-life mortality plateaus, as an inevitable consequence of redundancy exhaustion at extreme old ages. The theory explains why mortality rates increase exponentially with age (the Gompertz law) in many species, by taking into account the initial flaws (defects) in newly formed systems. It also explains why organisms prefer to die according to the Gompertz law, while technical devices usually fail according to the Weibull (power) law. Reliability theory allows specifying conditions when organisms die according to the Weibull distribution: organisms should be relatively free of initial flaws and defects. The theory makes it possible to find a general failure law applicable to all adult and extreme old ages, where the Gompertz and the Weibull laws are just special cases of this more general failure law. The theory explains why relative differences in mortality rates of compared populations (within a given species) vanish with age (compensation law of mortality), and mortality convergence is observed due to the exhaustion of initial differences in redundancy levels.

Mitohormesis

It has been known since the 1930s that restricting calories while maintaining adequate amounts of other nutrients can extend lifespan in laboratory animals. Recently, Michael Ristow's group has provided evidence for the theory that this effect is due to increased formation of free radicals within the mitochondria causing a secondary induction of increased antioxidant defence capacity.

Misrepair-Accumulation Theory

This very recent novel theory by Wang et al; suggests that ageing is the result of the accumulation of "Misrepair". Important in this theory is to distinguish among "damage" which means a newly emerging defect Before any reparation has taken place, and "Misrepair" which describes the remaining defective structure after (incorrect) repair. The key points in this theory are:

- There is no original damage left unrepaired in a living being. If damage was left unrepaired a life threatening condition (such as bleeding, infection, or organ failure) would develop.
- Misrepair, the repair with less accuracy, does not happen accidentally. It is a necessary measure of the reparation system to achieve sufficiently quick reparation in situations of serious or repeated damage, to maintain the integrity and basic function of a structure, which is important for the survival of the living being.
- Hence the appearance of 'Misrepair' increases the chance for the survival of individual, by which the individual can live at least up to the reproduction age, which is critically important for the survival of species. Therefore the 'Misrepair mechanism' was selected by nature due to its evolutionary advantage.
- However, since 'Misrepair' as a defective structure is invisible for the reparation system, it accumulates with time and causes gradually the disorganization of a structure (tissue, cell, or molecule); this is the actual source of ageing.

Ageing hence is the side-effect for survival, but important for species survival. Thus Misrepair might represent the mechanism by which organisms are not programmed to die but to survive (as long as possible), and ageing is just the price to be paid.

But, the most widely accepted structural damage theory - and the one theory that encompasses all of the previous theories - is the Free Radical Theory of aging.

Free-Radical Theory

The idea that free radicals (unstable and highly reactive organic molecules, also named reactive oxygen species or oxidative stress) create damage that gives rise to symptoms we recognize as ageing.

The Free Radical Theory of Aging was proposed in 1954 by University of Nebraska biochemist and professor emeritus of medicine, Dr Denham Harman. Like most bold scientific theories, Harman's ideas were largely ignored - even derided - until several investigations in the late 1960's overwhelmingly validated his brilliant insight.

According to Harman, aging occurs when cells become permanently damaged from the life-long and unrelenting attack of charged molecular fragments, known as free radicals. The cellular damage inflicted by this uncontrolled oxidative stress inexorably spreads outward to the level of tissues and organs, where it eventually manifests itself as some form of degenerative disease.

Over 80 degenerative diseases are now known to be linked to free radical-induced oxidative stress. An estimated 80 to 90 percent of all degenerative diseases are now believed to involve free radical activity. Which disease wounds you mortally depends much on the roll of the genetic dice, cast upon your conception, as well your individual lifestyle and life-long dietary choices.

Non-biological Theories

Disengagement Theory

This is the idea that separation of older people from active roles in society is normal and appropriate, and benefits both society and older individuals. Disengagement theory, first proposed by

Cumming and Henry, has received considerable attention in gerontology. The original data on which Cumming and Henry based the theory were from a rather small sample of older adults in Kansas City, and from this select sample Cumming and Henry then took disengagement to be a universal theory. There are research data suggesting that the elderly who do become detached from society as those were initially reclusive individuals, and such disengagement is not purely a response to ageing.

Activity Theory

In contrast to disengagement theory, this theory implies that the more active elderly people are, the more likely they are to be satisfied with life. The view that elderly adults should maintain well-being by keeping active has had a considerable history, and since 1972, this has become to be known as activity theory. However, this theory may be just as inappropriate as disengagement for some people as the current paradigm on the psychology of ageing is that both disengagement theory and activity theory may be optimal for certain people in old age, depending on both circumstances and personality traits of the individual concerned.

Selectivity Theory

Mediates between Activity and Disengagement Theory, which suggests that it may benefit older people to become more active in some aspects of their lives, more disengaged in others.

Continuity Theory

The view that in ageing people are inclined to maintain, as much as they can, the same habits, personalities, and styles of life that they have developed in earlier years. Continuity theory is Atchley's theory that individuals, in later life, make adaptations to enable them to gain a sense of continuity between the past and the present, and the theory implies that this sense of continuity helps to contribute to well-being in later life. Disengagement theory, Activity theory and Continuity theory, are social theories about ageing, though all may be products of their era rather than a valid, universal theory.

Measure of Age

The age of an adult human is commonly measured in whole years since the day of birth. Fractional years or months or even weeks may be used to describe the age of children and infants for finer resolution. The time of day the birth occurred is not commonly considered.

The measure of age has historically varied from this approach in some cultures. For example, in China, Korea, Japan and Vietnam, children were considered to be one year old at the moment of birth and two years old on the following New Year's Day. Thus, a child could be considered two years old several days after birth. In parts of Tibet, age is counted from conception i.e. one is 9 months old when one is born

Age in prenatal development is normally measured in gestational age, taking the last menstruation of the woman as a point of beginning. Alternatively, fertilisation age, beginning from fertilisation can be taken.

Dividing the lifespan

- Pre-conception: ovum, spermatozoon
- Conception: fertilization
- Pre-birth: conception to birth (pregnancy)
- Infancy: Birth to 1
- Childhood: 1 to 12
- Adolescence: 13 to 19
- Early adulthood: 20 to 39
- Middle adulthood: 40 to 64
- Late adulthood: 65+
- Death
- Post-death: decomposition

Geriatric Classification:

Person above 65 yrs is considered as Geriatric.
- 65 yrs to 74 yrs = Young old
- 75 yrs to 84 yrs = Older old
- 85 yrs above = Oldest
- UN - defines 60 +; developed nations 65+

Physiological Changes in Geriatrics

The various physiological changes which occur are:

Changes in the cardio-vascular system (Fig. 5.3): There is normal atrophy of the heart muscle, especially in the left ventricle, calcification of the heart valves, loss of elasticity in artery walls (arteriosclerosis) and intra-artery deposits (atherosclerosis). There is decreased cardiac output, baroreceptor sensitivity and SA node automaticity. The reduced blood flow results in reduced stamina reduced renal and hepatic function and less cellular nourishment. There is impaired blood pressure response to standing, volume depletion and heart blocks.

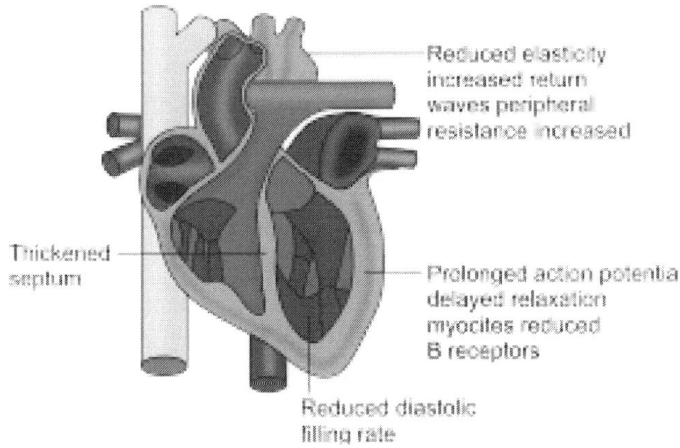

Fig. 5.3: Cardiovascular system

Changes in the respiratory system: The airways and lung tissue become less elastic with reduced cilliary activity. There is decreased oxygen uptake and exchange. The muscles of the rib cage atrophy, reducing the ability to breathe deeply, cough and expel carbon dioxide. There is ventilation/perfusion mismatch and decreased PO2.

Changes in musculo-skeletal system: There is generalized atrophy of all muscles accompanied by a replacement of some muscle tissue by fat deposits. This results in some loss of muscle tone and strength. Calcium is lost and bones become less dense. This can result in osteoporosis and a reduction of weight bearing capacity, leading to the possibility of spontaneous fracture. Thinning of the vertebrae also results in a reduction in height. In addition, the vertebrae can calcify, resulting in postural changes. The joints also undergo changes. In fact, arthritis, the degenerative inflammation of the joints, is the most common chronic condition in the elderly.

Changes in skin: The skin loses underlying fat layers and oil glands, causing wrinkles and reduced elasticity. There is increased susceptibility to cold, bruising and bedsores. In addition, the skin develops "age spots" due to deposits of melanin pigment. The hair gradually loses its pigmentation and turns gray. The nails become thicker due to reduced blood flow to the connective tissues. The skin becomes somewhat less sensitive to sensations including heat, cold and injury.

Changes in the gastrointestinal system: There is reduction in the production of hydrochloric acid, digestive enzymes and saliva. These changes may result in gastrointestinal distress, impaired swallowing and delayed emptying of the stomach. The breakdown and absorption of foods may also be impaired, sometimes resulting in deficiencies of vitamin B, C, and K or in extreme cases, malnutrition.

Changes in the metabolic system: The metabolic system is responsible for changing food into energy. After age 25, everyone experiences approximately a 1% decrease per year in their metabolic rate. This overall slowing results in food being less well absorbed and utilized. There is a decrease in the overall metabolism of drugs.

Changes in sexuality: Sexual desire and performance may continue well into an individual's eighth and ninth decade although frequency may diminish. Physiological changes in women include atrophy of the ovarian, vaginal and uterine tissues with decreased production of vaginal fluids. In men, sperm production is decreased and prostate enlarges. Both older men and women generally require more stimulation to become aroused and more time to reach orgasm.

Sensory changes with aging: Our special senses play a central role in our ability to gather information and to participate in social interactions.

These changes are:

- *Changes in vision:* In the fourth decade, the pupil begins to decrease in size and there is decreased response to light (see Fig. 5.4). Because of these changes, older people require three times the amount of illumination to see as compared to a younger person. Focusing takes longer with an increase in nearsightedness, making small print harder to read. There is loss of accommodation which makes reading and close work difficult. This condition, which is known as presbyopia, can be corrected by wearing glasses with convex lenses. There is thickening and yellowing of the lens of the eye. This results in light diffraction, increased sensitivity to glare, decreased depth perception and more difficulty distinguishing pastel colors, especially blues and greens.

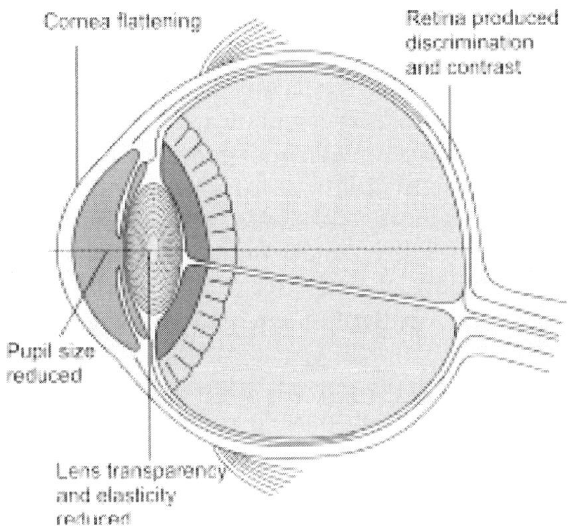

Fig. 5.4: Structure of eye with Agegins

Changes in hearing: There is a decrease in sensitivity to high frequency tones and decreased discrimination of similar pitches because of changes in the bones and cochlear hair cells of the inner ear. Approximately 30% of all elderly persons have some hearing impairment. It is an invisible disability which is often covered up or denied by a person who may then be mislabeled as senile, dumb or uncooperative.

- *Changes in taste and smell:* Taste and smell are interrelated and important for eating as well as checking for hazards in the environment such as spoiled food, smoke and fumes. Older adults experience some decline in the ability to taste resulting from a reduction in the total number of taste buds, especially after the age of 80.

Some individuals also experience a decline in their sense of smell, but this is usually because of abnormal conditions such as blockage or disease of the olfactory receptors in the upper sinus.

Cognitive changes associated with aging: After age 25, everyone loses nerve cells. Gradually over time, this results in a reduced efficiency of nerve transmission which affects response time and coordination. These changes may also affect sleeping patterns by decreasing the length of total sleep time and REM sleep. In spite of these anatomical and physiological changes in brain, studies have found evidence of limited impairment of actual intellectual functioning associated with the aging process.

Intellectual ability is one the factors affecting functioning in later life. The various changes in cognition are:

- *Effect on intelligence:* Intelligence generally is associated with a range of abilities that allow us to make sense of our experiences: the ability to comprehend new information, the ability to think abstractly, the ability to make rational decisions, spatial ability, numerical ability, verbal fluency, etc. Intelligence tests have demonstrated a pattern of age-related changes in intellectual functioning.

  The fact that older persons perform more poorly on tests of intelligence is due in part to reduced efficiency of nerve transmission in the brain, resulting in slower information processing and greater loss of information during transmission.
- *Effect on learning and memory:* Most persons experience a modest increase in memory problems as they get older, particularly with regard to the ability to remember relatively recent experiences. There is impairment of the ability to accumulate new information and to retrieve existing information from memory. There is little decline in the ability to store new information once it is learned.

Personality changes associated with aging: Whereas basic personality traits may remain rather stable throughout adulthood, relatively predictable shifts may occur in other aspects of a person's personality. One of the best documented personality changes in adulthood is an increased preoccupation with one's inner life, including greater attention to personal feelings and experiences and reduced extraversion. A second domain in which age-related changes have been reported is gender role identity. With advancing age, men and women appear to become more similar in terms of their values and personality styles. Studies in a number of different cultures have found that men tend to become more nurturing, expressive and affiliation-seeking as they grow older, whereas women tend to become more instrumental and achievement-oriented.

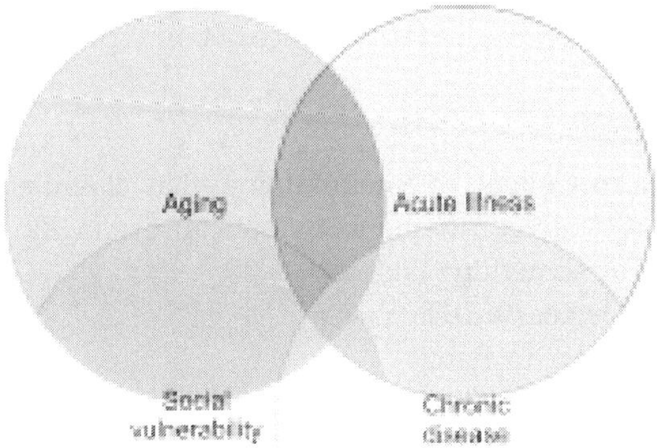

Fig. 5.5: Interaction of aging, environment and disease

OSTEOARTHRITIS (OA)

OA is the Degenerative Joint Disease

Osteoarthritis (OA) also known as **degenerative arthritis** or **degenerative joint disease** is a non inflammatory degenerative joint disease marked by degeneration of the articular cartilage, hypertrophy of bone at the margins, and changes in the synovial membrane. It is often associated with obesity, low bone density, repeated mechanical stress, and structural abnormalities of the joint. OA is a major contributor to functional impairment and reduced independence in older adults.

OA is characterized by joint pain, tenderness, swelling, and limitation in joint movement. The joints most often affected are the joints of the fingers, the base of the thumb, the hips, the knees, the neck (cervical spine), and the lower back (lumbar spine). Unlike some types of arthritis that affect multiple organ systems, any secondary inflammation associated with osteoarthritis is limited to the joints. *Pain after joint use that subsides with resting the joint is a classical sign of osteoarthritis.* As osteoarthritis worsens, pain may occur at rest or at night. Diagnosis of osteoarthritis is based on a history of joint symptoms, physical examination, and radiographic (X-ray) changes. X-ray changes may include joint-space narrowing, changes in the bones, and the presence of bony spurs.

Classification

The American College of Rheumatology has classified OA into PRIMARY (OA appears without obvious cause) and SECONDARY (OA caused by something known).

- **Primary Osteoarthritis:**
  - Occurs due to aging
  - Localized - of either hands, feet, knees, hips - one site affected, most common is knee.
  - Generalized - three or more of the above joint groups affected.
- **Secondary Osteoarthritis:**
  - Post-traumatic - after an accident or injury, especially if it affected the joint directly
  - Congenital Disorders - Congenital Hip Luxation, Abnormally formed joints (Hip Dysplasia)
  - Diabetes
  - Inflammatory Diseases (Perthes Disease, Lyme Disease)
  - Chronic forms of arthritis (Rheumatoid Arthritis, Costochondritis, Spondyloarthropathies)
  - Metabolic joint disease (Hemochromatosis, Acromegaly, Gout, Pseudogout, Wilson's Disease)
  - Joint Infection
  - Avascular Necrosis
  - Hormonal Disorders
  - Ligamentous deterioration or instability
  - Obesity
  - Sports injuries or similar injuries from exercise work
  - Pregnancy

- Alkaptonuria
- Vitamins D and C and estrogen deficiency
- Inherited Disorders or Genetic Mutation of Type 2 Collagen
- Occupational or Repetitive Joint use
- Quadriceps muscle weakness.

PATHOLOGY

The characteristic structural changes in OA include the progressive loss of articular cartilage, increased subchondral plate thickness, formation of new bone at the joint margins (osteophytes) and the development of subchondral bone cysts. In addition, at the junction of the articular hyaline cartilage and adjacent subchondral bone, in the region of the so-called tidemark, there is a remnant of calcified cartilage.

As OA progresses, there is evidence of vascular invasion and advancement of this zone of calcified cartilage into the articular cartilage that further contributes to a decrease in articular cartilage thickness. These structural alterations in the articular cartilage and peri-articular bone may lead to modification of the contours of the adjacent articulating surface. These changes, as well as the accompanying alterations in subchondral bone remodeling and modulus, may further contribute to the development of an adverse biomechanical environment and enhance the progression of the articular cartilage deterioration.

Changes in Articular Cartilage

Loss of Proteoglycans

Decrease in proteoglycans

Fibrillation

The first macroscopic change in the osteoarthritic joint is the fibrillation of the cartilage. Multiple, tiny surface cracks develop first in the superficial layer of the articular cartilage and gradually deepen. Synovial fluid flows into these cracks and, as deeper layers of cartilage fibrillate, pieces break off, lodging in the synovium and leaving the subchondral bone increasingly exposed.

Secondary Synovitis

Fragments of cartilage and bone join to form osteocartilaginous loose bodies in the joint.

Space

The presence of these bodies in the synovium elicits a foreign-body type inflammatory reaction, causing the synovium to become hyperemic and hypertrophied.

Changes in Subchondral Bone

In the region where the articular cartilage is cracked and fibrillated, the subchondral bone responds by forming new blood vessels (neovascularization). This process induces osteoclastic bone resorption and increased activity in adjacent osteoblasts, resulting in a thickening of the subchondral bone in the exposed area. Fibrocartilagenous plugs.

Eburnation

The subchondral bone becomes exposed such that it grinds against the opposite joint surface. As the joint moves, this grinding burnishes the exposed bone. It becomes eburnated - polished, shiny and smooth, with an appearance like ivory.

Subchondral bone cysts

These cysts form when synovial fluid flows into the bone marrow space following a crack in the eburnated subchondral bone.

Development of Osteophytes

In advanced OA, bony spurs called osteophytes develop when mesenchymal tissue of the synovium modulates into osteoblasts and chondroblasts to form a mass of bone and cartilage. Mechanially, osteophytes serve to increase the load-bearing area on the joint thus decreasing the load per unit area (i.e. stress). Osteophytes most often appear on the periphery of the joint.

PATHOGENESIS

Osteoarthritis attacks weakened joints. In idiopathic (primary) OA, hormonal, genetic, metabolic and mechanical factors appear to be implicated but the etiology remains unclear. In secondary OA, these entire factors one factor is identifiable as the primary cause. Often in secondary OA, mechanical causes are primary and the affected joints have been exposed to previous trauma involving repeated and/or excessive loading of the joints. Congenital and development deformities, neurologic disorder and pre-existing arthritis may also incite secondary OA.

Mechanically like all weight-bearing structures, articular cartilage has a critical stress which it can tolerate and above which, it begins to break down. When the joint is exposed to stresses above this critical value, the unit load on the chondrocytes becomes too high and overburdened chondrocytes begin to die. The death of chondrocytes cells weakens the matrix by stopping chondrocyte homeostasis in those cells; this leads to degradation of the articular cartilage. An increased unit load on the chondrocytes may also be the result of changes in the subchondral bone. In Paget's disease, for example, damage to the coarse cancellous bone of the epiphysis may cause an increase in the stiffness of the subchondral bone. This, in turn, increases the unit load on the chondrocytes and increases the likelihood that articular cartilage will eventually degrade and OA will develop.

Biochemical Abnormalities results in changes in composition of articular cartilage contribute to the development of OA. As healthy articular cartilage ages, its water content decreases. In osteoarthirtic cartilage, water content increases, contributing to the tendency for this cartilage to swell more than normal. Collagen fibres become thicker than normal and more water binds to these cllagen fibres. Proteoglycan content and aggregation are both decreased and the length of glycosaminoglycan chains is shortened. Chondrocytes bearing excessive loads eventually cease to respond to reparative stimuli, as a result protein synthesis by chondrocytes also decreases. Acid cathepsin attacks protein cores and is increased in OA cartilage.

Clinical Features

Symptoms

- Dull aching joint pain
  - Early Disease Condition - Gradual onset, mild in intensity, brought on by joint usage, and relieved with rest.
  - May be vague around joint
  - Self-limited or intermittent
  - Severe Disease Condition - pain at rest & during night
  - Severity of pain does not reflect the severity of the disease
- Joint stiffness < 30 minutes in the morning and becomes worse as the day goes on.
- Loss of normal function of the joint and the person as a whole.
- Advanced Condition - Sense of grinding or locking of a joint, and buckling or instability of joints during demanding tasks.
- Fatigue - if biomechanical changes lead to increased energy requirements for activities of daily living.
- Overuse of alternative muscle groups can lead to development of pain syndromes in other parts of the musculoskeletal system.

Signs

- Pain on movement
- Swelling of the joint
- Articular gelling - stiffness lasting short periods and dissipates after initial ROM.
- Spasm of periarticular muscles
- Bony enlargement of the joint
- Limitation of range of movement - End ROM mostly affected
- Crepitus when moved - loud cracks & crunches if the arthritis is severe.
- Tenderness to pressure
  - Around the joint margins
  - Very sore if knocked or injured in any way
- Joint Deformity or poor alignment
  - Genu Varum (Bow Legs)
  - Genu Valgum (Knock Knees).

LABORATORY AND RADIOGRAPHIC FINDINGS

- Radiographic findings:
  - Joint space narrowing
  - Subchondral bone sclerosis
  - Subchondralcysts
  - Osteophytosis
  - Change in contour due to bony remodling
  - Subluxation
- Laboratory testing (For secondary OA)
  - ESR
  - Serum chemistry
  - Blood counts
  - Urinalysis
  - Synovial fluid analysis
  - WBC < 2,000/mL
  - Mononuclear predominance.

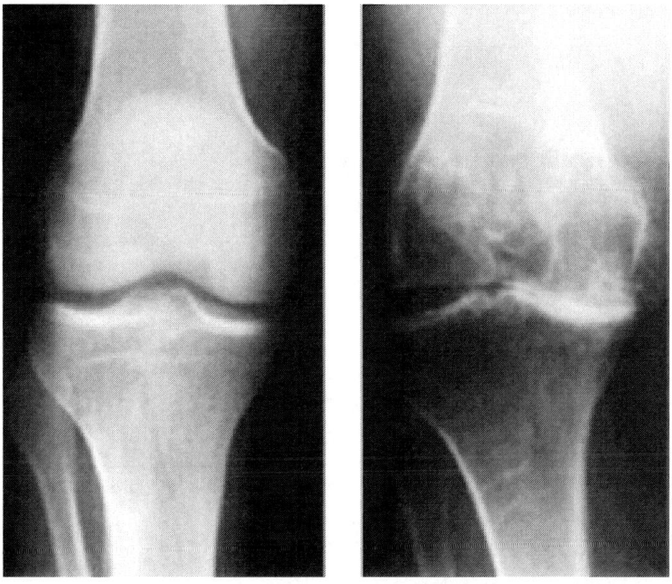

Normal knee in X-ray Arthritic knee in X-ray

Fig. 5.7:

EXAMINATIONS

Upon general examination, look for patients weight and fat proportion.

Hands

- Inspection.
  - Redness
  - Pattern of joint involvement
  - Heberden's and Bouchard's nodes
  - Squaring of hand (CMC)
  - Joint deformities (varus or valgus)
- Palpation.
  - bony swelling
- Also Notice
  - Crepitus: (cracking or grinding sound as bones rub) Particularly CMC joint.

Knee

- Inspection
  - Quads wasting
  - Valgus or varus deformity
  - Gait
- Palpation
  - Joint effusion
  - Bony swelling
- Also Notice
  - Crepitus
  - Reduced range of movement
  - Lateral instability.

Neck

- Inspection
  - Kyphosis or scoliosis
- Palpation
  - local tenderness

- Also Notice
  - Reduced range of movement.

Hip

- Inspection
  - usually nothing visible
  - Gait
- Palpation
  - Tenderness over the joint (mid-point inguinal ligament)
- Also Notice
  - Reduced range of movement (particularly rotation in flexion).

TREATMENT

Goals

- Reduce pain
- Maintain mobility
- Minimize disability.

Nonpharmacologic Management

Patient Education and Counseling.

Weight reduction reduces the risk of developing OA of the knees, and helps reduce pain and improve function in older women with knee OA.

Joint Protection

- Correction of poor posture.
- Support for excessive lumbar lordosis.
- Avoid excessive loading.
- Avoid prolonged standing, kneeling and squatting.
- Lose weight.
- Rest periods during the day.
- Thermoplastic splint blocks flexion can reduce pain, improve overall hand function and reduce muscle spasm.
- Use of cane/crutches or walker.

Patellar Taping

- For OA of patellofemoral compartment.
- Medial taping to reduce pain on kneeling, squatting or climbing stairs.

Exercise

- Multiple angle Isometrics to Quads and Hamstrings.
- Aerobic conditioning - Walking, cycling, aquatic exercises.
- Strengthening exercises to Lower limb for proper Gait.
- Stretching Exercises to Quads, Hams and Calf group of muscles.
- Range of Motion exercises.

Wedged Insoles/Orthoses

- For patients with medial compartment knee OA and medial tibial femoral compartment - Lateral wedge insoles.

Thermal Modalities

- **TENS**
- **IFT**
- **Cryotherapy**

Pharmacologic Therapy

- NSAIDs and Acetaminophen
- Selective COX-2 Inhibitors
- Glucocorticoid Injection
- Intraarticular Injection of Hyaluronan
- Opioids.

Orthopedic Surgery

- For patients with advanced OA in whom aggressive medical management has failed
- Arthroplasty: Relieve pain, increasing mobility
- Osteotomy: eliminate concentration of peak dynamic loads and provide effective pain relief.

Cartilage Regeneration

- Disadvantage: fibrocartilage that resurfaces is inferior to normal hyaline cartilage in its ability to withstand mechanical loads.

RATIONAL APPROACH TO NONSURGICAL MANAGEMENT OF OA

- Nonpharmacologic management: foundation of treatment of OA pain
- Pharmacologic management: adjunctive or complementary role in management of this disease
- Individualized approach.

DEMENTIA

Dementia is a syndrome of impaired cognition caused by brain dysfunction. It has been defined as "the development of multiple cognitive deficits that include memory impairment and at least one of the following: aphasia, apraxia, agnosia, or a disturbance in executive functioning" (American Psychiatric Association, 1994).

Most studies in the developed countries have reported the overall prevalence of dementia to be between 5% and 10% of the elderly. Dementia has become a major public health concern because it leads to serious physical, functional, and psychologic morbidity for the individual because it shortens life expectancy, and because caring for people with dementia exacts a heavy toll on the care providers over the course of the illness.

Types of dementia

1. Alzheimer's disease (60%; of cases)
2. Vascular dementia (30-40%; including about 20% where dual pathology exists)
3. Dementia with Lewy bodies (15% of cases)
4. Fronto-temporal dementia (5%)

Signs and Symptoms

- Duration of symptoms must normally exceed six months for a diagnosis of dementia or organic brain syndrome to be made.

- Memory impairment is generally a prominent early symptom of dementia.
- Poor judgment and poor insight are also common.
- Individuals have difficulty learning new material.
- Dementia is sometimes accompanied by motor disturbances, which may include gait difficulties, slurred speech, and a variety of abnormal movements.
- In more severe dementia, individuals also forget previously learned material, including the names of loved ones. Individuals with dementia may have difficulty with spatial tasks, such as navigating around the house or in the immediate neighborhood.
- Other symptoms of dementia include disinhibited behavior, including making inappropriate jokes, neglecting personal hygiene, suicidal behavior, exhibiting undue familiarity with strangers, or disregarding conventional rules of social conduct Anxiety is fairly common, depressed mood and sleep disturbances are also common. Other neurological symptoms, such as myoclonus and seizures, may also occur (American Psychiatric Association, 1997).

Examination in Dementia

Assessment of Daily Function

Careful and competent functional assessment identifies how to maximize patient autonomy. Functional assessment includes physical, psychological and socioeconomic domains. Standardized assessment instruments can provide information on the patient's capacity for self care and independent living. Physical functioning is measured along a continuum and may focus on basic Activities of Daily Living (ADL's) that include feeding, bathing, dressing, mobility and toileting. In addition, Instrumental (or intermediate) Activities of Daily Living (IADL's) assess more advanced self care activities, such as shopping, cooking, and managing finances and medications. A useful informant-based tool to assess dimensions of function is the Functional Activities Questionnaire.

Assessment of Cognitive Status

- Mini-mental state examination
- Modified Mini-mental state examination (3MS)
- Abbreviated mental test score.

Other Examinations

- Informant Questionnaire on Cognitive Decline in the Elderly (IQCODE).
- The General Practitioner Assessment of Cognition combines both, a patient assessment and an informant interview. It was specifically designed for the use in the primary care setting.
- Further evaluation includes retesting at another date, and administration of other (and sometimes more complex) tests of mental function, such as formal neuropsychological testing.

Laboratory Tests

- Routine blood tests are also usually performed to rule out treatable causes.
- Vitamin B12, folic acid, thyroid-stimulating hormone (TSH), C-reactive protein, full blood count, electrolytes, calcium, renal function, and liver enzymes.
- Abnormalities may suggest vitamin deficiency, infection or other problems that commonly cause confusion or disorientation in the elderly. The problem is complicated by the fact that these cause confusion more often in persons who have early dementia, so that "reversal" of such problems may ultimately only be temporary.
- Testing for alcohol and other known dementia-inducing drugs may be indicated.

Imaging

A CT scan or magnetic resonance imaging (MRI) scan is commonly performed.

Causes of Dementia

Fixed Cognitive Dementia

- Traumatic brain injury
- Neurosurgery
- Stroke
- Meningitis
- Hydrocephalus

Slowly Progressive Dementia

The causes of dementia depend on the age at which symptoms begin. In the elderly population (usually defined in this context as over 65 years of age), a large majority of cases of dementia are caused by Alzheimer's disease, vascular dementia or both. Dementia with Lewy bodies is another fairly common cause, which again may occur alongside either or both of the other causes.

Rapidly progressive dementia

- Dementia as a feature of other conditions
- Chronic neurodegenarative conditions of the brain may affect cognition in the long term.

Treatment

Medical Management

Pharmacological treatment:
- Risperidone
- Haloperidol
- Benzodiazepines
- Selegiline
- Beta-blockers
- Hormonal therapy.

Nonpharmacological Approaches to Treating Dementia

- Psychosocial interventions for treating the cognitive and noncognitive aspects of dementia are based on the fact that

neurological disease will affect each individual differently depending on the following:
- Individual's biography
- Individual's personality
- The presence of coexisting physical and mental health problems
- The person's social relationships
- The physical environment in which the person is living
- Community and cultural understandings of and tolerance for confusion and frailty
- The extent and location of the disease

Psychosocial Interventions

- Addressing the individual, social and environmental aspects of a person's life can prevent or minimize the disability associated with neurological impairment.
- Psychosocial approaches need to be individualized and tailored to the person's needs, personality, biography, goals, strengths, and preferences.
- The aim of psychosocial approaches should be to enhance the person's sense of self and quality of life.
- There is no single optimal psychosocial approach, there is a need to develop a range of flexible psychosocial approaches.
- Multidimensional assessment is essential to ensure effective interventions.

The psychosocial management of dementia includes social and environmental approaches to the care of patients with dementia, as well as psychosocial and behavioural approaches. A useful classification of behaviours has been devised, dividing them into three categories:

1. Physically aggressive
2. Verbally aggressive
3. Physically nonaggressive.

These have been linked to different causes. For example, physical aggression most commonly occurs during personal care and may be a function of the nature of the interaction between the carer and the person with dementia. Finding alternative approaches to personal care can prove useful.

In contrast, verbal agitation occurs most commonly when the person is alone or during personal care and, as such, may be linked to pain, discomfort or a need for social contact. The extent of undetected pain in people with dementia is well documented, so appropriate care for behaviour may include medical treatment for pain. Simulated presence therapy addresses the person's social need by providing an audio tape of a close relative talking about shared memories. This has led to decreased agitation for some patients.
Physically nonaggressive behaviours, such as wandering, are associated with stimulation seeking. Providing the person with something to do has been shown to reduce behavioural aspects of dementia.

Depression and Challenging Behaviours

A strong association exits between the lack of meaningful activity and the presence of depression and challenging behaviours.

Therapeutic activity programmes have been used to decrease disruptive behaviour by providing engagement in pleasant activities.In the treatment condition residents attended an activity programme where the goal was physical, mental and social stimulation which included exercise, music, crafts, relaxation and reminiscence

Physical designs - appropriate physical designs can minimize decline and improve functioning in patients with dementia. For example, low lighting has been linked to confusion and agitation, whereas noise is linked to agitation and poor functional performance. Changing these factors may improve the patient's condition. The potential exists to prolong independence, promote sense of safety and prevent development of 'challenging behaviours'.

Functional competence/daily living skills - there is a growing body of evidence that suggests that appropriate interventions can help maintain daily living skills, at least for those with mild to moderate impairments. For example, in a nursing home setting, residents get the most social contact from staff by exhibiting dependent behaviours and interventions have been designed to reverse this dynamicaly. Communication and social interaction - psychological, behavioural and environmental interventions are used to improve memory, communication, activities of daily living and emotional well being. Most of these interventions rely on carers to initiate or respond in ways that compensate for deficits and support the abilities of the person with dementia. There are several ways that families and carers can affect a person's quality of life. For example, encouraging carers to use memory books increases the amount and quality of social interaction with people, even those who have advanced dementia. Verbal prompts and cues can help people with dementia regain and maintain everyday abilities such as dressing. Using Reality Orientation (RO), where the carer provides the person with visual and verbal cues in order to help with orientation to time, place or person improves behaviour and cognition. This orientation can take place either in groups or in one-on-one interactions.

Carers can also assist people with dementia to recall events from their past, facilitated by the use of personalized aids, such as photos or memorabilia, either in one-to-one or in group sessions.

Helping caregivers is a critical component of comprehensive dementia care. Counselling, training programs and continued support can decrease caregiver's distress and depression and delay nursing home admission.

OLD AGE HOME

Many factors have contributed to the alienation of the elders. Migration of young couples from the rural areas to cities, elders who have been in control of the household for a long time are unwilling to give up the responsibility to their children, youngsters on their part are sometimes resentful of the attitude of their parents.

Elders are sometimes too incapacitated or unwell to look after themselves or get medical care especially in an emergency.

Condition Leading to Admission in Old Age Home:

- Lack of economic support
- Lack of affection in family/no familial support
- Self respect/peace of mind/away from familial conflict/more freedom/this is the best option at this age.
- Do not want to be a burden on any one
- Have no one to take care/absence of close family members
- Fulfillment of all needs/requirement/do not have to depend on any one.

The types of Old Age Homes

There are two types of Old Age Home:

- One is the "Free" type which cares for the destitute old people who have no one else to care for them. They are given shelter, food, clothing and medical care.
- The second type is the "Paid" home where care is provided for a fee. Nowadays, such "Retirement" homes have become very popular in India and they are well worth considering.
  - Services are free/at low cost
  - Food is good/wholesome food/find food suitable
  - Accommodation satisfactory
  - Good medical facility/medical care is good
  - Entertainment/library facility is good
  - Have freedom/facility to participate in religious activities
  - All services are good/good behaviour of the staff
  - Have no choice/have to be satisfied with services

SENIOR CITIZEN IN INDIA

Senior citizens are a treasure to our society. They have worked hard all these years for the development of the nation as well as the community. They possess a vast experience in different walks of life. The youth of today can gain from the experience of the senior citizens in taking the nation to greater heights. At this age of their life, they need to be taken care of and made to feel special. Indian Government provides several benefits through its schemes in various sectors of development.

With various tax benefits, travel and health care facilities provisioned for them, Indian Government has created reasons for Senior citizens to feel happy. This corner on Senior citizens is aimed at providing details on various aspects concerning them.

Constitutional Provisions

In the Constitution of India, entry 24 in list III of schedule VII deals with the Welfare of Labour, including conditions of work, provident funds, liability for workmen's compensation, invalidity and old age pension and maternity benefits. Further, Article 41 of Directive Principles of State Policy has particular relevance to Old Age Social Security.

Ministry Responsible for the Welfare of the Aged

Ministry of Social Justice and Empowerment, Under the ministry, special care is being taken for the welfare of the Aged.

Policies that facilitate the elderly

National policy on older persons

The Government of India announced a National Policy on Older Persons in January, 1999. In particular, the policy has identified a number of areas of intervention -- financial security, healthcare and nutrition, shelter, education, welfare, protection of life and property etc. for the well being of older persons in the country. Amongst others the policy also recognizes the role of the NGO sector in providing user friendly affordable services to complement the endeavors of the State in this direction.

National Council for Older Persons

A National Council for Older Persons (NCOP) has been constituted by the Ministry of Social Justice and Empowerment to operationalise the national policy on older persons. The basic objectives of the NCOP are to:

- Advice the Government on policies and programmes for older persons
- Provide feedback to the Government on the implementation of the National Policy on Older Persons as well as on specific programme initiatives for older persons
- Advocate the best interests of older persons
- Provide a nodal point at the national level for redressing the grievances of older persons which are of an individual nature
- Provide lobby for concessions, rebates and discounts for older persons both with the Government as well as with the corporate sector
- Represent the collective opinion of older persons to the Government
- Suggest steps to make old age productive and interesting
- Suggest measures to enhance the quality of inter-generational relationships.

- Undertake any other work or activity in the best interest of older persons.

Old age and Income Security

The Ministry has also launched a project called "Old Age Social and Income Security (OASIS)". An expert committee is constituted under the project. The first reports of the committee and the existing income security instruments available to older persons have been comprehensively examined. The report also contains detailed recommendations for enhancing the coverage, improving the rate of returns and for bringing about a qualitative improvement in the customer service of Public Provident Fund, the Employees Provident Fund, the Annuity Plans of LIC, and UTI etc.

Revision of the Schemes of the Ministry

In order to facilitate implementation of the National Policy, and to bring about a qualitative improvement in the programme intervention of the Ministry, both the on-going schemes were revised during 1998-99.

Scheme of assistance to Panchayati Raj Institutions/Voluntary Organizations/Self Help Groups for construction of old age homes/multi service centres for older persons. The scheme has been revised to enhance the one time construction grant for old age homes/multi service centres from Rs 5 lakh to Rs 30 lakh to eligible organizations.

An integrated programme for older persons has been formulated by revising the earlier scheme of Assistance to Voluntary Organizations for programmes relating to the welfare of the aged. With the aim to empower and improve the quality of older persons, the programmes hope to:

- Reinforce and strengthen the ability and commitment of the family to provide care to older persons.
- Foster amiable multi-generational relationships.
- Generate greater awareness on issues pertaining to older persons and enhanced measures to address these issues.
- Popularize the concept of Life Long Preparation for Old Age at the individual level as well as at the societal level.
- Facilitate productive ageing.

- Promote healthcare, Housing and Income Security needs of older persons.
- Provide care to the destitute elderly.
- Strengthen capabilities on issues pertaining to older persons of local bodies/state governments, NGOs and academic/research and other institutions.

Privileges and Benefits

Old age pension for the general public

National Old Age Pension (NOAP) Scheme

Under National Old Age Pension Scheme, Central Assistance is available on fulfillment of the following criteria:

- The age of the applicant (male or female) should be 65 years or more.
- The applicant must be a destitute in the sense that he/she has no regular means of subsistence from his/her own source of income or through financial support from family members or other sources.

The amount of old age pension is Rs 75 per month (see Table 5.6). This scheme is implemented in the State and Union Territories through Panchayats and Municipalities.

Table 5.3: Old Age Pension Amounts

Name of the State	*Current amount of pension (Rs per month)*	*Minimum age of eligibility (in years)*
Andhra Pradesh	75	65
Arunachal Pradesh	150	60
Assam	60	65 (males) 60 (females)
Bihar	100	60
Gujarat	200-275	60-65 +
Haryana	100	60
Himachal Pradesh	150	60
Jammu and Kashmir	125	60
Karnataka	100	65
Kerala	110	65

Contd...

Contd...

Name of the State	*Current amount of pension (Rs per month)*	*Minimum age of eligibility (in years)*
Madhya Pradesh	150	60 (males) 50 (females)
Maharashtra	100	65 (males) 60 (females
Mizoram	100	65 (males) 60 (females)
Orissa	100	65
Punjab	200	65 (males) 60 (females)
Rajasthan	200-300	58 (males) 55 (females)
Tamil Nadu	150	60
Uttar Pradesh	125	60
West Bengal	300	60
Chandigarh	200	65 (males) 60 (females)
Delhi	200	60

Annapurna

A new scheme called Annapurna has been recently initiated by the Government of India under which free food grains up to 10 kg per month will be provided to such destitute older persons who are otherwise eligible for old age pension under the National Old Age Pension Scheme but are not receiving it and whose sons are not residing with them. However, it is yet to be implemented.

(Ministry of Rural Development with the assistance of Ministry of Food and Civil Supplies)

Pension and Family Pension

For Central Government Employees

The revision of pension/family pension approved by the Central Government based on the 5th Pay Commission is given below:

Pension

People, who retired from service as on 1-1-96, will get their pension at 50 per cent of their basic pay. Pension of those who retired before 1-1-96 will be fixed based on 50 per cent of the minimum of the new scale applicable in place of old scale in which he/she retired. Special provision has been made for people retire before completing 10 months of service after 1 January 1999 (before 30 September 1996) and have opted to come over to the revised scales of pay are eligible weight age at 40 per cent on the existing basic pay for arriving at the average pay fixation of pension.

Family Pension

Family pension of people who retired from service as on 1-1-96 will be fixed at 30 per cent of the pay drawn by the deceased employee based on the new pension formula subject to his having put in 33 years of service. Family pension of people who retired before 1-1-96 will be fixed at 30 per cent of the pay drawn by the deceased employee based on the new pension formula subject to his having put in 33 years service.

Gratuity

- Minimum five years qualifying service and eligibility to receive service gratuity/pension is essential to get this on-time lump sum benefit.
- Retirement gratuity is calculated at the rate of one-fourth of month's basic pay plus dearness allowance last drawn before retirement for each completed six-monthly period of qualifying service.
- There is no minimum limit for the amount of gratuity.
- Maximum retirement gratuity payable is 16 1/2 times the basic pay limited to Rs. 3.5 lakhs.

(Ministry of Personnel, Public Grievances and Pensions, Department of Pension and Pensioners Welfare, New Delhi)

Taxation

- Income Tax Rebate (Section 88B of Finance Act, 1992).
- This provision provides for rebate of Income Tax to senior citizens.
- The rebate is available in the case of a resident individual (he may be an ordinary resident or a non-ordinary resident; he may be an Indian citizen or a foreign citizen) who has attained the age of 65 years at any time during the relevant previous year. From the assessment year 1998-99, tax rebate under section 88B shall be:

- the amount of income-tax before giving any rebate under sections 88, 88B and 89(1); or
- Rs 10,000 or 40 per cent, whichever is less.

The rebate will be available from the assessment year 1998-99, even if gross total income is above Rs 120,000.

(Ministry of Finance, Income Tax Act, 1961)

Deduction in respect of medical insurance premia (Sec. 80D)

An assessee is entitled to a deduction up to Rs. 15,000 with effect from the assessment year 2000-01, where the assessee or his/her spouse, or dependent parents or any member of the family is a senior citizen, (i.e. one who is at least 65 years of age at any time during the previous year), and the medical insurance premium is paid to effect or keep in force an insurance in relation to him or her.

(Ministry of Finance, Finance Bill, 1999)

Deduction in Respect of Medical Treatment (Sec. 80DDB)

Section 80DDB has been inserted to provide for a separate deduction to a resident assessee being an individual or a Hindu undivided family member for expenditure incurred for medical treatment for the individual himself or his dependent relative in respect of disease or ailments which may be specified in the rules. The deduction shall be limited to Rs 40,000. However, where the expenditure incurred is in respect of the assessee or his dependent relative or any member of a Hindu undivided family of the assessee and who is a senior citizen (one who is at least 65 years of age at any time during the previous year), a fixed deduction of Rs 60,000 will be available.

Insurance Schemes

Jeevan Dhara
Jeevan Akshay
Jeevan Suraksha
Bima Nivesh.

Senior Citizens Unit Plan (SCUP)

Senior Citizens Unit Plan is a scheme under which one has to make a one time investment depending on his/her age and have the benefit of medical treatment for self and spouse at any of the selected hospitals on completion of 58 years of age.

SCUP have special arrangements with New India Assurance Co. Ltd. (NIAC) under an exclusive medical insurance cover where by the bills from the hospitals in connection with all medical treatment by you will be settled directly by NIAC up to the prescribed limit. Age group of 18-54 years can join this Scheme. The person may be a resident or a non-resident Indian.

The person will be entitled for a medical insurance cover of Rs 2.5 lakh after he/she attains the age of 58 years. This insurance cover is available for both the citizen and his/her spouse. After the age of 61 years both of them are eligible for a cover of Rs 5 lakh after adjusting any claims made earlier.

The citizen can avail medical treatment in any of the hospitals under this Scheme. The Trust will call for all details about recent photograph, signature and address of the member and the spouse as soon as the member attains the age of 54 years so as to prepare an identity card cum log book, for the member and the spouse.

Medical Insurance Scheme

The Medical Insurance Scheme known as Mediclaim is available to persons between the age of 5 years and 75 years. Earlier, the sum insured varies from Rs 15,000 to Rs 300,000 and premium varies from Rs 175 to Rs 5,770 per person per annum depending upon the different slabs of sum insured and different age groups.

The cover provides for reimbursement of medical expenses incurred by an individual towards hospitalization/domiciliary, hospitalization for any illness, injury or disease contracted or sustained during the period of insurance.

Group Medical Insurance

Scheme The Group Mediclaim policy is available to any group/association/institution/corporate body of more than 100 persons provided it has a central administration point. The policy covers reimbursement of hospitalization and/or domicilary hospitalization expenses only for illness/diseases contracted or injury sustained by the insured person.

The basic policy under this scheme is Medi-claim only. This policy is also available to persons between the age of 5 years and 80 years. The sum insured varies from Rs 15,000 to Rs 500,000 and premium varies depending upon the different slabs of sum insured and different age groups.

Jan Arogya

Jan Arogya this scheme is primarily meant for the larger segment of the population who cannot afford the high cost of medical treatment. The limit of cover per person is Rs 5,000 per annum. The cover provides for reimbursement of medical expenses incurred by an individual towards hospitalization/domiciliary hospitalization for any illness, injury or disease contracted or sustained during the period of insurance. Age limit: 70 years.

Travel

By Road

Delhi: Fifty per cent discount on fare for travel on Delhi Transport Corporation buses to senior citizens who have attained the age of 65 years. Discount is applicable on Monthly Pass only.

(Letter No. TR/1/130/99/3568, Delhi Transport Corporation, Government of N.C.T of Delhi, dated 10-09-99)

Tamil Nadu: In Tamil Nadu Transport Corporation buses, two seats in the front exclusively for old people and handicapped.

Maharashtra: Best buses in Mumbai offer no concessions. However senior citizens can enter the bus from the front side. MSRTC (Maharashtra State Road Transport Corporation) buses provide 50 per cent concession if a person is 65 years and above and has an election identity card or a Tehsildar certificate. Local trains in Mumbai have around 8-10 seats for the senior citizens in one of the compartments.

Chandigarh: Senior citizens pass holders get 50 per cent travel concession for travelling in city buses in Chandigarh.

Punjab: Elderly women above 60 years enjoy free travel in Punjab

Rajasthan: RSRTC (Rajasthan State Road Transport Corporation) provides a concession of 25 per cent to a person of 65 years and above.

Kerala: Free passes are provided to old people who are freedom fighters to travel in fast and express buses.

By Train

Indian Railways provide 30 per cent concession in all classes and trains including Rajdhani/Shatabdi trains for citizens who have attained a minimum age of 65 years in case of men and 60 years in case of women. No certificate is required for booking but senior citizens must carry a documentary proof of their age during travel. In Tamil Nadu and West Bengal, lower berth for senior citizens is also provided on request.

By Air

Indian Airlines: Fifty per cent discount on the basic fare for travel on Indian Airlines domestic flights to senior citizens, who have attained the age of 65 years, in case of men and 63 years in case of women. Discount is applicable in economy class only.

Jet Airways: Fifty per cent discount on basic fare for travel on Jet Airways domestic flight to senior citizens who have attained the age of 65 years. Discount is applicable in economy class only.

Air Sahara: Fifty per cent discount on basic fare for travel on Air Sahara flight to senior citizens who have attained the age of 65 years. Discount is applicable in economy class only.

Special Counters

Railway Ticket Booking

Separate reservation counters are earmarked for Senior Citizens at various PRS (Passenger Reservation System) Centres, if the average demand per shift is more than 120 tickets. The position is reviewed from time to time for continuity of this facility. (Vide office memo of Government of India, Ministry of Railways (Railway Board), New Delhi, No. 96/TG-I/20/P dated 20.02.1996)

Income Tax Return

Separate counters are marked for Senior Citizens at the time of filing the income tax return. On the spot assessment: Person must 65 years or above as on 31st March of the assessment year, must be a pensioner and should come personally. (Directorate of Income Tax, Government of India)

Other Facilities

Priority is given to senior citizens while paying the electricity/ telephone bills as well as in the hospitals in Chandigarh and Haryana.

In Punjab, the Government provides priority to the senior citizens in paying the electricity/telephone bills, reservation of bus seats and separate OPD in the hospitals.

In Gujarat, all civil hospitals have separate counters for registration and separate queues for elderly.

In Delhi a separate counter has been opened to facilitate the senior citizens for submission of property tax bills.

(Vide circular No. A and C(PC)/SAU/PA(R)/IV-38/99-518 dated 24-6-99, Municipal Corporation of Delhi, Assessment and Collection Department, Special Assessment Unit)

Old Age Homes

Health Care

Sunday Clinics in Delhi

Sunday Clinics at various Hospitals of Delhi exist to enable senior citizens to get medical care easily. The aim is to provide OPD services/facilities on Sundays in the hospitals under Delhi Government so that the older patient's caregivers can also accompany them without having to take leave from their workplace.

Health Care in Maharashtra

Under District Blindness Control Scheme the state pays Rs. 600/- per IOL (Intra Ocular Lens) operation. In a few municipal hospitals there are geriatrics ward and they have OPD (out patient department) once in a week in the afternoons. They have separate queues for elderly.

Health Care in Gujarat

Free IOL (Intra Ocular Lens) is given to elderly for cataract surgery.

Health Care in Kerala

In Government Hospital, Trivandrum there is a geriatric ward having 12 beds (male -8, female - 4) and free treatment is provided to old people whose income is below Rs. 300/- per month. Medical College Hospital, Trivandrum has an Out Patient Wing on every Monday from 10.30 am to 12.00 noon for senior citizens.

Miscellaneous

Telephone

Telephone connection would be given on priority to senior citizens of age 65 years and above. They shall be entitled to registrer their demand for one telephone connection in their names. The telephones thus provided shall be transferable only in the name of spouse, if alive after death of the subscriber as a general category telephone and subsequent transfers shall be governed by prevailing telephone transfer rules.

(Vide office circular of Government of India, Ministry of Communications, Dept. of Telecommunications, New Delhi, No. 11/99 and. 1-12/99 PHA dated 05.10.1999)

Helpline

On the initiative and with the financial assistance of Ministry of Social Justice and Empowerment, Agewell Foundation, an NGO of Delhi, has started a Helpline for older persons. A centre named AADHAR is also being set up with the financial assistance of

Ministry of Social Justice and Empowerment to receive and process the representations/petitions of older persons pertaining to their various problems and to take follow up action there on.

Helpline telephone Nos. - 011-26836486, 011-26910484

[Vide letter of Government of India, Ministry of Social Justice and Empowerment (SD Section), New Delhi, F. No. 20-76/99-SD dated 03.11.1999]

Expeditious Disposal of Court Cases

The Hon'ble Chief Justice of India has advised Chief Justice of all High Courts in the country to accord priority to cases involving older persons and ensure their expededitious disposal.

[Vide letter of Government of India, Ministry of Social Justice and Empowerment (SD Section), New Delhi, F. No. 20-76/99-SD dated 03.11.1999]

Mumbai High Court has announced that it would give out-of-turn priority to hearing and disposal of petitions wherein litigants have crossed 65 years of age. The High Court decision would also be applicable to its benches at Goa, Aurangabad and Nagpur besides the subordinate courts in the State. It would extend to all the matters including civil or criminal pending in any court of law.

Mobile Medicare Unit Programme

The Mobile Medicare Unit (MMU) Programme is the only programme directly implemented by Help Age India to provide basic essential medicare at the door steps of needy and underprivileged elderly in India.

Presently Help Age India has a fleet of 20 directly controlled MMUs. These are at:

Table 5.4 HelpAge India MMUs

Lacation	*MMUs*
Delhi	2
Mumbai	2
Calcutta	2
Chennai	1

Contd...

Contd...

Lacation	*MMUs*
Bangalore	1
Hyderabad	1
Ahmedabad	1
Pune	1
Nagpur	1
Lucknow	1
Jammu	1
Faridabad	1
Chandigarh	1
Bhadohi	1
Bhubaneswar	1
Paradeep	1
Bikaner	1

Three more MMUs at Jaipur and Bhopal and Delhi-III/Gurgaon are to be launched within next two months or so and another at Coimbatore a little later. In addition, HelpAge India has provided about 80 MMUs to grass root NGOs for the similar services.

Banking

Indusind Bank Ltd. has launched a Senior Citizens Scheme - an investment option that gives you high returns with the assured security. It offers free ATM card, Telebanking, Internet banking and has 26 branches all over India. For more details visit www.ind usind.com or contact Indusind House, Dadasaheb Bhadkamkar Marg (limington Road), Mumbai - 400 004, Tel. : 91-22-385 6072/ Fax : 91-22-385 6037.

Magazines for the Elderly

There are two magazines specifically for elderly. Dignity Dialogue brought out by Dignity Foundation and Senior Heritage Selections by Heritage Medical Centre. Dignity Dialogue and Senior Heritage Selections are a refreshing social contribution and restore some balance to the otherwise distorted view society tends to have of old age.

The publications deal with a wide spectrum of issues, starting from the indignity of elder abuse to alternative medicine, to some philosophy and some inspirational material. Moreover, they provide a forum for the elderly to express their opinions and creativity.

REFERENCES

1. Bass, S.A. Gerontological Theory: The Search for the Holy Grail. The Gerontologist, 2006;46:139-44.
2. Bath, P.A. Differences between older men and woman in the Self-Rated Health/Mortality Relationship. The Gerontologist 2003; 43 387-94.
3. Charles S.T, Reynolds C.A., and Gatz M. Age-related differences and change in positive and negative affect over 23 years. Journal of Personality and Social Psychology, 2001;80:136-151.
4. Mather M, and Carstensen L. L. Ageing and motivated cognition: The positivity effect in attention and memory. Trends in Cognitive, Sciences 2005;9:496-502. PDF
5. Masoro E.J and Austad S.N (eds.). Handbook of the Biology of Ageing, Sixth Edition; Academic Press, San Diego, CA, USA, 2006. ISBN 0-12-088387-2
6. Moody, Harry R. Ageing: Concepts and Controversies. 5th ed. California: Pine Forge Press, 2006.
7. Zacks R.T, Hasher, L, and Li, K.Z.H. Human memory. In F.I.M. Craik and T.A. Salthouse (Eds.), The Handbook of Ageing and Cognition, 2000;pp. 293-357. Mahwah, NJ: Erlbaum .
8. Panek, Paul E.; Hayslip, Bert. Adult development and ageing. San Francisco: Harper and Row. ISBN 0060450126: (1989).
9. Sarah Harper. Ageing Societies: Myths, Challenges and Opportunities 2006.
10. Strawbridge WJ, Wallhagen MI, Cohen RD. Successful ageing and well-being: self-rated compared with Rowe and Kahn. Gerontologist 2002;42:6: 727-33. PMID 12451153.
11. Rowe JW, Kahn RL. Human ageing: usual and successful. Science 1987; 237 (4811):143-9. doi:10.1126/science.3299702. PMID 3299702.
12. Rowe JW, Kahn RL. Successful ageing. Gerontologist, 1997;37(4): 433-40. PMID 9279031.
13. Fentleman, DL; Smith, J and Peterson, J. Successful ageing in a post retirement society; in Baltes, Margret M; Baltes, Paul B. (1990). Successful ageing: perspectives from the behavioral sciences. Cambridge, UK: Cambridge University Press. ISBN 052143582X.
14. An Ageing Interventions Testing Program: study design and interim report. Ageing Cell. 2007 Aug;6(4):565-75. 2006;145:136-40.
15. Balcombe NR, Sinclair A. Ageing: definitions, mechanisms and the magnitude of the problem. Best Pract Res Clin Gastroenterol, 2001;15:835-49.

16. Laura H. Ageing research in the media. EMBO Rep 2005; 6: S81-S83.
17. Giacomoni PU.Ageing, science and the cosmetics industry. EMBO Rep 2005; 6:S45-S48.
18. Terman A, Brunk UT. The aging myocardium: roles of mitochondrial damage and lysosomal degradation. Heart Lung Circ 2005;14:107-14.
19. Levin DL, Buxton RB, Spiess JP, Arai T, Balouch J, Hopkins SR. Effects of age on pulmonary perfusion heterogeneity measured by magnetic resonance imaging. J.
20. Appl Physiol 2007;102:2064-70.
21. Dirks AJ, Hofer T, Marzetti E, Pahor M, Leeuwenburgh C. Mitochondrial DNA mutations, energy metabolism and apoptosis in aging muscle. Ageing Res Rev, 2006;5:179-95.
22. Goldspink DF. Ageing and activity: their effects on the functional reserve capacities of the heart and vascular smooth and skeletal muscles. Ergonomics, 2005;48:1334-51.
23. Calleja-Agius J, Muscat-BaronY, BrincatMP. Skin ageing. Menopause Int, 2007;13:60-64.
24. Newton JL. Effect of age-related changes in gastric physiology on tolerability of medications for older people. Drugs Aging ,2005;22:655-61.
25. Vaughan L, Zurlo F, Ravussin E. Aging and energy expenditure. Am J Clin Nutr, 1991;53:821-25.
26. Nusbaum MR, Lenahan P, Sadovsky R. Sexual health in aging men and women: addressing the physiologic and psychological sexual changes that occur with age. Geriatrics 2005;60:18-23.
27. Jaul E. The importance of increasing awareness of hearing and vision in the elderly population. Harefuah.
28. Schulz TJ, Zarse K, Voigt A, Urban N, Birringer M, Ristow M. "Glucose restriction extends Caenorhabditis elegans life span by inducing mitochondrial respiration and increasing oxidative stress. Cell Metab 2007;6(4):280-93. doi:10.1016/j.cmet.2007.08.011. PMID 17908557.
29. Roddy E, Zhang W, Doherty, M, Arden NK, Barlow J, Birrell F, Carr A, Et. Al. Evidence-based recommendations for the role of exercise in the management of osteoarthritis of the hip or knee- the MOVE consensus. Rheumatology, 2005; 44 67-73.
30. Conaghan PG. Update on osteoarthritis part 1: Current Concepts and the Relation to Exercise. British Journal of Sports Medicine, 2002; 36: 330-333.
31. Jyrki AK, Kujala UM. Exercise therapy for people with Rheumatoid Arthritis and Osteoarthritis. Scandinavian Journal of Medicine and Science in Sports, 2004;14:138-142.
32. Roddy E, Zhang W, Doherty M. et Al. Evidence-based recommendations for the role of exercise in the management of osteoarthritis of the hip or knee- the MOVE consensus. Rheumatology ,2005; 44: 67-73.

33. McEvoy GK, Editor. ACP's PIER: The Physicians' Information and Education Resource w/AHFS Dl Essentials (2005).
34. Wang J, Michelitsch T, Wunderlin A, Mahadeva R. Ageing as a Consequence of Misrepair -- a Novel Theory of Ageing. arXiv:0904.0575. http://arxiv.org/abs/0904.0575
35. Willis, Sherry L. Adult development and ageing. New York, NY: Harper Collins College Publishers. ISBN 0673994023: 1996.
36. Berrios GE. Dementia during the seventeenth and eighteenth centuries: a conceptual history. Psychological Medicine, November 1987;17(4):829-37. doi:10.1017/S0033291700000623. ISSN0033-2917. PMID 3324141.
37. Dementia definition. MDGuidelines. Reed Group. http://www. mdguidelines.com/dementia/definition. Retrieved 2009-06-04.
38. Gleason OC. Delirium. American Family Physician, March 2003; 67 (5): 1027-34. PMID 12643363. http://www.aafp.org/afp/20030301/1027.html. Retrieved 2009-06-04.
39. Calleo J, Stanley M. [http://www.psychiatrictimes.com/display/article/10168/1166976 Anxiety Disorders in Later Life Differentiated Diagnosis and Treatment Strategies. Psychiatric Times25 (8). http://www.psychiatrictimes.com/display/article/10168/1166976, 2008.
40. Shub, Denis; Kunik, Mark E. "Psychiatric Comorbidity in Persons With Dementia: Assessment and Treatment Strategies. Psychiatric Times, April 16, 200926 (4).http://www.psychiatrictimes.com/alzheimer-dementia/article/10168/1403050.
41. Drivers with dementia a growing problem, MDs warn, CBC News, Canada, September. 19, 2007
42. Teng EL, Chui HC. The Modified Mini-Mental State (3MS) examination. The Journal of Clinical Psychiatry, August 1987;48 (8): 314-8. ISSN 0160-6689. PMID 3611032.
43. Teng EL, Hasegawa K, Homma A, et al. The Cognitive Abilities Screening Instrument (CASI): a practical test for cross-cultural epidemiological studies of dementia. International Psychogeriatrics/IPA 6, 1994; (1): 45-58; discussion 62. doi:10.1017/S1041610294001602. PMID 8054493.
44. Royall D, Cordes, J Polk, M. CLOX: an executive clock drawing task". J Neurol Neurosurg Psychiatry, 1998; 64 (5): 588-94. doi:10.1136/jnnp.64.5.588. PMID 9598672.http://jnnp.bmj.com/cgi/content/full/64/5/588.
45. Boustani M, Peterson B, Hanson L, Harris R, and Lohr, K. Screening for dementia in primary care: a summary of the evidence for the U.S. Preventive Services Task Force". Ann Intern Med, 3 June 2003;138 (11): 927-37. PMID 12779304. http://www.annals.org/cgi/content/full/138/11/927.

46. Appendix: The Modified Mini-Mental State (3MS). http://www.cjns.org/27febtoc/predicting_appendix_.html. Retrieved 2007-09-06.
47. Cullen B, O'Neill B, Evans JJ, Coen RF, Lawlor BA. A review of screening tests for cognitive impairment. Journal of Neurology, Neurosurgery, and Psychiatry, August 2007;78(8):790-9.doi:10.1136/jnnp, 2006;095414. PMID 17178826.
48. Sager MA, Hermann BP, La Rue A, Woodard JL. Screening for dementia in community-based memory clinics (PF). WMJ : Official Publication of the State Medical Society of Wisconsin, October 2006;105 (7): 25-9. PMID 17163083. http://www.wisconsinmedicalsociety. org/_WMS/publications/wmj/issues/wmj_v105n7/sager.pdf. Retrieved 2009-06-04.
49. Fleisher A, Sowell B, Taylor C, Gamst A., Petersen R, Thal L. Clinical predictors of progression to Alzheimer disease in amnestic mild cognitive impairment. Neurology, 2007; 68(19):1588. doi:10.1212/01.wnl.0000258542.58725.4c. PMID 17287448.
50. Karlawish, J. and Clark, C. Diagnostic evaluation of elderly patients with mild memory problems. Ann Intern Med, 2003;138(5):411-9. PMID 12614094.http://www.annals.org/cgi/content/full/138/5/411.
51. Jorm AF. The Informant Questionnaire on cognitive decline in the elderly (IQCODE): a review. International Psychogeriatrics / IPA September, 2004;16 (3): 275-93.doi:10.1017/S1041610204000390. PMID 15559753.
52. Bonte FJ, Harris TS, Hynan LS, Bigio EH, White CL 3rd. Tc-99m HMPAO SPECT in the differential diagnosis of the dementias with histopathologic confirmation. Clinical Nuclear Medicine, July 2006;31 (7): 376-8. doi:10.1097/01.rlu.0000222736.81365.63. PMID 16785801.
53. Dougall NJ, Bruggink S, Ebmeier KP. Systematic review of the diagnostic accuracy of 99mTc-HMPAO-SPECT in dementia. The American Journal of Geriatric Psychiatry, Nov-December 2004;12 (6): 554-70. doi:10.1176/appi.ajgp.12.6.554. PMID 15545324.
54. An Alternative Route to Maintenance of Licensure, Manitoba Health Emergency Services, March 2001.
55. National Occupational Competency Profiles, Paramedic Association of Canada, C, June 2001 last revision.
56. Emergency Medicine, version 2.0, CD, Tintinalli, Kelen, Stapczyski, McGraw-Hill Publishing, C, 2000
57. Mosby's Paramedic Textbook, Second edition, Mick J. Saunders, Mosby Inc. C, 2000
58. Mosby's The Basic EMT, Second edition, CD, Norman E. McSwain, James L. Paturas,

59. Geriatric Education for Emergency Medical Services, American Geriatrics Society, David R. Snyder, Jones and Bartlett Publishers, C 2003
60. Emergency Treatment Guidelines, Manitoba Health Emergency Services, July 2001.
61. Bullough PG. The geometry of diarthrodial joints, its physiologic maintenance, and the possible significance of age-related changes in geometry-to-load distribution and the development of osteoarthritis. Clin Orthop Relat Res, 1981;156:61-66.
62. Buckland-Wright JC, Lynch JA, Macfarlane DG. Fractal signature analysis measures cancellous bone organisation in macroradiographs of patients with knee osteoarthritis. Ann Rheum Dis 1996; 55:749-755.
63. Burr DB. Subchondral bone. In: Brandt KD, Lomander S, Doherty M (eds). Osteoarthritis. Oxford University Press, Oxford, UK; 1998:144-156.
64. Li B, Aspden RM. Mechanical and material properties of the subchondral bone plate from the femoral head of patients with osteoarthritis or osteoporosis. Ann Rheum Dis 1997; 56:247-254.
65. Altman R, Asch E, Bloch D, Bole D, Borenstein, D Brandt K, et al. Development of criteria for the classification and reporting of osteoarthritis. Classification of osteoarthritis of the knee. *Arthritis & Rheumatism*;1986, 29, 1039-1049.
66. Altman R, Alarcon G, Appelrouth D, Bloch D, Borenstein D, Brandt K, et al. The American College of Rheumatology criteria for the classification and reporting of osteoarthritis of the hand. *Arthritis & Rheumatism*, 1990, 33, 1601-1610.

Six

Amputation Rehabilitation

An amputation is the removal, usually by surgery, of a limb or part of a limb.

The term limb difference is used for the congenital malformation of a limb or congenitally missing limbs. Amputations may involve the upper extremities, the lower extremities or both. Following amputation, most individuals will go through a period of grieving and adjustment of body image. In addition to physical and occupational rehabilitation, counseling may be involved in recovery. For major amputations (removal of a foot, leg, hand, arm, etc. as opposed to a finger or toe), individuals will usually be fitted for a prosthetic replacement soon after surgery.

There are many physiological, psychological, ADL and livelihood issues. can vary tremendously, depending on the extremities involved and whether the amputation is bilateral or not, and the type of prosthesis.

INDICATIONS FOR AMPUTATION

- **PVD** (Peripheral Vascular Disease)
  - Dysvascular Related Amputations is the leading cause (82% of limb loss)
  - Men more than women 2-3:1 and African American
  - Infections can be a complication ie. Staph, Osteomyelitis
  - Ninty seven percent of PVD account for lower limb amputations

- **Trauma** is the second leading cause of amputation
  - 68.6% are upper extremity amputations
  - MVA or gunshots
  - Leading cause in 20-30 age group
  - Men more than women 9-10:1
- **Tumor** is the third leading cause
  - Leading cause in 10-20 age groups
- **Congenital limb deformities** or absence of limb is a possible cause, but more rare.
  - *Transverse-* Limb ends at location of deficit
  - *Longitudinal-* a total or partial absence of a structure along the long axis of a segment, beyond which normal skeletal elements may exist. (ie- absence of a tibia with a normal foot)
  - *Amelia-* absence of a whole limb
  - *Apodia-* absence of a hand or foot
  - *Adactylia-*absence of fingers or toes with MC or MT
  - *Aphalangia-* absence of finger or toes
  - *Phocomelia-* *flipper* limb due to absence of a limb segment.

TYPES OF AMPUTATIONS

- Open
  - Infection remove part most infected and leave open 3-7 day, with aggressive treatment. Drain with soft dressing.
- Closed or Flap
  - Use bottom portion for flap with no evidence of infection with no drain if small

Level of Amputation – Upper Limb (see Fig 6.1)

- Forequarter : Clavicle and scapula involved
- Shoulder disarticulation
- Transhumeral (above-elbow amputation): Short, standard A/E
- Elbow disarticulation
- Transradial (below elbow amputation): Very short, short, long B/E (Fig 6.2)
- Wrist disarticulation:
- Transcarpal.

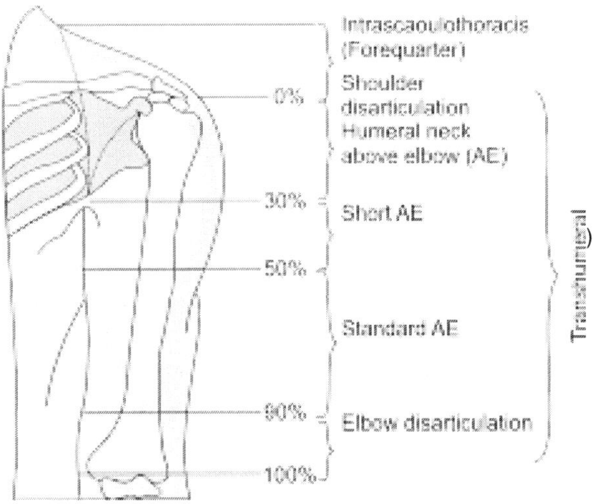

Fig. 6.1: Level of Amputation in Upper Limb (Below Elbow)

- Transmetacarpal amputation : Partial hand
- Finger amputation

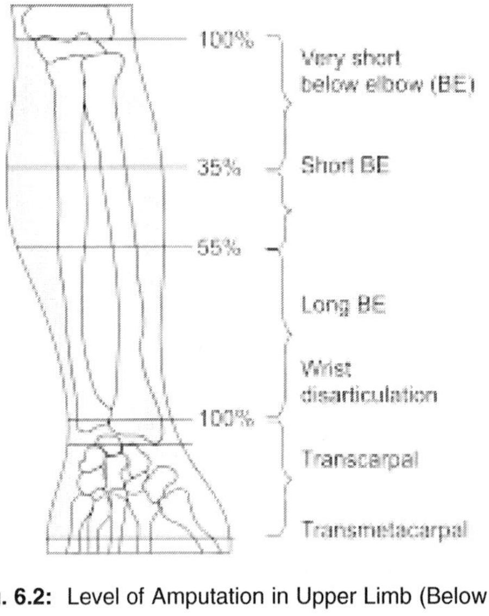

Fig. 6.2: Level of Amputation in Upper Limb (Below Elbow)

Level of Amputation – Lower Limb (see Fig 6.3)

- Knee disarticulation: Through knee joint, femur intact
- Long transfemoral: >60% femoral length
- Transfemoral: between 35-60% femoral length
- Short transfemoral: <35% femoral length
- Hip disarticulation: Through hip joint, pelvis intact
- Hemipelvectomy: resection of lower half of the pelvis
- Hemicorporectomy: Both LE and pelvis below L4-L5
- Syme's: (Named for James Symes, 1800) Ankle disarticulation with attachment of heel pad
- Long transtibial: >50% tibial length
- Transtibial: between 20-50% tibial length
- Short transtibial: <20% tibial length trauma
- Partial toe: any part of one or more toes
- Toe disarticulation: at the MP joint
- Partial foot/ray resection:3, 4,5 metatarsal and digits
- Transmetatarsal: midsection of all metatarsals
- Lisfranc-disarticulation of all metatarsals and digits
- Chopart-disarticulation at the midtarsal joint leaving calcaneus and talus.

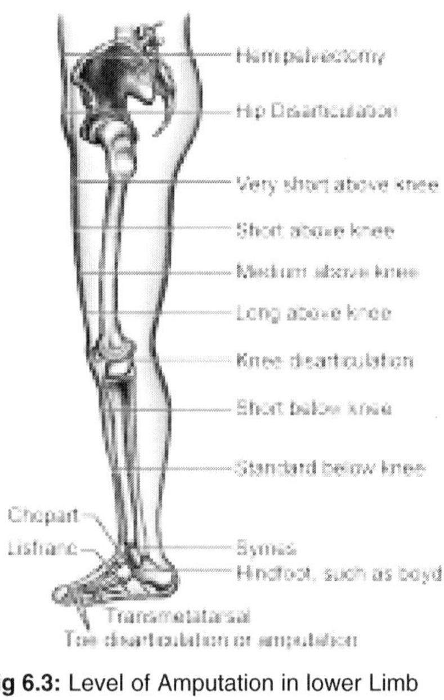

Fig 6.3: Level of Amputation in lower Limb

Surgical Management for Amputation

- Preserve as much tissue as possible
- Blood vessels and nerves are severed
- Allow to retract to reduce stump pain
- Bone beveling
- Smooth the rough edge and prevent spur development
- Muscle
- Sutured to the bones distally (myodesis)
- Close or open surgical procedure
- *Open :* Allow drainage, minimize infection
- *Close:* Reduce the days of hospitalization, but increase infection.

Special Considerations and Problems after Limb Amputation

- *Skins:* Delay healing, skin break down, stump corn
- *Stump edema:* Compression wrapping, rigid dressing
- Extensive skin graft
- Skin adhesion to the bone
- Daily gentle massage of the adhesive tissue is necessary
- Sensory problems
- Loss of sensory feedback
- Stump hypersensitive
- Neuroma
- A small ball of nerve tissue, excessive growth of axons attempting to reach the distal portion of the stump (2.5~5 cm proximal to the end of the residual limb)
- Phantom sensation, phantom pain
- Bone and joint problems
- Bone spurs formation and cause pain.

Phantom Sensation and Phantom Pain

- Most in crush injuries, in distal parts
- The neural system exists within the brain even when, the body input is cut off by amputation.
- Phantom limb sensation often never subsides and is ordinarily accepted by the patient

- Pain is experienced as more intense with stress increases
- Peripheral nerve irritation, abnormal sympathetic function, and psychological factors are thought to be contributory factors of phantom pain.

Treatment of Phantom Pain

- Avoid emphasizing the issue of pain when possible
- Severe pain
- Analgesics have been used as well as surgery such as nerve blocks and neurectomies
- Limb rubbing and tapping, ultrasound, and transcutaneous electrical nerve stimulation (TENS), acupuncture and biofeedback:
- Psychotherapy, hypnotherapy, and relaxation techniques.

Psychological Reaction to Amputation

- Shock, self-pity, suicidal impulses
- Fear for the future, anger, grief
- Depression
- Personality of the person determines the severity and duration of the reactions to amputation.

Possible Functional Issues

- Upper Extremity Amputation:
- Lifting, reaching
- Fine motor coordination
- Gross motor coordination
- Eye-hand-foot coordination
- Work tolerance (strength, holding objects)
- Writing, signing documents
- Heat tolerance.

Lower Extremity Amputation

- Walking, climbing
- Balancing
- Stooping, kneeling, crouching,

- Lifting
- Twisting
- Eye-hand-foot coordination
- Work tolerance (stamina, strength, carrying heavy objects)
- Heat tolerance.

Post-surgical Assessment

- Patient History
- Social History
- Prior level of activity/employment
- Living environment/community Access
- General health
- Health behaviors
- Medical History
- Chief complaints
- Medications
- Communication, affect, cognition, language and learning style.

Impairments

Losses or abnormalities of anatomic, physiologic, psychologic or mental structure or function.

Physical impairments

- Aerobic capacity and endurance
- Anthropometric measurements
- Circumference in cm
- Document anatomical landmarks
- Skin assessment
  - Warm
  - Cool
  - Abnormally warm.

Post-surgical Treatment Objectives

- Emotional supports, facilitate psychological adjustments
- Instruct limb hygiene, wound healing care

- Control edema and shaping of the stump
- Elastic bandage, elastic shrinker
- Removable rigid dressing
- Immediate postoperative prosthesis
- Early postoperative prosthesis
- Desensitize the residual limb
- Percussion or weight bearing
- Tapping and rubbing, applying a vibrator
- Wrapping
- Massage is useful as a desensitizing technique but is primarily used to prevent or release adhesions and soften scar tissue
- Maintain and regain ROM
- Strengthening of all remaining muscles
- Increase one hand skill, independence in ADL
- Discuss the prosthetic choice
- Demonstrate the prostheses to help the patient establish realistic expectations
- Arrange a meeting with the patient and former patient with a similar level of amputation
- Choosing a myoelectrically controlled prosthesis
- Conduct muscle site testing
- Provide visual and auditory feedback for muscle reeducation training
- Train the patient to control the intensity of the muscle contractions and relaxation, and help him to isolate the contractions of different muscle groups.

Early Postsurgical Fitting of U/E Amputees

- Within the first 30 days postsurgery
- Strong recommend for bilateral amputation
- Decrease rejection rate of U/E prosthetics
- Encourage early use of bilateral activities with prosthesis
- Control edema and accelerate stump shaping
- Prevent or reduce phantom pain
- Early prosthetic training
- Better psychological adaptation
- Higher rates of return to work

Factors of Prescribing the Prosthesis

- Patient's preferences for cosmesis and function
- Life activities at work, home, and school
- Physical attributes of the residual limb
- Length of limb, ROM, strength, and skin integrity
- Financial coverage for the prosthesis
- Third-party payment
- Patient's motivation and attitude
- Patient's cognitive abilities to learn and grasp concepts of prosthetic component controls.

REHABILITATION CONSIDERATIONS

A. Skin Care

- Patients must learn to care for their limbs once the sutures are removed. A daily hygiene routine with mild soap and tap water is usual. The stump needs to be dried completely before any shrinkage devices are applied to prevent skin problems.
- Gentle massage to the residual limb helps to decrease sensitivity and increases tolerance to pressures.
- Any open area should be aired for short periods daily (e.g., one hour four times per day), or as ordered by physician. To protect open areas or sutures, Telfa pads are used under the shrinkage device.

B. Positioning

- Positioning is an essential part of patient's program as it assists in the prevention of adaptive shortening of soft tissue as well as prevention of joint contractor. It must be consistently stressed to the amputee the recommended postures and exercises that they should do to maintain the residual limb fully mobile.
- Use of a pillow under the hip or knee of the residual limb is not recommended for it develops flexion contractors.

C. Residual Limb Shrinkage

- When the residual limb has started to heal, bandaging is important to prevent swelling and ensure that the residual limb is properly shaped. A cylindrical shaped residual limb is easier to fit with a prosthesis and therefore is desirable. The limb is usually rewrapped every three to four hours in order to allow the residual limb to be exposed to fresh air and to adjust the bandage's tension.

- PostsurgicalDressings:
  Just after surgery any or all of three basic types of dressings may be used.

  Rigid Dressing: As per physician order many patients are fitted with a rigid dressing (cast) to ensure control of swelling and to provide comfort. The end of the cast is made to take a simple training prosthesis (usually called a "pylon") so training in standing and walking can be started immediately.

  Ace Wrap: Wrapping with an elastic bandage is still the most frequently used shrinkage method. Careful patient and family instruction is necessary because poor wrapping leads to skin problems and a poorly shaped residual limb. With any patient who fails to learn the technique, who has visual or sensory deficits, or who lacks the use of one upper extremity, and alternative shrinkage method needs to be provided.

  JOBST Compression Pump: These air-filled sleeves place constant, equal pressure on all sides of the residual limb to shrink it rapidly and to shape it appropriately.

  Residual Limb Shrinkers:

  a. Shrinker socks are usually used after the final prosthesis is made and adjusted. Residual limb shrinkers are frequently worn at night as well as during the day when the patient is not wearing the prosthesis.
  b. A series of gradually smaller sizes will be employed to encourage consistent, even shrinkage. Shrinkage and shaping of the residual limb take about six weeks to three months, depending on the patient's response and condition.

D. Prosthetic Fitting

- When the residual limb has healed and is relatively stable in size and shape, the patient will be measured for a prosthesis, as ordered by the surgeon. The first fitting is for a Temporary Prosthesis", about six weeks after the amputation, barring no complications. This prosthesis will be used through the interim shaping period (3 to 6 months post surgery).

REHABILITATION GOALS

- Phase I: Acute Hospital
- Phase Ii: Inpatient Rehab.

PRE-PROSTHETIC PROGRAM

Goals

- To gain the ability, safety and independence to perform Activities of Daily Living (ADL's).
- To achieve maximum independence with bed mobility activities to prevent bed-rest hazards (e.g. thrombophlebitis, pulmonary embolism, decubitus ulcer, pneumonia).
- To achieve independence for proper care of the residual limb.
- To gain full range of motion in all joints to prevent contractures.
- To gain flexibility of major muscle groups.
- To gain functional strength of all muscle groups on both lower extremities to prevent significant muscle weakness that will have implications for prosthetic prescription, prosthetic fitting, and prosthetic training.
- To gain upper extremities/upper body (trunk) strengthening to facilitate mobility, transfers and walking.
- To educate on residual limb sensory expectations i.e., phantom sensation and phantom pain.
- To teach independent and safe transfers to all surfaces.
- To train patient for functional walking with assistive device as appropriate.
- To maximize endurance and cardiopulmonary fitness.
- To maximize independence in wheelchair mobility skills and wheelchair parts management.
- To ensure optimal residual limb shrinkage and shaping in preparation for prosthetic fitting.

- To educate patient and family as needed to ensure independence and safety. Providing written instructions for positioning, stump wrapping and specific home exercise programs.
- To assess equipment needs prior to discharge.
- To ensure patient's safety at discharge. Home Evaluation as appropriate.
- To make arrangements for outpatient physiotherapy or occupational therapy as needed or assist with other arrangements as per patient's needs.
- To help amputees regain their normal functional independence so they can return to their home, to their work, and to their place in the community participating in the activities that are important to them.
- To assist the patient in understanding phantom sensation and pain.
- To administer prescribed analgesics to reduce pain
- To encourage the patient and family to express and examine feelings about body changes.
- To instruct and assist the patient in ways of enhancing his or her appearance.
- To support the patient during the grieving process related to changes in the body.

AMPUTEES TREATMENT PROTOCOL

I. PHASE ONE (ACUTE CARE HOSPITAL)

A. Post-Operative Day 1 - 10

Activities

- Begin bed mobility skills
- Begin training on Activities of Daily Living
- Begin transfers training
- Start education on positioning to prevent contractures
- Begin education on Active Range of Motion Exercises to upper and lower extremities.

II. PHASE TWO (INPATIENT REHABILITATION PRE-PROSTHETIC TRAINING)

A. Nursing Focus

Activities

1. Skin Care for the other limbs and areas at risk for breakdown.
2. Nutrition which promotes healing and prevention of further breakdown.
3. Patient education about causative disease processes such as:
   - Diabetic Daily Self-Management skills including:
     a. Administration of insulin and other anti-diabetic agents
     b. Self-blood glucose monitoring
     c. Diabetic emergencies
     d. Foot/nail care practices
     e. Managing blood sugar how-to's
     f. Chronic complications prevention/management
   - Peripheral Vascular Disease
     a. Detection and response to emergencies
     b. Use of medications
     c. Positioning and prevention of vascular constriction/occlusion
   - Pain Management Modalities
   - Psychological Impact of Amputation
     a. Emotional Support during the grieving process
     b. Self-Esteem and Body Image Disturbances
     c. Practical suggestions about dressing and improved appearance.

B. Functional Activities

- Activities of Daily Living Training.
- Bed mobility skills training.
- Transfers training to all surfaces: bed, wheelchair, mat, toilet, tub, shower, upholstered sofa or chair, car, floor as indicated.
- Positioning techniques and education to patient and family to prevent contractures on the residual limb as well as on the uninvolved extremities. (Proper positioning in sitting, supine, prone and standing.) (see Fig 6.4)

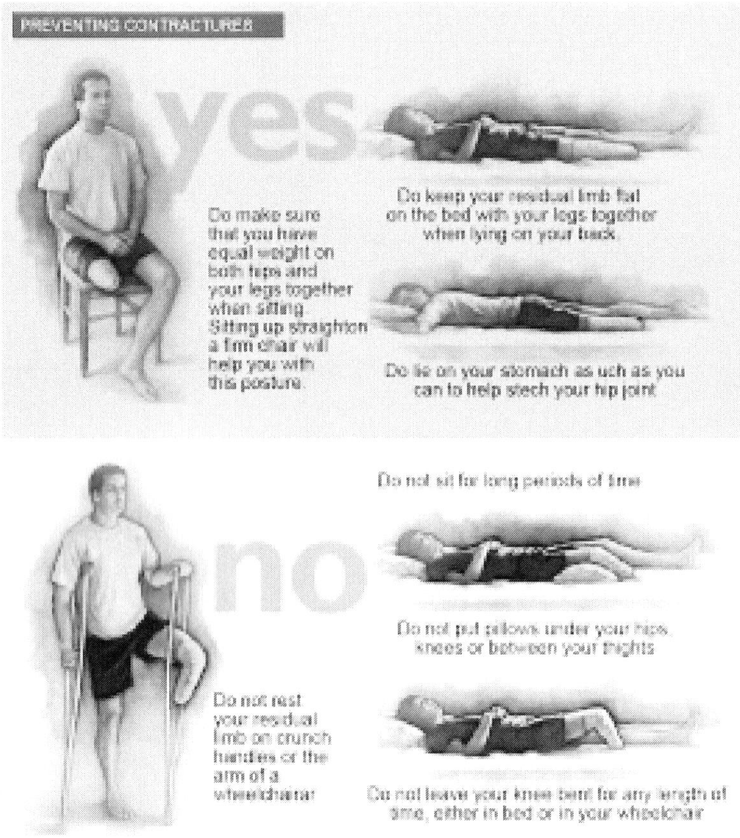

Fig. 6.4: Do's and Don'ts in Amputees

- Education on care of the residual limb including desensitizing techniques, awareness of appropriate skin integrity to prevent skin breakdown and residual limb wrapping.
- Education on stump sensory expectations (phantom sensation/ phantom pain)
- Pressure Relief Techniques training.
- Wheelchair mobility/training including propulsion on different surfaces indoors/outdoors, maneuvering wheelchair in narrow/ small places and safe management of wheelchair parts and maintenance.

- Sitting and standing balance training.
- Endurance training in sitting and standing.
- Gait training with assistive device as applicable (Include safety issues and safety awareness to prevent falls as possible).

C. Range of Motion Therapeutic Exercises

Activities

- Upper Extremities (working on all planes and all joints).
- Lower Extremities (working on the residual limb and uninvolved leg on all planes and all joints).

D. Strengthening Therapeutic Exercises

Activities

- Upper Extremities (to achieve maximum strength for transfers and use of a walker or crutches).
- Lower Extremities (to achieve maximum strength possible in all muscle groups of the residual limb and the uninvolved lower extremity).
- Upper body strengthening to improve trunk stability to facilitate transfers and walking.

E. Patient and Family Education

Provided within instructions for appropriate care of the residual limb, positioning and patient's Home Exercise Program. Addressing psychosocial issues.

F. Home Safety Evaluation as applied

G. Order patient's equipment as indicated

H. Follow-up Recommendations

If the patient is unable to perform functional activities safely and independently outpatient rehabilitation is highly recommended.

III. PHASE THREE (OUTPATIENT REHABILITATION)

A. Pre-prosthetic Training: (Post-Operative Week 4-6)

Recommended for patients who have been discharged from Inpatient Rehabilitation, but still need more therapy "to achieve maximum independence and safety" with transfers and functional ambulation activities without the prosthesis. To maximize balance, endurance and strength of upper body and all four extremities.

B. Prosthetic Training

Time for prosthetic training varies depending on patient's status, healing of the residual limb and surgeon's orders.Frequency of Therapy-therapy will be administered in a clinic model with the following team members:

- Patient
- Family
- Physiatrist
- Prosthetist
- Physiotherapist
- Occupational Therapist
- Case Manager (consult as needed)
- Occupational Therapy per physician's orders for patients with upper extremities amputations.

C. Prosthetic Training:

- Prosthetic checkout of the Below Knee Prosthesis Therapy for prosthetic training: includes:
  - Fitting of prosthesis.
  - Education to patient on appropriate use of prosthetic socks.
  - Education on skin care (awareness of appropriate pressure points and gradual increased use of prosthesis).
  - Education/training for proper independence in application and removal of prosthesis.
  - Activities of Daily Living Skills with the prosthesis. (Donning and Doffing of prosthesis).

- Educate patient on proper care of prosthesis and prosthetic socks. Teach inspection of socket for: cracks, missing rivets, cracked bumpers.
- Transfers training to all surfaces wearing the prosthesis. (Transfers to the toilet, to the bed, to regular furniture, to the car and to the floor).
- Balance training with prosthesis.
- Gait training with prosthesis. (Evaluate for appropriate assistive device) Indoors/Outdoors.
  - Educate on appropriate prosthetic component control
  - Training on all surfaces (smooth to rough and uneven)
  - Ambulation and maneuvering in narrow places.
  - Training on: Stairs, ramps, curbs, elevators, escalators
  - Training on ability to "fall safely", if indicated
  - Reevaluate ambulation skills periodically and "upgrade" assistive device as applicable
- Family training as necessary/Include education on skin (stump) care, prosthesis care and Home Exercise Program.
- Home/work place evaluation as applicable.
- Driving evaluation and referral for training as appropriate.

Seven

Prosthetics and Orthotics

In a simple language a prosthesis is an artificial substitute for a missing body part.

> ***Prosthesis** (see Fig. 7.1) is a device or an artificial substitute designed to replace, as much as possible, the function or appearance of a missing limb or body part.*
>
> ***Orthosis** is a device designed to supplement or augment the function of an existing limb or body part.*

Prosthesis is often also referred to as a prosthetic device. Similarly, an orthosis is often referred to as an orthotic device.

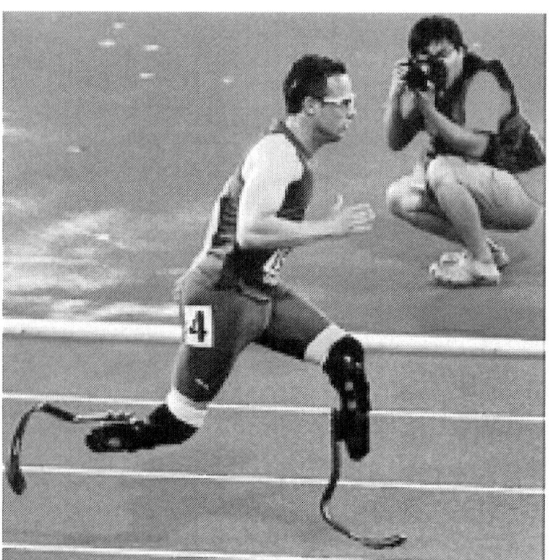

Fig. 7.1: All Athelete with lower limb prosthesis

PRINCIPLES IN PROSTHETICS

Objectives

- To transfer body weight comfortably to the prosthetic socket.
- To achieve alignment stability.
- To stimulate normal locomotion.

The prosthesis should have following features:
- Durable, comfortable, easy for patients to use and maintain
- Easy for technicians to learn, use and repair
- Standardized but compatible with the climate in different regions of the world
- Low-cost but modern and consistent with internationally accepted standards
- Easily available.

DIFFERENT TYPES OF PROSTHESIS

- Cosmetic Prosthesis
- Body powered Prosthesis
- Externally powered Prosthesis
- Hybrid Prosthesis.

Important Points to be Considered in Choosing Prosthesis.

- Amputation level
- Expected function of the prosthesis
- Cognitive function of the patient
- Patient's vocation (desk job vs. manual laborer)
- Patient's avocational interests (i.e., hobbies)
- Cosmetic importance of the prosthesis
- Patient's financial resources (e.g., medical insurance, worker's compensation).

Prosthesis Care

Prosthesis is a mechanical device and as such requires regular maintenance and care. If there is any unusual sign (visible, audible or functional) it should be inspected by a prosthetist as soon as possible. The prosthesis is designed for use in normal conditions and environments.

It has not been designed for use in:

- Wet environments
- Activities that will include unusually high impacts
- Chemical environments that may alter the structural integrity of the prosthesis.

The Socket

For optimum function of the prosthesis, daily cleaning of the interior of the socket is required. Clean with a sponge or soft cloth and a little mild soap. Inaccessible points can be reached with an old toothbrush. Push toweling in to dry inside. Leave to dry thoroughly overnight. Clean the exterior in a similar way when necessary.

Limb Socks

Are indicated for protection of the skin, for greater comfort and to absorb perspiration. Change daily and wash by hand with mild soap (not deter gent) and water. Any soap left in the sock may irritate the skin. The sock must fit snugly, without wrinkles, to avoid pressure points on the residual limb.

Silicone Socks/ Liners

Avoid contact with ball point pens, newsprint; vegetable dyes etc which will leave a permanent stain. Follow manufacturers' instructions for cleaning (this differs for manufacturers). If the silicone liner is of the type that has an attachment or locking mechanism at the bottom or distal end, regularly inspect attachment points for signs of wear and tear.

Leather Parts

Keep clean and dry. Use saddle soap to clean any leather parts.

Webbing

Wash straps with soap and warm water.

Valves in Suction Socket

Clean the base of the valve and the opening into the socket with a soft brush to remove any accumulation of powder or other substance. The valve is very important to the functioning of the prosthesis particularly, if it is the only mechanism providing the suspension of the prosthesis. The valve may function incorrectly if it fills with talc or other substances. It needs to always be secured properly in its outer housing and if it has a button, this should work positively. Prosthetist should show you how to check that valve is secured properly, how it can be cleaned and what is acceptable in terms of air leaking through the valve.

Mechanical Parts/Components

1. A frequent maintenance check-up with prosthetist is essential for maintenance and optimal function.
2. Do not adjust screws, hinges or other parts of prosthesis.
3. Any excessive noise or grating during use should be reported to prosthetist.
4. Any dust (often black) should be reported to prosthetist.
5. Where prosthesis is fitted with a hydraulic knee joint, store in upright position only.

Prosthetic Wrist Units

- Wrist units are used for attaching terminal devices to prostheses as well as providing pronation and supination to place the terminal device in its proper position.
- The rotation function is passive; the amputee rotates the terminal device in the wrist unit with his sound hand or by pushing against a part of the body or other surface to produce either pronation or supination. The wrist unit also permits interchange of the terminal devices.
- Two types of wrists: friction or locking
  - Friction wrists permit pronation and supination of the terminal device and hold it in a selected position by means of friction derived from a compressed rubber washer or from forces applied to the stud of the terminal device.

- Locking wrists permit manual rotation and then lock the terminal device in its fixed position.
- *Advantage:* The locking mechanism prevents inadvertent rotation of the TD in the wrist unit when a heavy object is grasped.

- Two types of wrist-flexion units are also available: add-on and combination
  - Add-on is worn between the wrist and the terminal device and allows manual positioning of the terminal device in either the straight or the flexed position.
  - Combination type combines a friction wrist and a wrist-flexion component in one and provides for setting and locking in one position.
  - Electric wrist rotator units are also available and are generally considered for bilateral upper-extremity amputees.

Transradial / Below-Elbow (BE) Amputation Prostheses

In addition to the components discussed above, a transradial amputee needs a socket, elbow-hinge, an upper arm cuff, and a harness and control system (see Fig. 7.2).

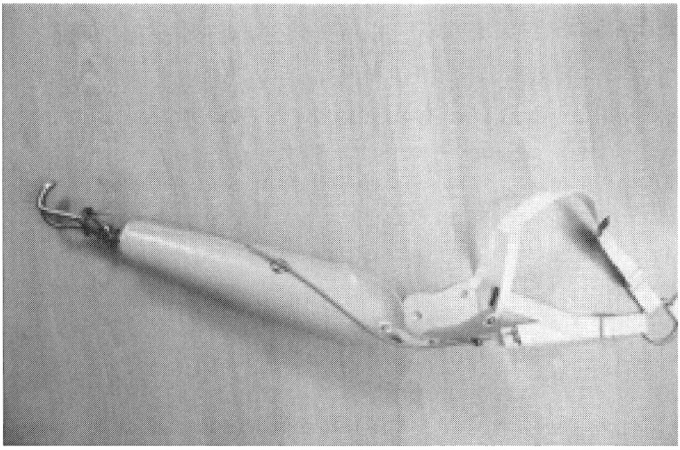

Fig. 7.2: Transradial / Below-Elbow (BE) Amputation Prostheses

BE Sockets

- The socket must provide a comfortable but stable, total contact interface with the residual limb (avoiding inadvertent motion and precluding uncomfortable concentrations of pressure), efficient energy transfer from the residual limb to the prosthetic device, secure suspension and adequate appearance.
- To accomplish these goals, most sockets are double walled with the inner wall giving total contact fit and the outer wall matching the contour and the length of the contra lateral forearm.
- Proximally, the socket extends posteriorly to the olecranon and anteriorly to the elbow crease. The shorter the residual limb, the closer is the trimline to the crease.

Split Socket

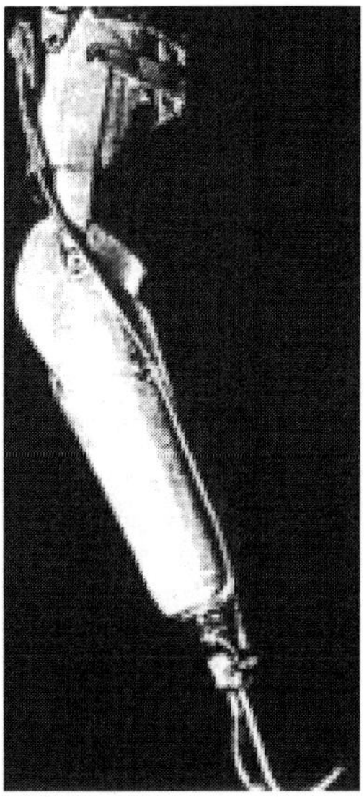

Fig. 7.3: Split socket

Split socket consists of a total-contact segment encasing the residual limb and connected by hinges to a separate forearm shell to which the wrist unit and the terminal device are attached. It is sometimes used in patients who have very short stumps, so that the special elbow hinges can be used to increase available joint range of motion or to incorporate an elbow-lock mechanism in the prosthesis.

Muenster Socket (self-suspended socket)

- An alternative to the split socket (for short transradial amputees) is the Muenster-type socket design (see Fig. 7.4). In this, the socket and forearm are set in a position of initial flexion and the socket encloses the olecranon and the epicondyle of the humerus. The intimate stump encapsulation, flexion attitude, and high trimlines provide excellent retention and security. Although there is some limitation in the range of flexion-extension this may be compensated by preflexing.

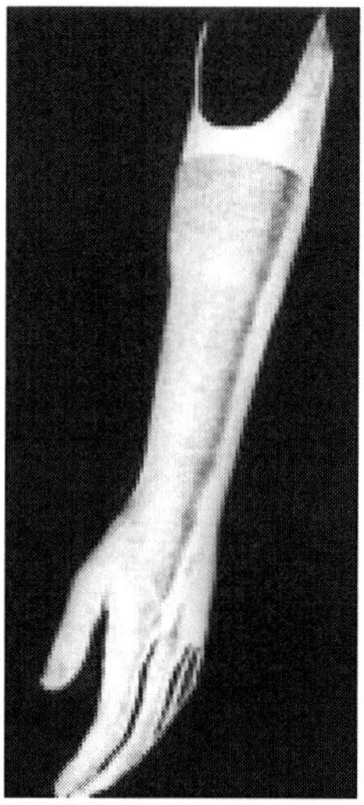

Fig. 7.4: Muenster-type socket

- When this type of suspension is used, a figure nine harness can be used for control purposes only.
- With these prostheses the patient can operate his terminal device in common positions and still apply full torque about the elbow. Although these techniques yield less elbow flexion than the split socket, the reduction in force requirements and the ease of use more than compensate for this limitation.
- Northwestern University socket is another example of a self-suspended socket design.

Elbow Hinges

Transradial amputation prosthesis hinges connect the socket to a cuff on the upper arm and are important for suspension and stability.

Types

1. Flexible elbow hinge:
   - Used primarily to suspend the forearm socket
   - Permits active pronation and supination of the forearm
   - Used where sufficient voluntary pronation and supination are available to make it desirable to maintain these functions: wrist-disarticulations and long transradial amputations
2. Rigid elbow hinge:
   - Used in short transradial amputations when normal elbow flexion is present but there is no voluntary pronation-supination and more stability is needed.
   - Types:
     - single axis
     - polycentric
     - Step-up design-used with split-socket prosthesis, in very short transradial amputation where flexion is limited. By virtue of a gear or double-pivot arrangement, these hinges permit the stump to drive the prosthetic forearm through an increased range of motion. Disadvantage is that it takes twice the force (energy cost doubles) to provide the same amount of flexion than is the case with no step-up design.
3. Residual limb-activated locking elbow.

Cuffs and Pads

Except in the Muenster socket, a half-cuff or a triceps pad, with appropriate elbow hinge, is used on the upper arm to connect the socket to the harness and help furnish socket suspension and stability. It also serves as an anchor for the cable control action point. The half-cuff is used in the majority of short transradial fittings. The triceps pad is used with long trans-radial, wrist-disarticulation, and transmetacarpal prostheses.

Transradial Harness Suspension and Control Systems

- The functions of the below-elbow harness: to suspend prosthesis from the shoulder so the socket is held firmly on the residual limb, utilize body motions as sources of power or force, and transmit this force via a cable system to operate the terminal device.
- Three types:
  - Figure-eight (see Fig. 7.5)
  - Figure-nine
  - Chest-strap with shoulder saddle.
- **Figure-eight** (O-ring harness)
  - Most commonly used harness. The axilla loop, worn on the sound side, acts as a reaction point for the transmission of body force to the terminal device.

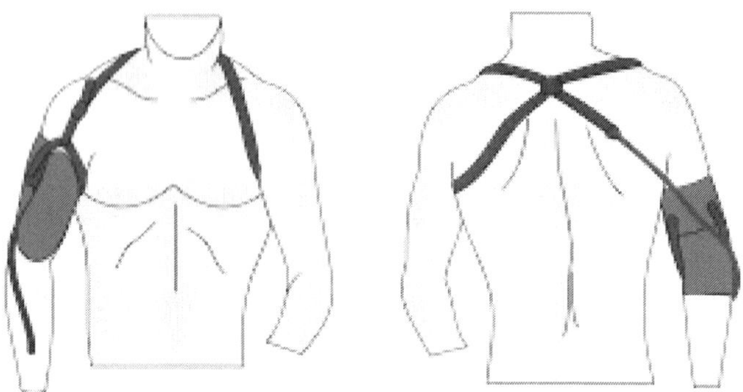

Fig. 7.5: Figure-Eight harness

- **Figure-nine**
  - Figure-nine harness is often employed with a self-suspended transradial socket (e.g., Muenster socket) that requires a harness only for controlling the TD
  - Consists of an axilla loop and a control attachment strap
  - Pros: is lighter and provides a greater freedom and comfort by the elimination of the usual front support strap and triceps pad or cuff.
- **Chest-strap with shoulder saddle**
  - Chest-strap with shoulder saddle is used if the patient cannot tolerate the axilla loop. Also used with those who will be doing heavy lifting.

Transhumeral/Above-Elbow (AE) Prostheses

- Transhumeral prostheses (see Fig. 7.6) consist of a terminal device, wrist unit, forearm, elbow unit, an upper arm, a socket, and a harness and control-cable system.
- The terminal devices and wrist units are the same as those used for the transradial prostheses, but the sockets, elbow unit, and harness and control systems differ in several respects from those used in the transradial prostheses.

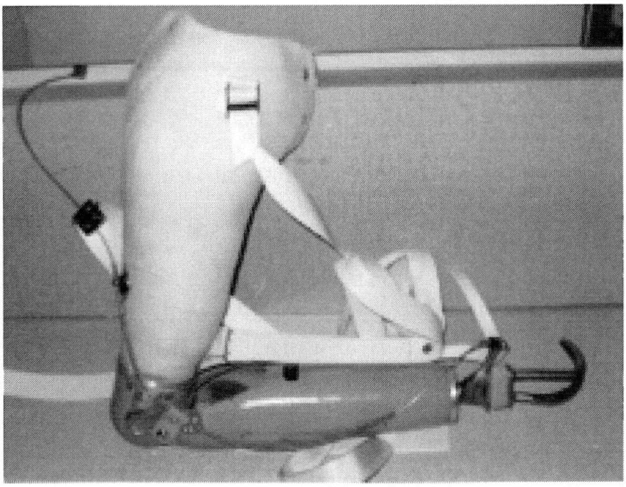

Fig. 7.6: Transhumeral prostheses

AE Sockets

As in transradial prostheses, the transhumeral socket is usually of double-wall construction, with the inner wall providing a snug, total contact fit and the outer shell providing appropriate length and shape. The lateral socket wall extends to the acromion and the medial socket wall is flattened below the axilla to help prevent inadvertent socket rotation.

Elbow Units

- When an amputation occurs at or above the elbow joint, elbow function is supplied by the use of an elbow unit, which provides for elbow flexion and for locking in various degrees of flexion.

- Elbow-locking systems are divided into two types:
  - External (outside) locking elbow
  - Internal locking elbow.
- The former is used with elbow-disarticulations because there is not enough space for the internal locking mechanism, and the latter is used with transhumeral and shoulder prostheses
  - Internal elbow joint.
- Preferred because of greater mechanical durability
- Used in level of amputation 4 cm or more proximal to the level of the epicondyles.

External Elbow Joint

- Used when the residual limb extends more distally than 4 cm to the level of the epicondyles to maintain the elbow joint center equal to that in the nonamputated side.
- Both types of elbows are flexed by means of the control cable of the dual-control system and locked at the desired flexion angle by a separate elbow-lock control cable, which is attached at one end to the elbow mechanism and at the other end to the harness
- The lock mechanism operates on the alternator principle, that is, locking and unlocking actions alternate with each control-cable cycle of tension and relaxation.
- For amputees who have difficulty flexing their prosthetic forearm, an accessory in the form of a spring-assist for elbow flexion may be provided for the use with the internal elbow.
- In transhumeral and shoulder prostheses, passive humeral rotation is accomplished by means of a turntable between the elbow unit and the upper arm shell or socket. As in the case of a wrist unit, friction between the elbow unit and the turntable permits control of the rotation to maintain the desired plane of elbow operation.

Shoulder Prostheses

- All shoulder prostheses consist of a terminal device, a wrist unit, a forearm section, an elbow unit, humeral and shoulder sections, and a harness and cable-control system.

- The terminal device, wrist unit, forearm section, and elbow unit are identical to those used in the transhumeral prosthesis
- The shoulder section includes a socket, which provides:
  - A comfortable, stable bearing on the residual shoulder elements and thorax, and
  - A means of utilizing whatever mobility remains in the shoulder girdle for control of the prosthesis
- Several components are available for the socket allowing ROM.

Prosthesis Prescription and Component Parts by Site at Amputation

Partial Foot Amputations

- Small-toe amputations do not affect ambulation and usually require no replacement
- Partial foot prostheses are used to restore foot function (particularly walking) and forefoot contour.
- Amputation of the great toe reduces push-off force, thus requiring resilient toe filler and also a molded insole with arch support to maintain the alignment of the amputated foot.
- Partial foot amputations involving the forefoot, such as ray resections and trans-metatarsal amputations generally require only shoe fillers or shoe modifications. The shoe modifications required may include a stiff sole, the addition of a spring steel shank extending to the metatarsal heads, a rocker sole and/or padding of the tongue of the shoe to help hold the hind foot firmly in the shoe.
- Transtarsal amputations, such as Chopart, Lisfranc, and Boyd, are not the most desirable levels of elective amputation, but they will have better functional results if there is an active balanced dorsiflexion and plantar flexion with normal skin and heel pad present. The best prosthetic option for a hindfoot amputation is the use of a custom prosthetic foot with a self-suspending split socket, which allows a regular low quarter shoe to be worn. A posterior leaf spring ankle-foot orthosis is another alternative.

Syme Amputation

- In the Syme amputation, preservation of the articular cartilage covered by the heel pad allows direct end bearing on this residual limb.
- The patient can stand easily and walk on the end of the residual limb without wearing a prosthesis for short household distances.
- Prosthesis: Canadian Syme socket (either posterior or medial opening).
  - Both require removal of a portion of the socket wall to get bulbous stump in
  - Major disadvantage: poor cosmesis.
- Newer socket designs that incorporate an expandable air suspension chamber inside the socket or a thin removable expandable inner socket liner provide a more cosmetically acceptable prosthetic design.
  - Pros: thinner, tighter, and stronger prosthetic socket (there is no need to remove a section from the socket wall maintaining the structural integrity of the prosthesis).
- Prosthetic feet available: for Syme's Amputation
  - Syme solid ankle cushion heel (SACH)
  - Syme SAFE (stationary ankle flexible endoskeleton)
  - Seattle Syme foot
  - Syme flex foot
  - Carbon copy Syme foot
  - No STEN (stored energy) available for Syme's amputees.

Transtibial (TT) Amputation/Below the Knee Amputation

- The components in BKA prosthesis include the socket, the shank, the suspension, and the prosthetic foot.

Socket for BKA

- **Patellar tendon bearing (PTB) socket**
  - The standard socket used for the average below-the-knee amputee is the total contact patellar tendon bearing (PTB) socket.

- PTB socket is (see Fig. 7.7 and Fig. 7.8) a custom-molded plastic socket that distributes weight through convex buildups (bulges) over pressure-tolerant areas; it provides concavities (relief areas) on pressure-sensitive areas.
- Characterized by bar in anterior wall designed to apply pressure on patellar tendon.
- The trimline extends anteriorly to the midpatellar level, may extend medially and laterally to the femoral condyles, and extends posteriorly to below the level of the PTB bar.
- Despite name, pressure should be equally distributed over pressure-tolerant areas, with more weight bearing in the area of the patellar tendon and the tibial flare and reduced weight bearing over the bony prominences, such as the tibial crest, distal end of the tibia, and head of the fibula.

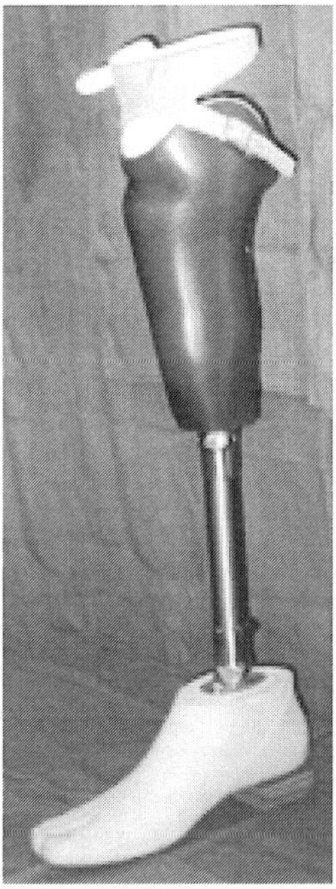

Fig. 7.7: Patellar tendon bearing (PTB) socket

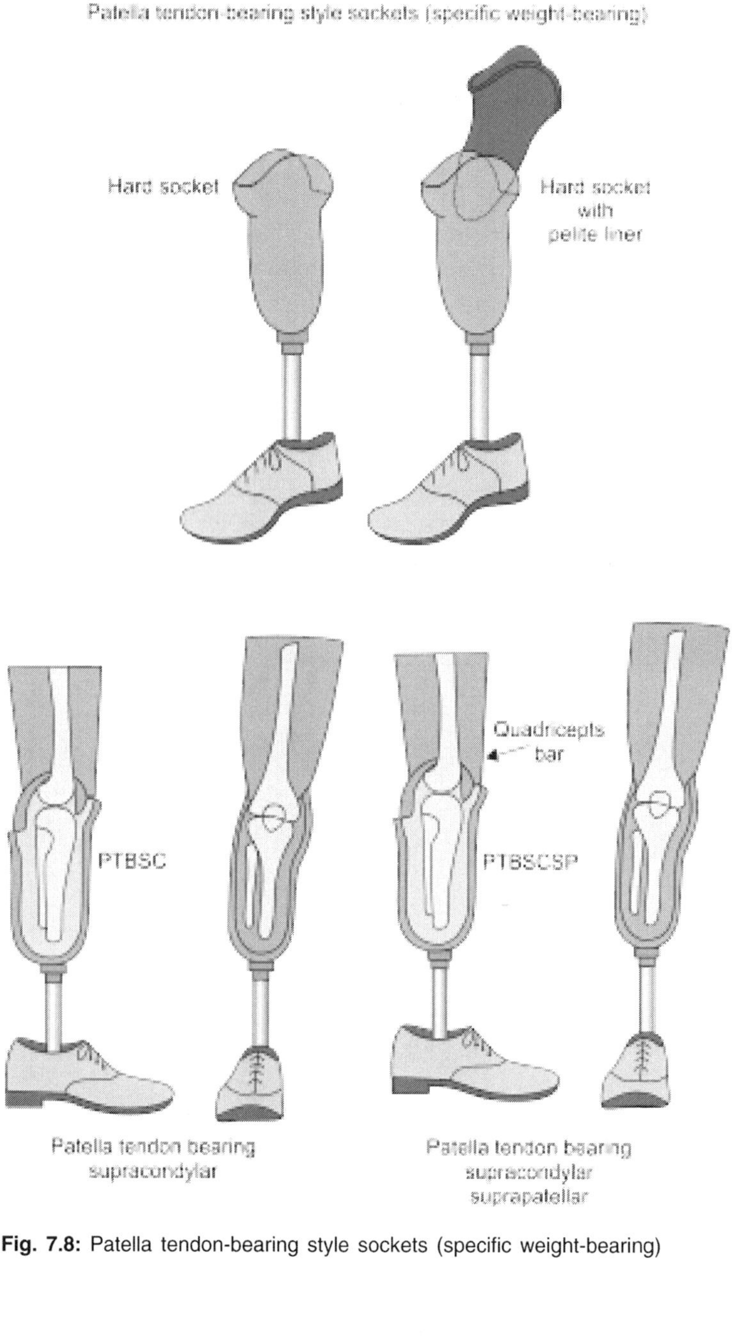

Fig. 7.8: Patella tendon-bearing style sockets (specific weight-bearing)

Some Commonly Used Suspension Systems for BKA

- Supracondylar cuff suspension socket
- Brim suspension
- Rubber or neoprene sleeve
- Silicone suction suspension
- Thigh corset.

Prosthetic Feet

1. *Solid ankle cushioned-heel (SACH) (see Fig. 7.9) foot*–most commonly used prosthetic foot.

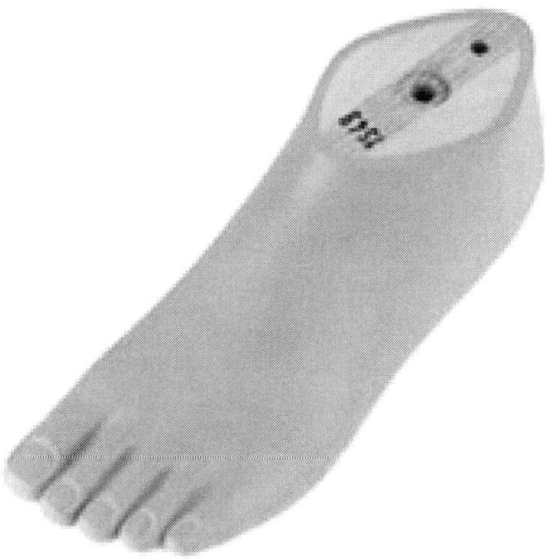

Fig. 7.9: SACH foot

   a. Durable, lightweight, inexpensive, and easily interchanged to accommodate shoes of different heel height
   b. Compressible heel and wooden keel in this design allow it to simulate the motions of the ankle in normal walking without actual ankle movement occurring
   c. Accommodates partially for uneven terrain, but this foot is best suited for flat, level surfaces.
2. *Single axis foot*–permits movement of the foot ankle complex in one plane.

a. Movement occurs in the plantar flexion dorsiflexion axis. The movement is controlled by the use of adjustable internal rubber bumpers that provide resistance to dorsiflexion and plantar flexion.
b. This foot is heavier than the SACH foot, and the internal components need periodic adjustment or replacement.
c. Typically used for more proximal amputations that requires additional knee control or stability. Can relieve pressure on distal tibia for BKA.

3. *Multi-axis prosthetic foot*–for the amputee who is involved in athletic activities or who walks on uneven terrain
   a. Some controlled movement in the normal anatomic planes of the ankle dorsiflexion, plantar flexion, inversion, eversion, and rotation
   b. A number of different foot designs are available to provide this motion
   c. Some of the feet accomplish this movement without the use of mechanically moving parts. They rely on the inherent flexibility of the materials and design of the foot. Other multi-axis feet use mechanical systems
   d. The additional mechanical components necessary for the movement of these feet add to their overall weight and may require frequent maintenance, especially in the very active amputee
   e. For the active amputee, however, the improved balance, coordination, and function provided by these feet outweigh the disadvantages of increased weight and more frequent maintenance.
4. *Flexible keel prosthetic foot*
5. *Energy storing/dynamic response prosthetic foot*
   - Major advances in lower-extremity component design continue in the development in dynamic-response prosthetic feet such as the Flex foot, the spring-light foot, Seattle foot, Endolite foot, and the Carbon copy II and III feet. The design of these feet incorporates the use of resilient, flexible, energy-storing materials. Energy is stored in the foot at the time of heel strike, as the weight of the body compresses or flexes the resilient

material within the foot and is returned to the amputee at the time of push off. Resiliency of these feet makes them particularly suitable for amputees involved in activities that require running and jumping. Many amputees report they believe they are more functional with prosthesis with a dynamic response foot. It has been assumed, thus, that these prosthetic designs make ambulation more efficient and require less energy consumption. The flex foot and spring-light foot have the added advantages of reducing energy expenditure because they are lightweight.

6. *Jaipur foot*
   - Jaipur foot (see Fig. 7.10 and Fig. 7.11) is an improved version of a conventional SACH (Solid Ankle Cushion Heel) foot rather to say a dynamic foot with shorter/flexible keel. It is basically a soft multi axial foot, meaning that it is flexible along multiple axes. The greatest advantage of Jaipur foot over SACH foot is that it allows all natural movement of the foot including dorsiflexion movement and looks like a natural

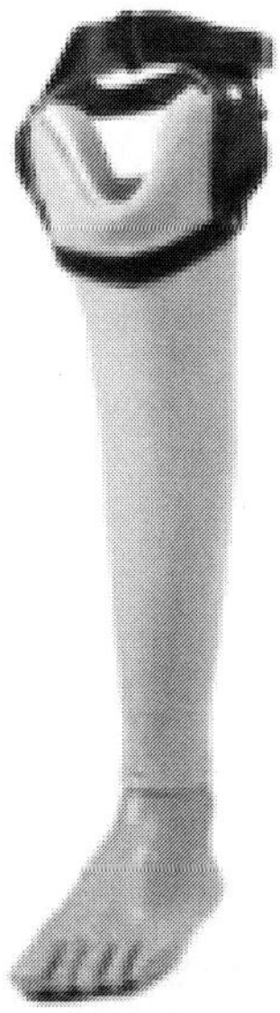

Fig. 7.10: Jaipur foot

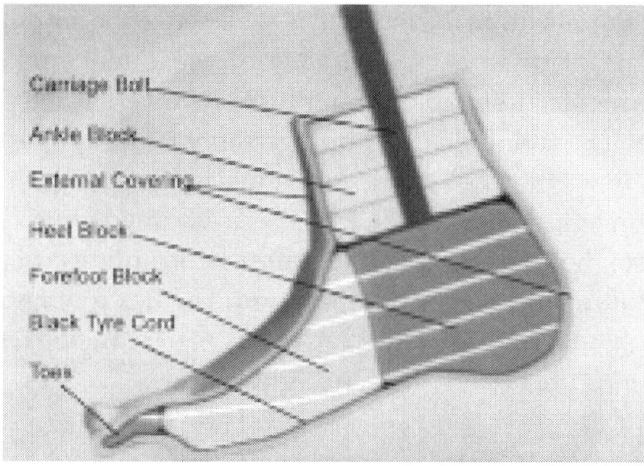

Fig. 7.11: Components of Jaipur foot

foot. Jaipur foot means a glimmer of hope for millions who have paused in their journey due to amputation and helps them to take - A Step forward Every Day

It is the cheapest prosthetic feet in the globe.

Ankle Units

- Seattle ankle
- Endolite Multiplex Ankle: component of the Endolite foot-ankle system, which is a multi-axis foot, can be used separately in conjunction with a different foot , i.e., with Seattle lite foot
- Ankle requires increased maintenance

Knee Disarticulation

- The socket in a knee disarticulation is usually a modified quadrilateral socket with some ischial weight bearing, and a soft socket liner with supracondylar build ups to provide suspension. Proximal socket trimlines prevent socket rotation on the limb, though ischial weight bearing is not an absolute requirement, as the femoral condyle provides suspension. The problem with prosthetic fitting of a knee disarticulation is that the prosthetic knee's center of rotation needs to go through the distal residual limb. Fitting a knee unit distal to the residual limb has caused problems in the past, but the four-bar polycentric knee has helped to solve the problem. *The polycentric knee, unlike the single-axis knee, has an instantaneous center of rotation that changes, and is proximal and posterior to the knee unit itself. This allows greater knee stability, a more symmetrical gait, and equal knee length when sitting.*

Transfemoral (TF) amputation/Above-knee amputation (AKA) (see Fig. 7.12)

Sockets for AKA

- The initial design developed specifically for the AKA socket was the total contact quadrilateral socket. This design replaced the plug fit socket as the standard for above-the-knee prosthesis. In the past, the quadrilateral socket was the only socket design

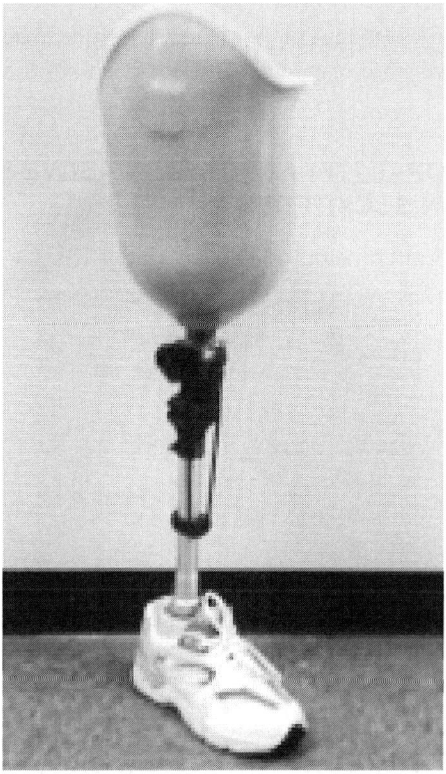

Fig. 7.12: Transfemoral prostheses

used for above-the-knee prosthesis. Now, more recent socket designs are being used; these are the ischial containment socket with narrow mediolateral configuration, and the above-knee frame socket with a flexible liner known is the ISNY.

- Ischial containment, narrow mediolateral design, also known as Normal Shape Normal Alignment (NSNA) or contoured adducted trochanter-controlled alignment method (CAT-CAM) was developed to provide for a more normal anatomic alignment of the femur and for the prosthesis. It also stabilizes the relationship between the pelvis and proximal femur because the ischial tuberosity is controlled inside the socket, rather than just sitting on top of the posterior brim as the tuberosity does in the quadrilateral socket. To control the pelvis, the trim line of the socket brim is brought more proximally than that of the quadrilateral socket. A higher trim line results in better control of the residual limb, especially for short above-the-knee amputations.

TRANSFEMORAL (TF) AMPUTATION/ABOVE-KNEE AMPUTATION SOCKET DESIGN

1. Quadrilateral Transfemoral Socket (Fig. 7.13)

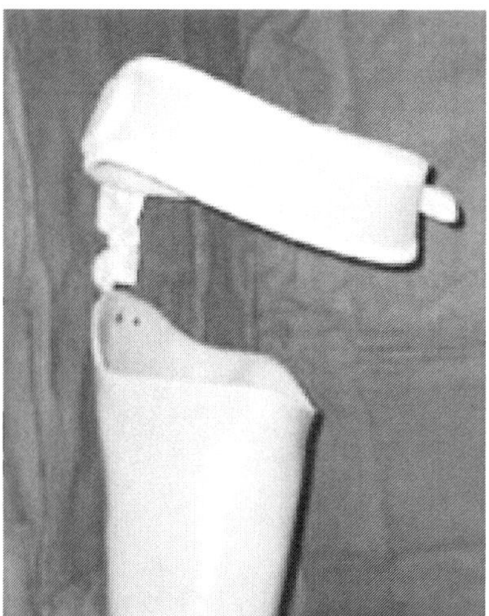

Fig. 7.13: Quadrilateral transfemoral socket

2. Narrow mediolateral (narrow ML) socket/Ischial containment (IC) socket/Contoured adducted Trochanteric-Controlled Alignment Method (CAT-CAM) socket.

Suspension of AKA Prosthesis

- Suction Socket
- Silesian Belt
- Total Elastic Suspension (TES) Belt
- Pelvic Band and Belt with Hip Joint.

Knee Units

- All knee units, except for the hydraulic stance control units, attempt to keep the knee flexion and extension fixed at one angle throughout the stance phase.
- Provide stability during walking, particularly during early knee stance, to prevent knee from buckling, and allow the knee to bend when the patient sits and, in most cases, during swing phase (to allow easy clearance of the toes).
- Most are single axis; some are multi-axis
- *Conventional single-axis knees*
  - Light, durable, and inexpensive
  - Rely on alignment for stability and work best at one speed
  - Excessive heel rise in the early swing phase, as well as terminal swing impact in the late swing phase, may occur at faster cadences
  - Amputee must prevent knee buckling by activating hip extensors
  - The debilitated amputee or amputee with a short residual limb cannot adequately contract the hip extensors, and requires a knee that is set posterior to the trochanter knee angle line. This alignment has a disadvantage of causing difficulty in flexion of the knee for the swing phase that causes increased energy expenditure compared to other units.
- *Manual locking knee*
  - Maximum stability for the debilitated or elderly amputee
  - Worst gait efficiency and increased energy consumption

- *Stance control knee*
  - Weight-activated stance-controlled knee or safety knee may provide a stable stance for up to 20 degrees of flexion by producing friction when the weight increases during stance
  - Design is for amputees with weak hip extensors or for geriatric amputees
  - Stance control is not automatic, and the amputee must be able to initiate and maintain control of the knee.
- *Four-bar* polycentric works well for patients with very long residual limbs, as well as for those with poor stability due to short residual limbs, poor balance, or weak hip extensors. Fluid control can be added and some polycentric knees can be manually locked.
- *Hydraulic and pneumatic control knee units are* cadence responsive through cadence dependence resistance.
  - Pneumatic units are air-filled and are lighter in weight, but they cannot support the heavier or more athletic amputee as well as the hydraulic units can.
  - Hydraulic/fluid-controlled knees (oil) are helpful for the active amputee who varies cadence and who can tolerate the extra weight and expense.
  - Most fluid-controlled knees control the knee velocity during swing phase only, although hydraulic stance-controlled knees give gradually yielding resistance to knee flexion during the late stance phase as well.
  - When weight is applied to the slightly flexed knee, the unit allows a slow yielding action instead of a precipitous collapse. This permits the young, agile amputee to descend ramps and stairs in a step-over-step manner.
  - The Endolite pneumatic intelligent prosthesis has a computer-controlled valve that adjusts knee swing phase speed based on cadence.
  - The hydro cadence knee is unique, in that it also hydraulically controls ankle dorsiflexion and plantarflexion.

SOCKET DESIGN-TRANSTIBIAL AND TRANSFEMORAL AMPUTATIONS

Flexible Socket

- Provide softer, thermoplastic material for weight transmission
- Sits in rigid frame.

Advantages

- Comfort
- Better sense of outer objects through socket
- Often translucent or transparent
- Feels cooler
- Rapidly fabricated and modified
- Suction suspension if desired.

Disadvantages

- Expensive
- Imprecise fit secondary to linear shrinkage of thermoplastic material.

SILICONE GEL LINER/SUCTION SUSPENSION

Properties Similar to Human Adipose Tissue

Advantages

- Able to distribute shear forces generated at socket interface
- Assists vascular inflow by creating a negative pressure
- Can provide suction suspension.

Disadvantages

- Not always tolerated, excessive sweating
- Need constant volume to ensure suction fit
- Expensive.

Laminated Socket

Advantages

- Cheaper
- Durable.

Disadvantages

- Less comfortable
- Less total contact
- Not easily modified.

Hip Disarticulation/Hemipelvectomy

Amputees with less than five centimeters of residual femur usually are fitted as hip disarticulation level amputees.

- Canadian hip disarticulation prosthesis is the standard prosthesis for a hip disarticulation.
  - Socket of this prosthesis encloses the hemipelvis on the side of the amputation and extends around the hemipelvis of the nonamputated side, leaving an opening for the nonamputated lower extremity.
  - There is a flexible anterior wall with an opening that allows the prosthesis to be donned. Weight bearing is on the ischial tuberosity of the amputated side
  - Endoskeletal prosthetic components are preferred for this level of amputation to reduce the overall weight. The endoskeletal hip joint has an extension assist as does the knee unit, which usually is a constant friction knee.
  - Endoskeletal components may be made from aluminum, titanium, or carbon graphite composite.
  - Single axis foot or SACH foot with a soft heel used most. The newer lightweight foot-ankle combination may be even a better option. The prosthesis for a hemipelvectomy resembles that for the hip disarticulation socket except in the interior configuration of the socket. In the hemipelvectomy, most of the weight bearing is by the soft tissues of the amputated side, with some of the weight bearing by the sacrum on the opposite ischial tuberosity.

AMBULATION AIDS

- Assistive devices for mobility/ambulation can be referred to as ambulatory aids.

- Ambulatory aids (canes, crutches, walkers) are used to provide an extension of the upper extremities to help transmit body weight and provide support for the patient.
- The type of ambulatory aid needed depends on how much balance and weight-bearing assistance is needed. Generally, the more disabled the individual is, the greater the complexity required in the walking device. A walker supplies the most support, and a standard cane or crutch provides the least.

Uses of assistive devices include the following:
- Redistribute and unload a weight-bearing lower limb
- Improve balance
- Reduce lower limb pain
- Provide sensory feedback.

Batavia and Hammer identified 4 key evaluation and selection criteria for long-term users of assistive devices:
- *Effectiveness:* The extent to which the function of the device improves one's living situation, functional capability, or independence.
- *Affordability:* The extent to which the purchase, maintenance, or repair of the device causes financial difficulty.
- *Operability:* The extent to which the device is easy to operate and adequately responds to demands.
- *Dependability:* The extent to which the device operates with repeatable and predictable levels of accuracy under conditions of reasonable use.

Assistive Devices and their Use for Impairments

- Moderate-to-severe unilateral weakness/hemiplegia - (Walk cane/ hemi-walker)
- Bilateral lower extremity weakness/paralysis - Bilateral crutches or walker (pickup or front-wheeled)
- Severely impaired stability - Walker (pickup or front-wheeled) Impaired wrist or hand function - Platform forearm walker Difficulty climbing stairs - Stair-climbing walker

Canes

When properly used canes will:
- Increase base of support

- Decrease loading and demand on the lower limbs
- Provide additional sensor information
- Assist acceleration/deceleration during locomotion.

Prescribed in various disabilities to:

- Improve balance
- Decrease pain
- Reduce weight-bearing forces of injured structures
- Compensate for weak muscles
- Scan the immediate environment.

Components

- Handle
- Adjusting knob for handle
- Shaft
- Adjusting mechanism for height
- Rubber tip.

C-handle or Crook Top Cane (see Fig. 7.14)

Advantages: Inexpensive

Disadvantages: uncomfortable, difficult to grasp (i.e., RA patient), weight-bearing line falls behind the shaft of the cane reducing support, not adjustable.

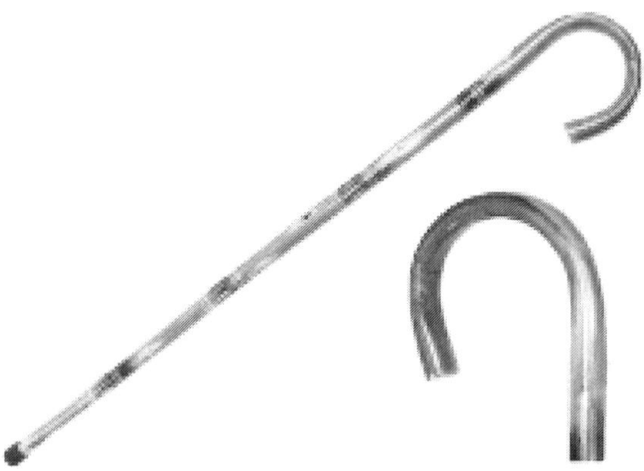

Fig. 7.14: C-Handle cane

Adjustable Metal Cane

- Advantages: inexpensive, adjustable
- Disadvantages: same as above.

Functional Grip Cane (see Fig. 7.15)

Advantages: handle fits the grip, conforms to natural angle of hand. and is more centered over the shaft of the cane, provides more support. **Disadvantages:** More expensive

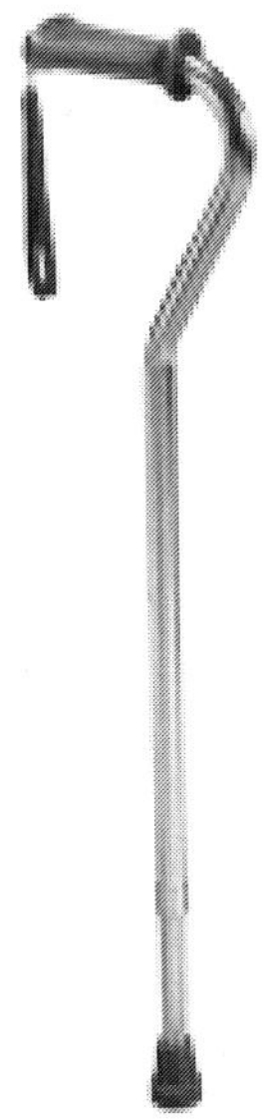

Fig. 7.15: Functional grip cane

Wide-based or Quadruped Cane (see Fig. 7.16)

Advantages: More Support

Disadvantage: Heavy, awkward appearance, WBQC does not fit on stairs

- Difference between crutch and a cane:
- Cane has one point of contact with the body
- Crutch has 2 points of contact with the body

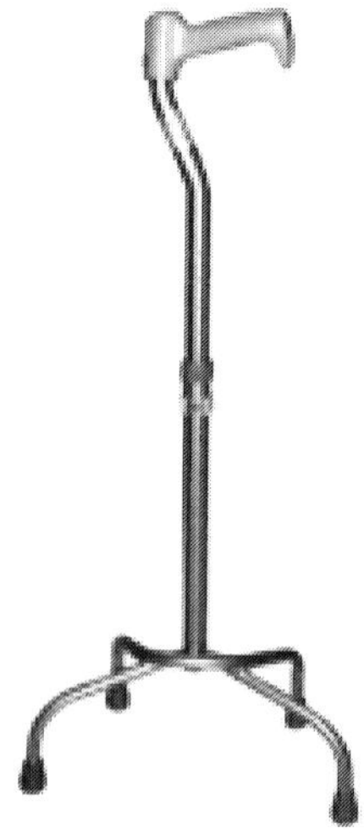

Fig. 7.16: Quadraped cane

Cane Measurement/Prescription

- 20° elbow flexion or height of greater trochanter
- Crutches

Axillary Crutches (see Fig. 7.17)

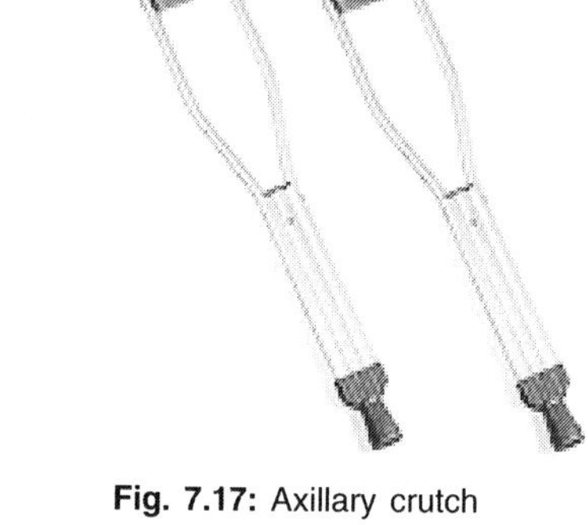

Fig. 7.17: Axillary crutch

Components

- Padded axillary piece (on top)
- Two upright shafts
- Handpiece (in middle)
- Extension piece
- Rubber tip.

Advantages: Inexpensive, adjustable, easier to use

Disadvantages: need good strength and ROM in upper limbs, ties up hands. Increased cardiac/metabolic demand.

Forearm Crutches/Lofstrand Crutches (see Fig. 7.18)

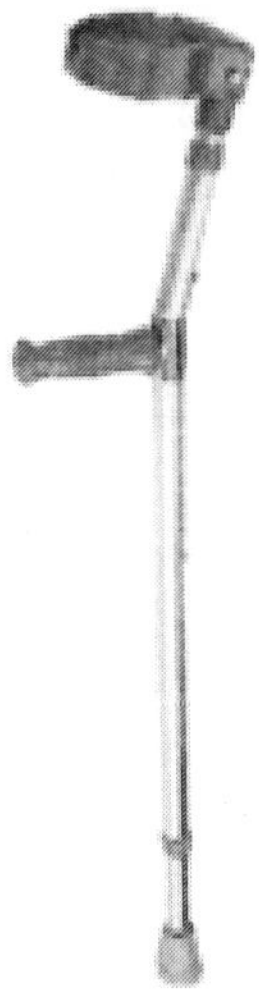

Fig. 7.18: Forearm crutch

Components

- Forearm cuff with narrow anterior opening
- Forearm piece bent posteriorly and adjustable (extends to 2 inches below elbow)
- Molded handpiece
- Single aluminum tubular shaft
- Rubber tip.

Advantages: lightweight, easily adjustable, freedom for hand activities.

Disadvantages: needs more strength, requires more skill, and better trunk balance.

Platform Crutches (see Fig. 7.19)

Advantages: Do not need weight bearing through wrist and hand (i.e., fractures, arthritis of wrist or hand. or weakness triceps or grasp).

Disadvantages: awkward, heavy.

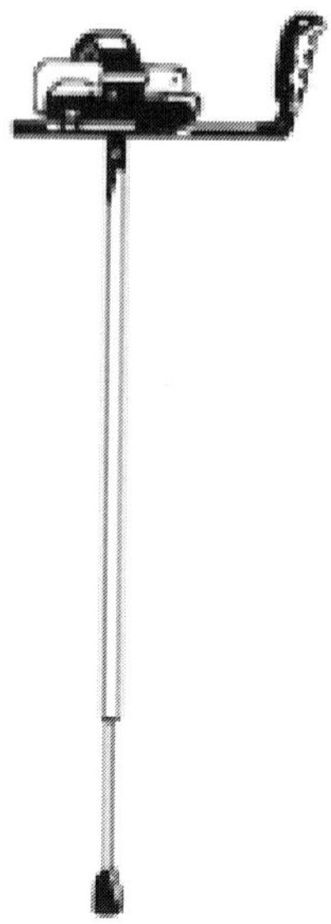

Fig. 7.19: Platform crutch

Walkers

Indications

1. Bilateral weakness and/or incoordination of the lower limbs or whole body, whenever a firm, free standing aid is appropriate (i.e., multiple sclerosis or Parkinsonism) to increase balance.
2. To relieve weight bearing either fully or partially on a lower extremity (allow the upper extremities to transfer body weight to the floor)

3. Unilateral weakness or amputation of the lower limb where general weakness makes the greater support offered by the frame necessary (i.e., osteoarthritis or fractured femur).
4. General support to aid mobility and confidence (i.e., after prolonged bedrest and sickness in the elderly).

Advantages

- Provide a wider base of support
- More stable base of support
- Provide a sense of security for patients fearful of ambulation

Disadvantages

- More conspicuous in appearance
- Interfere with development of a smooth reciprocal gait pattern (e.g., increase step length with step-to-gait pattern)
- Interfere with stair negotiation/difficult to maneuver through doorways or bathrooms.

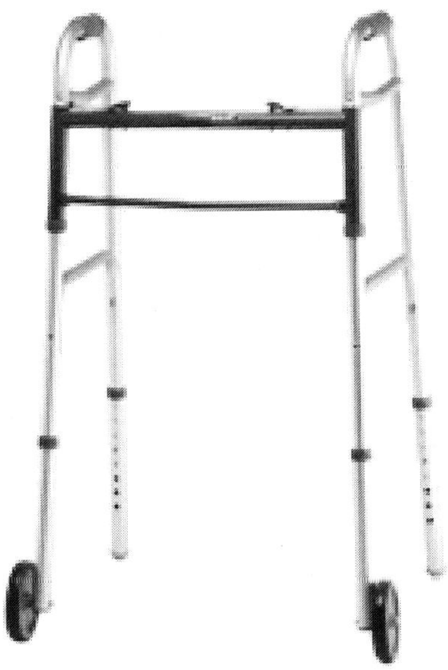

Fig. 7.20: Walker

Types

- Lightweight walking frame
- Folding walking frame
- Rolling walking frame
- Forearm resting walking frame
- Hemi-walking frame

PRINCIPLES IN ORTHOTICS

An orthotic device (commonly just referred to as an orthotic) is an external device applied on the body to limit motion, correct deformity, reduce axial loading, or improve function in a certain segment of the body.

Design characteristics of an orthotic device are crucial to function. Most important features include the following:

- Weight of the orthosis
- Adjustability
- Functional use
- Cosmesis
- Cost
- Durability
- Material
- Ability to fit various sizes of patients
- Ease of putting on (donning) and taking off (doffing)
- Access to tracheostomy site, peg tube, or other drains
- Access to surgical sites for wound care
- Aeration to avoid skin maceration from moisture.

Indications for recommending orthotic devices include the following:

- Pain relief
- Mechanical unloading
- Scoliosis management
- Spinal immobilization after surgery
- Spinal immobilization after traumatic injury
- Compression fracture management
- Kinesthetic reminder to avoid certain movements.

Duration of orthotic use is determined by the individual situation:

- In situations where spinal instability is not an issue, recommend use of an orthosis until the patient can tolerate discomfort without the brace.
- When used for stabilization after surgery or acute fractures, allow 6-12 weeks to permit ligaments and bones to heal.

Use of an orthotic device is associated with several drawbacks, including the following:

- Discomfort
- Local pain
- Osteopenia
- Skin breakdown
- Nerve compression
- Ingrown facial hair for men
- Muscle atrophy with prolonged use
- Decreased pulmonary capacity
- Increased energy expenditure with ambulation
- Difficulty donning and doffing orthosis
- Difficulty with transfers
- Psychological and physical dependency
- Increased segmental motion at ends of the orthosis
- Unsightly appearance
- Poor patient compliance

Success of the orthosis may lead to any of the following:

- Decreased pain
- Increased strength
- Improved function
- Increased proprioception
- Improved posture
- Correction of spinal curve deformity
- Protection against spinal instability
- Minimized complications
- Healing of ligaments and bones

Physiotherapist must understand the biomechanics of the spine and each individual orthosis. The cervical spine is the most mobile spinal segment with flexion greater than extension. The occiput and C1 have significant flexion and extension with limited side bending and rotation. The C1-C2 complex accounts for 50% of rotation in the cervical spine. The C5-C6 region has the greatest amount of flexion and extension. The C2-C4 region has the most side bending and rotation.

When compared to the cervical and lumbar spine, the thoracic spine is the least mobile. The thoracic spine has greater flexion than extension. Lateral bending increases in a caudal direction, and axial rotation decreases in a caudal direction.

The lumbar spine has minimal axial rotation. The greatest movement in the lumbar spine is flexion and extension. Immobilization of the spine increases erector spinae muscle activity since normal rotation that occurs with ambulation is limited by the orthosis.

The biomechanical principles in orthotic design include balance of horizontal forces, fluid compression, distraction, construction of a cage around the patient, placement of an irritant to serve as a kinesthetic reminder, and skeletal fixation. Construction of a cage around the patient, like a thoracolumbar brace, increases intra-abdominal pressure. Increased intraabdominal pressure converts the soft abdomen into a semirigid cylinder, which helps to relieve part of the vertebral load. In general, structural damage to posterior elements of the spine creates more instability with flexion, whereas damage to anterior elements creates more instability with extension.

Orthotic devices (orthoses) are generally named by the body regions that they span. For example, a CO is a cervical orthosis, while a CTLSO is a cervicothoracolumbosacral orthosis, spanning the entire length of the spine. Many of these devices are also known by eponyms.

Several drawbacks to Cervical Orthotic (CO) use have been noted. The soft tissue structures around the neck (eg, blood vessels, esophagus, and trachea) limit application of aggressive external force. The high level of mobility at all segments of the cervical spine makes it difficult to restrict motion. Cervical orthoses offer no control for the head or thorax; therefore, motion restriction is minimal. Cervical orthoses serve as a kinesthetic reminder to limit neck movement.

Observe appropriate precautions associated with orthotic use.

Keep in mind that continued long-term use has been associated with decreased muscle function and dependency.

SPINAL ORTHOSIS (SEE FIG. 7.21)

The soft collar is a common orthotic device made of light weight material, polyurethane foam rubber, with a stockinette cover. It has Velcro closure strap for easy donning and doffing. Patients find the collar comfortable to wear, but it is soiled easily with long-term use.

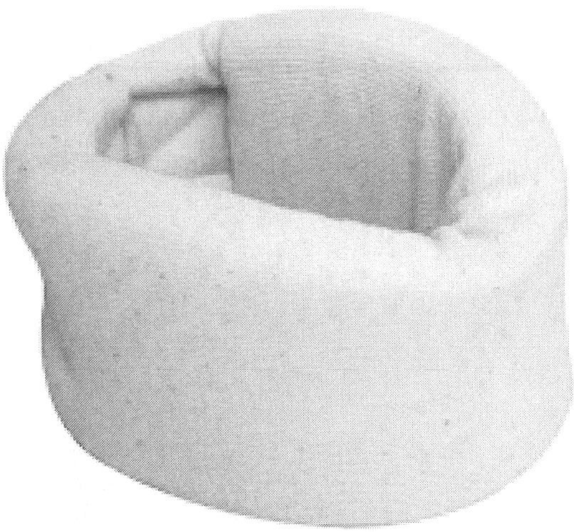

Fig. 7.21: Soft collar

Indications for use of the soft collar include the following benefits for the patient:

- Warmth
- Psychological comfort
- Support to the head during acute neck pain
- Relief with minor muscle spasm associated with spondylolysis
- Relief in cervical strains.

The soft collar provides some limitations of motion for the patient, including the following:

- Limits full flexion and extension by 5-15%
- Limits full lateral bending by 5-10%
- Limits full rotation by 10-17%

The Hard cervical collars (see Fig. 7.22) are similar in shape to a soft collar but are made of Plastizote, a rigid polyethylene material shaped like a ring with padding. Height can be adjusted in certain designs to fit patients better. Velcro straps are used for easy donning and doffing. The hard collar is more durable than a soft collar with long-term use. Several problems can be alleviated with use of a hard collar. The indications include the following:

Support to the Head During Acute Neck Pain

- Relief of minor muscle spasm associated with spondylosis
- Psychological comfort
- Interim stability and protection during halo application

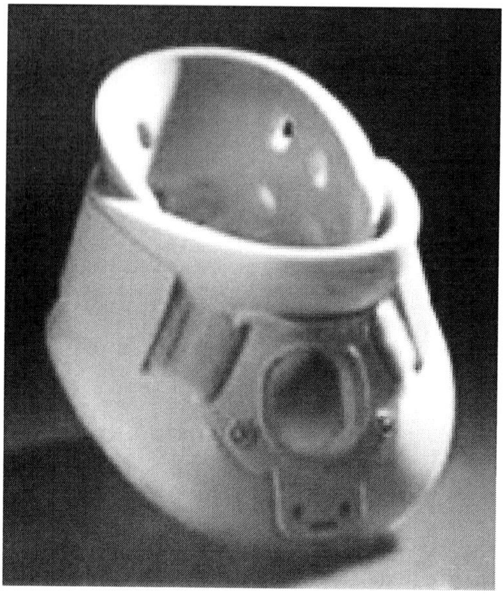

Fig. 7.22: Hard collar

Motion restrictions for the hard collar include the following:

- Limits full flexion and extension by 20-25%
- Less effective in restricting rotation and lateral bending
- Better than a soft collar in motion restriction

Several drawbacks to cervical orthotic (CO) use have been noted.

The soft tissue structures around the neck (e.g., blood vessels, esophagus, trachea) limit application of aggressive external force. The high level of mobility at all segments of the cervical spine makes it difficult to restrict motion. Cervical orthoses offer no control for the head or thorax; therefore, motion restriction is minimal. Cervical orthoses serve as a kinesthetic reminder to limit neck movement. Observe appropriate precautions associated with orthotic use. Keep in mind that continued long-term use has been associated with decreased muscle function and dependency.

Head cervical orthotics (HCOs) includes the occiput and chin to decrease range of motion (ROM). Supported chin area is a common place for skin breakdown and in grown hair for men. The clavicle is another area for skin breakdown and discomfort with HCOs. HCOs generally are used in stable spine conditions. Like in the case of cervical orthotics, continued long-term use of HCOs has been associated with decreased muscle function and dependency.

The **Philadelphia collar** (see Fig. 7.23) is a semirigid HCO with a 2-piece system of Plastizote foam. Plastic struts on the anterior and posterior sides are used for support. The upper portion of the orthosis supports the lower jaw and occiput, while the lower portion covers the upper thoracic region. The Philadelphia collar comes in various sizes and is comfortable to wear, improving patient compliance. Velcro straps are used for easy donning and doffing. The

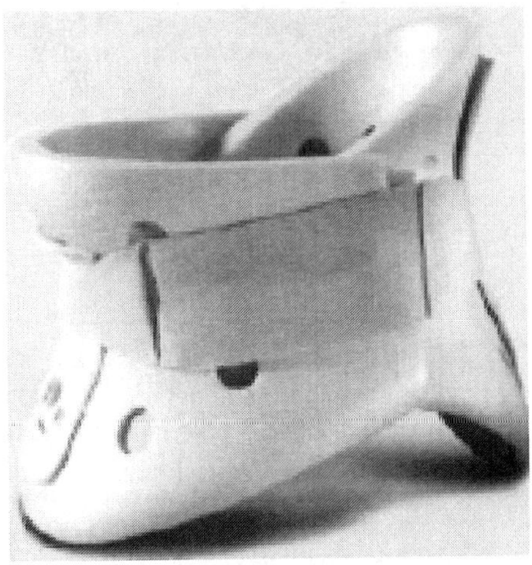

Fig. 7.23: Philadelphia Collar

Philadelphia collar is difficult to clean and becomes soiled very easily. An anterior hole for a tracheostomy is available. A thoracic extension can be added to increase motion restriction and treat C6-T2 injuries. Motion restrictions for the Philadelphia collar include the following:

- Limits flexion and extension by 65-70%
- Limits rotation by 60-65%
- Limits lateral bending by 30-35%.

The goal of the Philadelphia collar is to provide immobilization and is indicated after the following:

- Anterior cervical fusion
- Halo removal
- Dens type I cervical fracture of C2
- Anterior diskectomy
- Suspected cervical trauma in unconscious patients
- Tear-drop fracture of the vertebral body (Note: Some tear-drop fractures require anterior decompression and fusion.)
- Cervical strain

The **Miami J collar** (see Fig. 7.24) is another cervical orthotic device in common use. The Miami J collar has a 2-piece system made

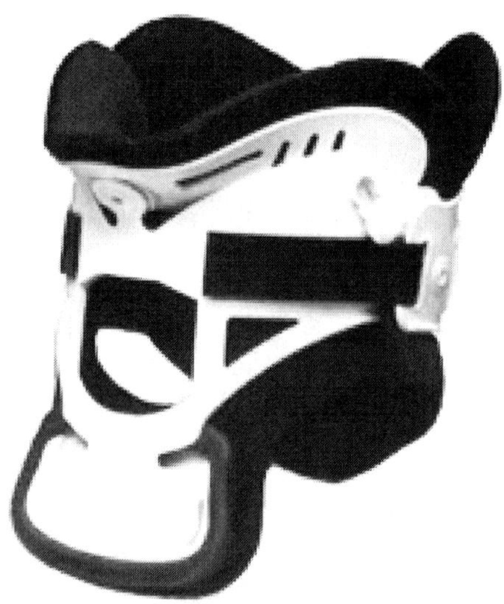

Fig. 7.24: Miami J collar

of polyethylene and a soft washable lining. The anterior piece has a tracheostomy opening similar to that in the Philadelphia collar. Velcro straps provide easy donning and doffing. The Miami J collar is a semi-rigid HCO. A thoracic extension can be added to increase support and treat C6-T2 injuries. The Miami J collar is available in various sizes and can be heated and molded to a contoured fit.

Motion restrictions with the Miami J collar include the following:

- Limits flexion and extension by 55-75%
- Limits rotation by 70%
- Limits lateral bending by 60%.

Indications for use of a Miami J collar are the same as the Philadelphia collar. (See indications for Philadelphia collar.)

The **Malibu collar** (see Fig. 7.25) is similar to the Philadelphia collar as it is a semi-rigid orthosis designed in a 2-piece system with an anterior opening for a tracheostomy. The Malibu collar comes in only one size, but it is adjustable in multiple planes to ensure proper fit. Anterior chin support height is also adjustable. Straps around the chin, occiput, and lower cervical area provide for tightening. Padding around the chin can be trimmed to ensure proper fit. Thoracic extension can be added to increase support and treat C6-T2 injuries.

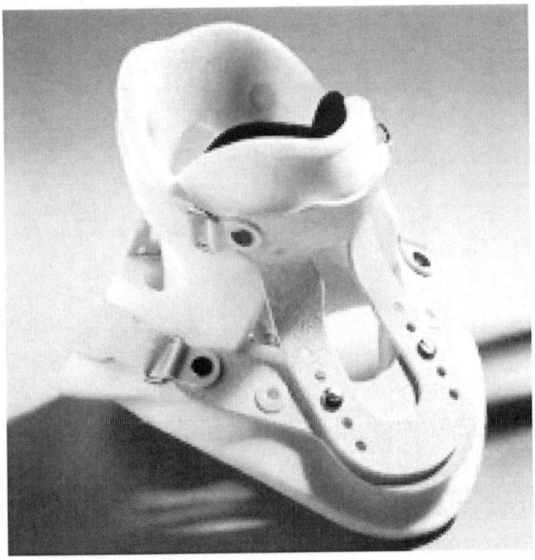

Fig. 7.25: Malibu Collar

Motion restrictions for the Malibu collar include the following:

- Limits flexion and extension by 55-60%
- Limits rotation by 60%
- Limits lateral bending by 60%

Indications for use of a Malibu collar are similar to those for the Miami J and Philadelphia collars. (See indications for Philadelphia collar.)

The **Aspen Collar** (see Fig. 7.26) has a 2-piece system made of polyethylene with soft foam liner with an anterior opening for a tracheostomy. The Aspen collar is a semi-rigid HCO with Velcro straps for easy donning and doffing.

Motion restrictions mirror those of the Miami J collar and include the following:

- Limits flexion and extension by 55-60%
- Limits rotation by 60%
- Limits lateral bending by 60%.

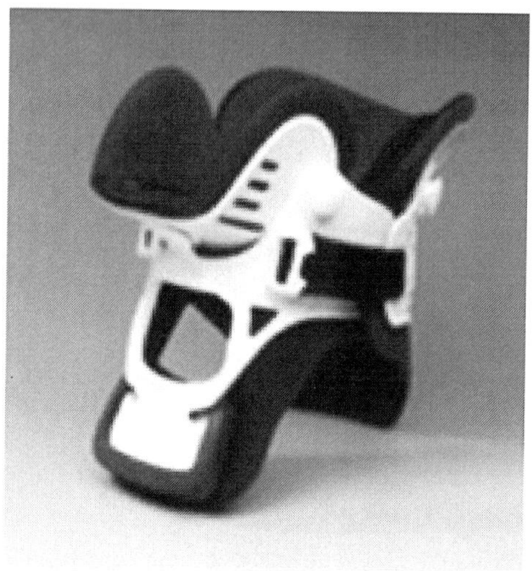

Fig. 7.26: Aspen collar

Indications for use of the Aspen collar include the same as the HCOs discussed above. (See indications for Philadelphia collar.) The Jobst Vertebrace is made of high-density polyethylene with soft polyethylene foam liner. The Jobst Vertebrace is a semi-rigid HCO designed for use in emergent transport situations, and it is similar to the Yale or Philadelphia collar in restricting motion. The Jobst Vertebrace provides full contact along its costal ends to the sternum and cradles the mandible for stability.

Motion restrictions for the Jobst Vertebrace are similar to those of the Yale and Philadelphia collars, including the following:

- Limits flexion and extension by 55-60%
- Limits rotation by 60%
- Limits lateral bending by 60%.

Cervical thoracic orthotics (CTOs) (see Fig. 7.27) provides greater motion restriction in the middle to lower cervical spine from the added pressure on the body. The upper cervical spine has less motion restriction. CTOs are used in minimally unstable fractures.

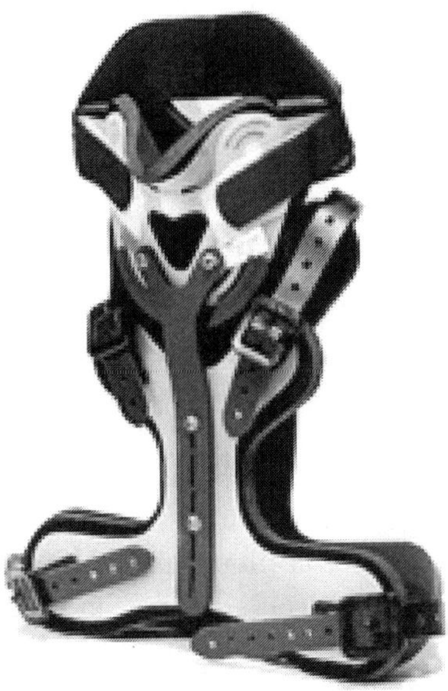

Fig. 7.27: Cervical thoracic orthotics (CTOs)

The Sternal-Occipital-Mandibular Immobilizer (SOMI) (see Fig. 7.28) is a rigid three-poster CTO with anterior chest plate that extends to the xiphoid process and has metal or plastic bars that curve over the shoulder. Straps from the metal bars go over the shoulder and cross to the opposite side of the anterior plate for fixation. A removable

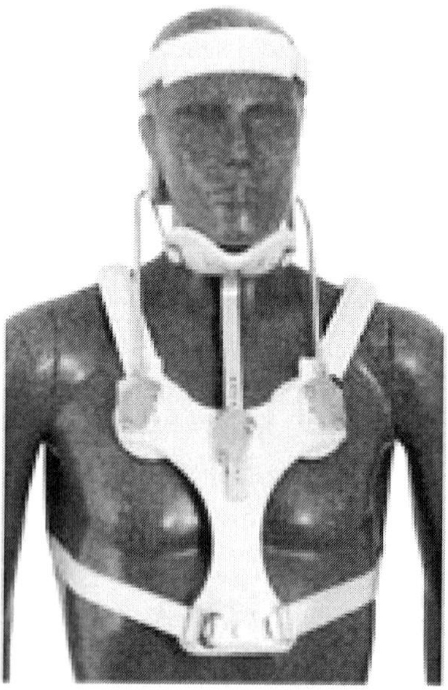

Fig. 7.28: SOMI brace

chin piece attaches to the chest plate with an optional headpiece that can be used when the chin piece is removed for eating. The two-poster CTOs start from the chest plate and attach to the occipital component. The SOMI is ideal for bedridden patients since it has no posterior rods.

The SOMI is relatively comfortable to wear. Proper adjustment is crucial for motion restriction; in fact, motion restriction may be minimal with incorrect application. The SOMI is less effective compared to other braces in controlling extension, but it is very effective in controlling flexion at the atlantoaxial and C2-C3 segments. The SOMI is better than the cervicothoracic brace in controlling flexion in the C1-C3 segments.

Indications for use of the SOMI include the following:

- Immobilization in atlantoaxial instability because of rheumatoid arthritis (Note: Ligamentous disruption in rheumatoid arthritis affects flexion more than extension since extension is held in check by the intact dens).

- Immobilization for neural arch fractures of C2 since flexion causes instability

Motion restrictions with the SOMI include the following:

- Limits cervical flexion and extension by 70%-75%
- Limits lateral bending by 35%
- Limits rotation by 60-65%

The Yale orthosis is a modified Philadelphia collar with thoracic extension made of fiberglass extending anteriorly and posteriorly with mid-thoracic straps on the sides connecting the 2 thoracic extensions. The thoracic component helps to treat C6-T2 injuries. The occipital piece extends higher up on the skull posteriorly. Increased contact surface area improves stability of the brace. Patients find the Yale orthosis comfortable to wear.

Various indications for use of the Yale orthosis include the following:

- Immobilization to C1 fractures with intact transverse ligament
- Immobilization after surgical fixation of Dens Type III fractures
- Immobilization to Dens type I fractures
- Immobilization to Hangman fractures (traumatic spondylolisthesis of C2)
- Immobilization to Jefferson fractures (multiple fractures of C1 ring with spreading due to axial loading)
- Provide immobilization to postoperative fixation.

Motion restrictions for the Yale orthosis include the following:

- Limits flexion and extension by 85%
- Limits rotation by 70% to 75%
- Limits lateral bending by 60%.

The four-poster brace is a rigid orthosis with anterior and posterior chest pads connected by a leather strap. Molded occipital and mandibular support pieces connect to the chest pads and have adjustable struts. Straps connect the occipital and mandibular support pieces. The mandibular plate can interfere with eating. This brace uses shoulder straps, but it has no underarm support. Open design allows heat loss from the neck. The brace is as effective as the cervicothoracic brace in controlling flexion in the mid-cervical area and is better than the Philadelphia collar. The four-poster design limits lateral bending and rotation better than the two-poster brace.

Motion restrictions provided by the four-poster orthosis include the following:

- Limits flexion and extension by 80%
- Limits lateral bending by 55%-80%
- Limits rotation by 70%.

The Guilford brace is a rigid CTO with a two-poster design with anterior chest plate and shoulder straps that connect to the posterior plate. Chin plate and occipital piece connect to the anterior and posterior struts. Underarm straps circle the lower chest wall for stability. The brace has poor control of flexion, extension, rotation, and lateral bending at C1-C2.

Motion restrictions afforded by the Guilford brace include limitation of flexion and extension from C3-T2.

Indications for use of the Guilford brace include the following:

- Immobilization to minimally unstable fractures from C3-T2
- Immobilization after postoperative internal fixation from C3-T2

The Halo device is the most common device for treatment of unstable cervical and upper thoracic fractures and dislocations as low as T3. The halo provides maximum motion restriction of all cervical orthotics. The halo ring is made of graphite or metal with

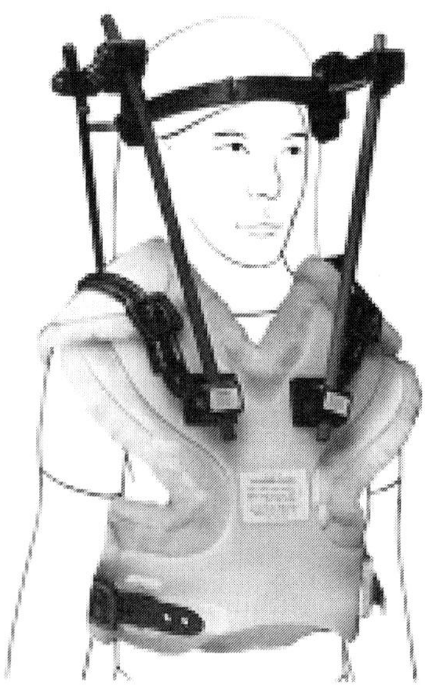

Fig. 7.29: Helo device

pin fixation on the frontal and parietal-occipital areas of the skull. Development of lightweight composite material led to design of radiolucent rings compatible with magnetic resonance imaging (MRI). The halo ring attaches to the vest anteriorly and posteriorly via 4 posters.

The halo vest has shoulder and underarm straps for tightening and usually is made of rigid polyethylene and extends down to the umbilicus. Restriction in cervical motion depends on the fit of the halo vest since improper fit can allow 31% of normal spine motion. The halo vest is the weak link in terms of motion control. Compressive and distractive force can occur with variable fit of the vest.

Multidirectional shear forces can cause increased pinhole size with crater like enlargement. Pin loosening occurs twice as frequently with a heavier halo vest. Generally, upper cervical spine injuries are treated best with a full-length vest to the iliac crest.

Indications for use of a halo device are for immobilization in the following cases:

- Dens type I, II, and III fractures of C2 (Note: Dens type III fractures of C2 are treated more successfully with surgery).
- C1 fractures with rupture of the transverse ligament
- Atlantoaxial instability from rheumatoid arthritis with ligamentous disruption and erosion of the dens
- C2 neural arch fracture and disc disruption between C2 and C3 (Note: Some patients may need surgery for stabilization)
- Bony single column cervical fractures
- Following cervical arthrodesis
- Following cervical tumor resection in an unstable spine
- Following debridement and drainage of infection in an unstable spine
- Following spinal cord injury (SCI).

Contraindications for use of the halo device include the following:

- Concomitant skull fracture with cervical injury
- Damaged or infected skin over pin insertion sites

The relative contraindications for use of the halo device include the following:

- Cervical instability with ligamentous disruption

- Cervical instability with 2 or 3 column injury
- Cervical instability with rotational injury involving facet joints.

The application process for the halo device consists of several steps. Optimal placement for the anterior pins is the anterolateral aspect of the skull 1 cm above the orbital rim on the lateral part of orbit since this prevents penetration into the orbit. Avoid placing pins in the temporalis muscle and through the zygomaticotemporal nerve, which supplies sensation to the temporal area. Pins inserted into the temporalis muscle affect mandibular motion and cause pain. Placement away from the medial one third on the orbital rim preserves the supraorbital and supratrochlear nerves and decreases risk of entering the frontal sinus.

Insertion of posterior pins on the posterolateral aspect of the skull is less crucial. Skin incisions are not necessary prior to pin placement. The halo ring should be 1 cm above the top of the ear. Place all pins perpendicular to the skull, and allow 1-2 cm clearance with the halo ring along the skull perimeter.

In adults, pin insertion requires a torque wrench set at 8 inches per pound since this lowers incidence of pin infection and loosening. In children, set the torque wrench between 2-5 inches per pound since the skull is too weak to sustain heavier forces. Use multiple pin sites in children because of the weaker skull.

Determine the halo vest size by measuring chest circumference at the xiphoid process. Elevate the patient at 30-40° for vest placement. Secure the posterior portion to the halo first, then to the anterior part of the vest. Tighten the bolts on the vest to a torque setting of 28 feet per pound. Tools for the vest sometimes are taped to the anterior part of the vest in case of emergency.

At 24-48 hours after placement, recheck all pins for loosening. Clean the pin sites with saline or soap and water on a sterile swab. Take X-rays immediately after halo placement and after any adjustment to check spinal alignment. Shaking of the cervical spine because, of forced movement against the orthosis or changes in pin tightening can cause some segmental motion. Symptoms of dysphagia may result from placement of the neck in too much extension. Repositioning of the halo, if possible, can eliminate dysphagia.

Motion restrictions provided by the halo include the following:

- Limits flexion and extension by 90-96%
- Limits lateral bending by 92-96%
- Limits rotation by 98-99%.

Various complications associated with halo placement include the following:

- Neck pain or stiffness 80%
- Pin loosening 60%
- Pin site infection 22%
- Scars 30%
- Pain at pin sites 18%
- Pressure sores 11%
- Redislocation 10%
- Restricted ventilation 8%
- Dysphagia 2%
- Nerve injury 2%
- Dural puncture 1%
- Neurological deterioration 1%
- Avascular necrosis of the dens
- Ring migration
- Inadequate bony healing
- Inadequate ligamentous healing.

In use of the halo device, keep in mind the following important considerations:

- The halo fixation device is used for 3 months to allow adequate time for bone healing.
- Use of an HCO after removal of the halo provides some support for the head, as the neck muscles are weak and stiff.
- Approximately 40-45% of patients with facet joint dislocations achieve stability with the halo vest, whereas 70% of patients without facet joint dislocations achieve stability.
- Nearly 75% of patients without facet joint dislocation achieve good anatomic results.
- Surgical stabilization in cases of facet joint dislocation improves outcome.
- Patients with facet joint dislocation have higher likelihood of spinal cord injury.

- Thorough neurologic examination before and after reduction of facet joint dislocation is important.

The best orthotic device to control various cervical regions is indicated as follows:

- All orthotics tend to control flexion better than extension.
- The halo is the most effective in controlling flexion and extension at C1-C3, followed by the four-poster brace, and then the cervicothoracic orthotics.
- The cervicothoracic orthotics are best at controlling flexion and extension at C3-T1, while the SOMI brace is best at controlling flexion from C1-C5.
- The SOMI is less effective in controlling extension compared to other orthotics.
- The halo is the best at controlling rotation and lateral bending from C1-C3.
- The cervicothoracic brace is second best at controlling rotation and lateral bending in the cervical spine.
- The four-poster brace is slightly better at controlling lateral bending compared to the cervicothoracic brace in the cervical spine.

Thoracolumbar orthotics (TLOs) (see Fig. 7.30) are used mainly to treat fractures from T10-L2 since their mobility is not restricted by the ribs, unlike fractures from T2-T9. Immobilization from T10-L2 helps prevent further collapse.

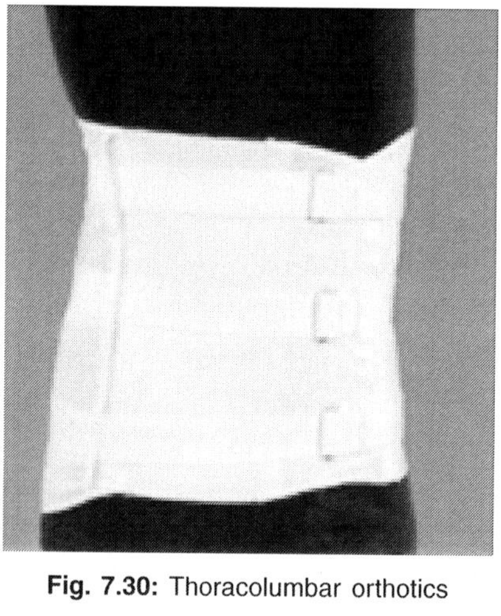

Fig. 7.30: Thoracolumbar orthotics

The **Cruciform anterior spinal hyperextension (CASH) brace** (See Fig. 7.31) features anterior sternal and pubic pads to produce force opposed by the posterior pad and strap around the thoracolumbar region. Sternal and pelvic pads attach to the anterior metal cross-shaped bar, which can be bent to reduce excess pressure on the chest and pelvis. The brace is easy to don and doff, but it is difficult to adjust. Compared to the Jewett brace, it provides greater breast and axillary pressure relief. Two round upper chest pads can be used instead of the sternal pad to decrease discomfort around the breast area.

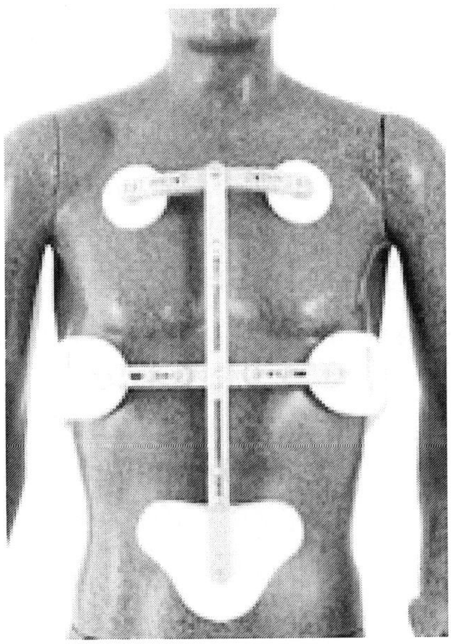

Fig. 7.31: CASH Brace

Indications for the CASH brace include the following:

- Flexion immobilization to treat thoracic and lumbar vertebral body fractures
- Reduction of kyphosis in patients with osteoporosis.

Motion restrictions provided by the CASH brace include the following:

- Limits flexion and extension from T6-L1

- Ineffective in limiting lateral bending and rotation of the upper lumbar spine

Contraindications to use of the CASH brace include the following:
- Three-column spine fractures involving anterior, middle, and posterior spinal structures
- Compression fractures due to osteoporosis.

The Jewett hyperextension brace (see Fig. 7.32) uses a 3-point pressure system with 1 posterior and 2 anterior pad. The anterior pads place pressure over the sternum and pubic symphysis. The posterior pad places opposing pressure in the mid-thoracic region. The posterior pad keeps the spine in an extended position, and it has a lightweight design that is more comfortable than the CASH brace. Pelvic and sternal pads can be adjusted from the lateral axillary bar where they attach. The pads can cause discomfort from pressure applied to small surface area. No abdominal support is provided with this device. When the patient is seated, the sternal pad should be half an inch inferior to the sternal notch, and the pubic pad should be half an inch superior to the pubic symphysis. Indications for use of the Jewett brace include the following:
- Symptomatic relief of compression fractures not due to osteoporosis

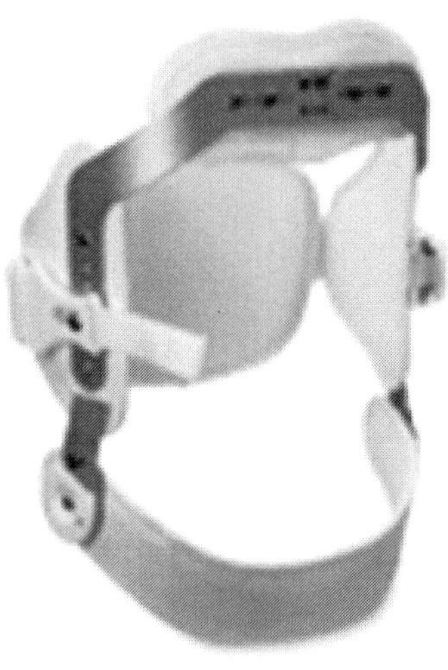

Fig. 7.32: Jewett Hyperextension Brace

- Immobilization after surgical stabilization of thoracolumbar fractures.

Motion restrictions provided by the Jewett brace include the following:

- Limits flexion and extension between T6-L1
- Ineffective in limiting lateral bending and rotation of the upper lumbar spine.

Contraindications to use the Jewett brace include the following:

- Three column spine fractures involving anterior, middle, and posterior spinal structures
- Compression fractures above T6 since segmental motion increases above the sternal pad
- Compression fractures due to osteoporosis.

One important consideration in use of the Jewett brace is that it is more effective than the CASH brace. **The Korsain brace** is a modification of the Jewett brace with added abdominal support for increased rigidity.

Indications for the Korsain brace include the following:

- Symptomatic relief of compression fractures not due to osteoporosis
- Immobilization after surgical stabilization of thoracolumbar fractures
- Flexion immobilization to treat thoracic and lumbar vertebral body fractures.

Motion restrictions and contraindications of the Korsain brace are similar to the Jewett brace. (See Jewett brace motion restrictions). **The Knight–Taylor** brace features a corset type front with lateral and posterior uprights and shoulder straps to help reduce lateral bending, flexion, and extension. Shoulder straps may cause discomfort in some patients. The brace can be prefabricated and made with polyvinyl chloride or aluminum. The posterior portion of the brace has added cross supports below the inferior angle of the scapula and a pelvic band fitted at the sacrococcygeal junction. The anterior corset is made of canvas and provides intracavitary pressure. The anterior corset is laced to the lateral uprights. The brace is indicated to provide flexion immobilization to treat thoracic and lumbar vertebral body fractures.

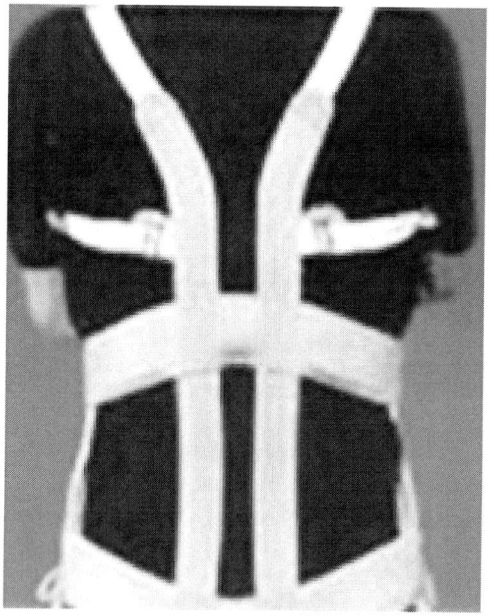

Fig. 7.33: Knight-Taylor brace

Motion restrictions of the Knight-Taylor brace include the following:

- Poor rotation control
- Limits flexion, extension, and lateral bending.

Custom-molded plastic body jacket or thoracolumbosacral orthosis (TLSO) (see Fig. 7.34) is fabricated from polypropylene or plastic and offers best control in all planes of motion and increases intra-cavitary pressure. This orthosis has a lightweight design and is easy to don and doff. The material is easy to clean and comfortable to wear. This brace sometimes is referred to as the clamshell. The TLSO provides efficient force transmission as pressure is distributed over wide surface area, which is ideal for use in patients with neurologic injuries. The brace may have a tendency to ride up on the patient in a supine position. Plastic retains heat, so an undershirt helps to absorb perspiration and protect the skin. Frequent checks to ensure proper fit help prevent pressure ulcers. Velcro straps are used to tighten the brace. Indications for the TLSO include the following:

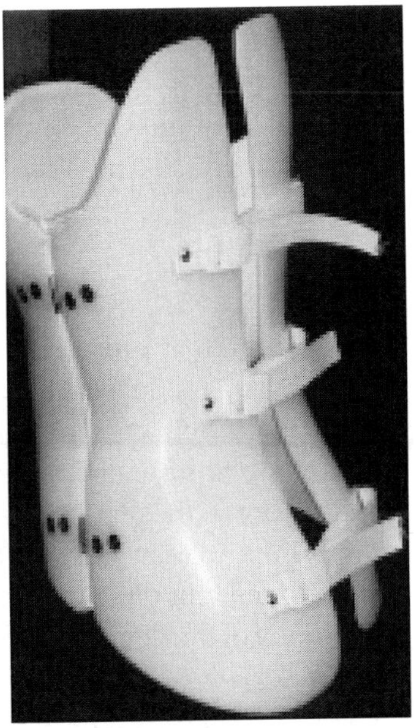

Fig. 7.34: TLSO

- Immobilization for compression fractures from osteoporosis
- Immobilization after surgical stabilization for spinal fractures
- Bracing for idiopathic scoliosis
- Immobilization for unstable spinal disorders for T3 to L3.

Motion restrictions for the TLSO include the following:

- Limits sidebending
- Limits flexion and extension
- Limits rotation to some extent

Clinical information on the custom-molded TLSO suggests that it is more effective in preventing idiopathic scoliosis curve progression than the Milwaukee and Charleston braces. The mean curve progression with TLSO is less than 2° while the Charleston and Milwaukee braces have a curve progression greater than 6°. Fewer than 18% of patients treated with TLSO brace required surgery for scoliosis compared to 23% for patients treated with a Milwaukee brace.

LOWER LIMB ORTHOTIC PRESCRIPTION (AFO, KAFO, HKAFO)

Ankle-Foot Orthosis (AFO): Commonly prescribed for weakness affecting the ankle and subtalar joints. These can be made of plastic, metal, or a hybrid of both.

Plastic AFO

Plastic ankle foot orthoses are either prefabricated out of thermal plastic or custom molded over a model of the patient's limb taken from a casting. Generally they would encompass the posterior calf area with anterior Velcro® strap closure continuing down posteriorly by the ankle and extending down the plantar surface of the foot to assist in dorsiflexion and limit plantar flexion. The design of the trim lines and the design of the foot plate will help determine the structural support and rigidity of the device. The following includes typical designs:

1. Posterior Leaf Spring-PLS design is the most flexible plastic AFO with a very thin plastic band behind the ankle allowing the patient to overpower the brace during the push-off or plantar flexion phase and yet allowing dorsiflexion position of the foot during swing phase. This design is typically used for flaccid foot drop.
2. Semi-rigid plastic AFO with trim lines just behind the malleoli will allow for increase of support and provide both dorsiflexion positioning of the foot and mediolateral stability of the ankle. Much less motion is allowed with this brace design and the patient cannot easily propel during push-off. This design is most commonly used for patients that have foot drop with some extensor tone and/or with mediolateral instability of the ankle.
3. Rigid or solid plastic AFO used most commonly for patients that have the highest levels of spasticity or tone, when complete immobilization of the ankle is necessary. In this case the plastic trim line may be at the malleoli or anterior to the malleoli with no motion allowed at the tibiotalar or subtalar joint. The standard plastic AFO would typically have a foot plate extending through the metatarsal heads, but if the toes are also spastic and claw

into a flex position, then a full foot plate should also be incorporated into this type of solid plastic AFO. Inhibitory foot plate designs are commonly used, which may put the toes into extension to help reduce tone throughout the entire limb. This brace design is typically used for patients with the highest levels of spasticity, early to moderate Charcot joint, and for postoperative immobilization of the foot or ankle.

Plastic vs. Metal AFO

Plastic design AFOs are most desirable due to their light weight, intimate fit, cosmetic appeal, and lack of attachment to the shoe. However, in some cases, the selection of plastic materials may be inappropriate due to risk of excessive pressure or skin breakdown on the leg or foot. Commonly patients with insensate foot due to peripheral neuropathy or peripheral nerve injury should be considered candidates for metal AFOs rather than plastic. Also patients with fluctuating edema that is not managed with compression stockings should be considered most appropriate for metal AFOs rather than plastic AFOs.

AFOs with Hinged Ankle Joint

1. **Paralysis of Dorsiflexion, Plantarflexion, Inversion, Eversion**
   Most mechanical ankle joints prevent mediolateral instability and either control or assist dorsiflexion and plantar flexion by means of stops or assists (springs).
   a. **Plantar flexion control:**
      - May use plantar flexion stop-angulation of the top of the stirrup posteriorly that restricts plantarflexion but allows unlimited dorsiflexion. Substitutes for paralyzed foot dorsiflexors during swing phase. Prevents rapid foot flat after heel strike and maintains the ground reaction force posterior to the knee joint.
   b. **Dorsiflexion control:**
      - May use dorsiflexion stop-anterior angulation that allows full plantar flexion while limiting dorsiflexion. Substitutes for paralyzed gastroc-soleus muscles during push-off.

Allows center of gravity and the ground reaction force to move forward to the metatarsal head area, and creates a moment arm in front of (anterior to) the knee, which promotes knee extension and stability.

c. **Dorsiflexion-assist spring joint (Klenzak joint):**
   - Uses coils located posteriorly that are compressed following heel (or foot) strike (in stance phase). At heel strike, the springs also yield slightly into plantar flexion and help prevent inadvertent knee flexion. During swing phase, the spring rebounds to aid dorsiflexion.

d. **Dorsiflexion/plantar flexion assist joint:**
   - Has an anterior spring that is compressed at midstance and as it recoils, it helps to plantarflex the ankle into push-off. It is used in flail ankle.

e. **Bi-channel adjustable ankle lock (BICAAL) joint:**
   - Have anterior and posterior receptacles with springs that can be compressed to assist motion. The springs can be replaced by pins to alter the alignment of the joint and thus convert it into adjustable stops.

2. **Prevention and Correction of Deformities**
3. **Reduction of Weight Bearing.**

(a) Patellar Tendon Bearing (PTB) Orthosis

- For reduction of weight transmission through the mid or distal tibia, ankle and foot.
- E.g., healing of os calcis fracture, postoperative ankle fusion, heel with refractory pain, delayed unions or nonunions of fractures or fusions, avascular necrosis of the talar body, DJD of the talar or ankle joint, osteomyelitis of the os calcis, and diabetic ulceration/Charcot joint.
- Supports weight on the patellar tendon or tibial flares with the load being transmitted to the shoe via the metal uprights.
- To bypass the lateral aspect of the foot in patients with Charcot joints
- May have plastic bivalve design or calf corset if the patient has fluctuating edema.

- Because little or no ankle motion is allowed, a cushion heel or a rocker bottom is added to provide smoother gait pattern.

(b) Ischial Weight-Bearing Orthosis

- Quadrilateral brim or an ischial (Thomas) ring to relieve weight from the femur or knee.

(c) Patten-Bottom Orthosis

- Uses uprights with no ankle joint that terminate in a floor pad distal to the shoe so the foot is freely suspended in midair. A shoe lift is needed in the opposite side to equalize leg length.

(d) Fracture Orthosis

- Stabilize the fracture site and help promote callus formation by allowing weight bearing and joint movement after initial rest period to allow pain and edema to subside. Minimize joint stiffness and reduce complications such as nonunions. Circumferential compression of the soft tissue can be used to prevent undue bony motion at the fracture site.

4. Reduce the energy cost of ambulation, e.g. in patients with spastic diplegia (CP), LMN. weakness (poliomyelitis), and spastic hemiplegia (stroke).

Knee-Ankle/Foot-Orthosis (KAFO)

Represents extensions of the AFO proximally to control knee motion and alignment:

1. Control genu recurvatum, genu valgum and varum. Used with free-motion knee joints. Free-motion knee joint or polycentric knee joint provides unlimited flexion and extension but usually has a stop to prevent hyperextension. For patients with genu recurvatum but with enough strength to control the knee in stance and ambulation.
2. To provide skeletal support following surgery or nonunion fracture.
3. Knee-flexion contractures. Locked knee joints are usually used for these applications. Adjustable knee lock:

- Serrated adjustable keen joint permits locking in almost any degree of flexion
- Useful in a patient with a knee flexion contracture which is diminishing with treatment.

4. Locked knee joints-to prevent knee buckling. To be able to lock the joint, the patient must be able to fully extend the knee, either actively or passively. Contraindicated in patients with knee contracture (use an adjustable knee lock instead)
   - Drop-ring locks-rings drop over the joints in extension, locking them. They are designed to either drop by gravity, or with assistance from the patient.
   - Pawl lock with bail release-engages when knee is fully extended, but easier to release because of the semicircular lever (bail) attached posteriorly, which unlocks the joint with an upward pull on the bail (either manually or by backing up to sit down on a chair).
   - Disadvantages: The bail is bulky and can be accidentally released, if hits a rigid object.
   - Trick knee allows 0-25 degree of measurement while in the locked position to normalize gait. Free knee when unlocked.
   - Offset knee joint-hinge is placed posterior to the knee joint so the patient's weight line falls anterior to the offset joint, stabilizing the knee during early stance on level surfaces. It is free to flex during swing phase, and allows sitting without the need to manipulate the lock. Should not be used in patients with knee- or hip-flexion contracture, or with plantar flexion stop at the ankle. The patient must be careful when walking on a ramp as the knee may flex inadvertently.

Hip-Knee-Ankle-Foot Orthosis (HKAFO)

- Hip joint and pelvic band attached to the lateral upright of a KAFO converts it to a HKAFO.
- Indications:
  - Hip flexion/extension instability
  - Hip adduction/abduction weakness
  - Hip internal rotation/external rotation instability.

Example

- Scott-Craig orthosis (Scott-Craig long leg brace)
- Reciprocal Gait Orthosis (RGO).

Knee Orthoses

Flexible Knee Orthosis

- Made from an elastic material or rubber
- May include hinged metal knee joints, patellar pads, adjustable straps to change tension, and anterior cutout to relieve pressure on the patella when the knee is flexed
- Function:
  - Provide comfort for patients with osteoarthritis, minor knee sprains, and mild edema
  - Proprioceptive feedback/kinesthetic reminder
  - Minimal mechanical support
  - Can retain body heat
  - Stabilize patellar tracking with patellofemoral dysfunction.

Knee orthoses (KOs): Rehabilitative, Functional, and Prophylactic

- Generally prescribed to prevent genu recurvatum and to provide mediolateral stability. Prophylactic KOs, theoretically, are designed to prevent injury to the knee or at least to reduce the degree to which the knee is injured in athletic activities.
- KOs may be used during sports and other physical activities to provide functional support for unstable knees or during rehabilitation after injury or surgery of the knee. The use of KOs for the prevention of knee injuries in sports is controversial.
- Numerous designs of KOs available; most consist of two uprights, free or adjustable knee joints, and thigh and calf cuffs.

Upper Limb Orthotics

Static Upper-Limb Orthoses

a. **Indications**
   - Immobilize, stabilize, and support a joint in a desired position

- Protect weak muscles from overstretch
- Prevent contractures
- Support structures following surgical repair
- Facilitate the healing of soft tissue injuries and fractures.

b. **Complications associated with use of static orthoses**
- Skin breakdown
- Contractures
- Infection.

Wrist, Hand, and Finger Static Orthoses

Positional Orthoses

Opponens orthoses: primarily used to immobilize the thumb to promote tissue healing and/or protection or for positioning of the weak thumb in opposition to other fingers to facilitate three-jaw-chuck pinch.

- Stabilization of the first MCP joint

Basic Opponens Orthoses

- Thumb orthoses that consist of a dorsal and a palmar bar encircling the mid palm, with a thumb abduction bar projecting from the palmar bar.
- Examples: short opponens splints, C-bar splints, cone splints, static thumb splints.

Opponens Orthoses with Wrist Control Attachments

- Similar to basic opponens orthosis with a forearm bar and proximal and distal crossbars for wrist control
- *For example,* long opponens splints and thumb spica splints
- In addition to the benefits already mentioned for opponens orthoses (stabilizes first MCP), forearm bar maintains wrist in extension and prevent radial and ulnar deviation deformities.

Opponens Orthoses with Lumbrical Bar

- Finger orthosis that prevents metacarpal phalangeal joint hyperextension but allows full MCP flexion
- Prevents claw hand deformity (in addition to the benefits already mentioned for opponens orthoses).

Opponens Orthoses with Finger Extension Assist Assembly

- Similar to basic opponens orthoses plus finger orthosis that assist proximal interphalangeal and distal interphalangeal extension
- Used for interphalangeal flexion contracture, boutonnière deformity, or postsurgical release of Dupuytren's contracture.

Protective orthoses: used to protect wrist, hand, and/or fingers from potential deformity or damage by restricting active function/limiting motion.

Digital Stabilizers

Finger Stabilizers/static Finger Orthoses (FOs)

Interphalangeal stabilizers (DIP, PIP, and DIP+PIP gutter splints, static finger splints, stax or stack splints, egg-shell finger casts, etc.)

- FOs used to restrict motions at the PIP and DIP
- Generally, IPs maintained in full extension to keep the collateral ligaments stretched and to prevent IP flex contracture (unless condition dictates otherwise)
- Used to promote healing (e.g., phalanx fx, PIP/DIP dislocation, etc.) and to provide prolonged finger stretch (e.g., burns and contractures).

Ring Stabilizers

- Swan neck ring-FO that prevents hyperextension of the PIP joint (via three point pressure system) but allows full IP flexion
- Boutonnière ring-FO that immobilizes the PIP in extension (prevents flexion) through a three point pressure system.

Wrist-hand-finger Stabilizers

Resting hand splints:

- Static wrist-hand finger orthosis (WHFOs) used to immobilize the wrist, fingers, and thumb
- Usually applied to the volar surface (can be dorsally applied or circumferential)
- Extend from the fingertips to two-thirds of the distal forearm

- Hand usually placed with wrist in neutral to slight extension and the digits in an intrinsic plus position (MCPs flexed 70-90°, IPs in full extension, thumb CMC in palmar abduction and thumb MCP/IP in full extension.
- Immobilization in this position preferred because metacarpophalangeal joint and Interphalangeal collateral ligaments are kept stretched, minimizing future joint capsule contractures.
- In addition, it provides functional thumb position for opposition and three-jaw chuck pinch.

Wrist-hand Stabilizers

Volar wrist-hand stabilizers/wrist cock-up splint

- Wrist-hand orthosis (WHO) extending from distal two-thirds inch of forearm to about one-quarter proximal to the distal palmar crease to allow full metacarpophalangeal flexion while maintaining the functional position of the wrist and hand.
- Uses: include resting wrist and hand in acute arthritis (RA), wrist sprain/contusion, flexor/extensor tendinitis, carpal tunnel syndrome, postsurgical wrist extensor tendon repair, wrist fusion, and skin grafting, contractures prevention, reduce pain, reduce spasticity, prevent ulnar/radial deviation wrist/hand (e.g., RA).

Dorsal wrist-hand stabilizers

- WHO are used to provide the same functions of the volar WHO as well as greater stabilization because of rigid dorsal hand section.
- More difficult to fabricate and fit than the volar WHO

Dynamic (Functional) Orthoses: Upper Limb

Elbow Orthoses-assist in Flexion or Extension

- Dynamic elbow splints, static progressive elbow splints, turnbuckle elbow splints-gently elongate the soft tissues over a long period to attempt to reverse joint malalignment (contractures, burns, and late phase of fracture). They are not used in spastic muscles as they may further increase tone:
  - Dorsal elbow-extension mobilization orthosis-extend the elbow as well as provide mediolateral elbow stability and rotational forearm stability

– Dorsal elbow-flexion mobilization orthosis-flex the elbow and provide mediolateral stability and rotational forearm stability

Forearm Orthosis

Forearm mobilization (corrective) orthosis-dynamic supination/pronation splints Used to increase supination or pronation in forearm rotational contracture, or to increase passive or active-assisted ROM in upper trunk.

Indications

Brachial plexus lesions, or Erb's palsy, and spinal cord injury.

Finger Orthoses

1. **Thumb Mobilization Orthoses:**
   a. *Thumb extension-mobilization orthosis*-dynamic thumb IP extension splints. Use: thumb IP flexion contracture.
   b. *Thumb flexion-mobilization orthosis*-dynamic IP flexion splints *Use:* Thumb IP flexion contractures.
   c. *Thumb abduction-mobilization orthosis*-dynamic thumb abduction splint.
   Use: Thumb-adduction contracture.
2. **Finger mobilization orthosis:**
   a. *Interphalangeal extension-mobilization orthoses*-passively extend the PIP joints
      - Uses: Finger IP flexion contracture, Boutonnière deformity, and postsurgical release of Dupuytren's contracture
      - Examples: Dynamic IP extension splints, reverse finger knuckle benders, Capener splints, safety-pin splints, spring coil assist, eggshell finger extension casts, buddy splints.
   b. *Interphalangeal flexion mobilization orthoses*-passively flex PIP joints
      - Use: Finger IP extension contracture
      - Examples: Dynamic IP flexion splints, finger-knuckle benders, fingernail book orthoses, buddy splints.

Metacarpophalangeal (MCP) mobilization orthoses

a. *MCP- extension mobilization orthoses:*
   - Uses: extend MCP joints in MCP-flexion contractures, burns, and post ORIF of metacarpal fracture, patients with weak finger extension (e.g., radial nerve lesion and brachial plexus lesion).
   - Examples: Reverse MCP knuckle benders, dynamic MCP extension splints with dorsal outrigger, MCP extension assists; radial nerve splints

b. *MCP-flexion mobilization orthoses:*
   - Uses: used to flex MCP joints in MCP collateral ligament contractures, extensor tendon shortening, median/ulnar lesion, claw hand, postcapsulotomy, post ORIF of metacarpal fracture.
   - Examples: MCP knuckle benders, dynamic MCP flexion splints with volar outrigger and fingernail hooks, MCP flexion assists.

SHOES AND LOWER LIMB ORTHOSES

Shoe Component (see Fig. 7.35)

A shoe consists of the upper, the sole, and, in most cases, an added heel.

Upper–Part of Shoe above the Sole

- The shoe upper is made of a flexible material-leather, woven fabrics, or synthetic materials such as urethane or vinyl
- In the oxford style shoe, the upper consists of three basic parts:
  - Vamp (one piece)-anterior part covering the instep and toes
  - Quarters (two pieces sewn together)-the pieces that make up the posterior part; laterally, the quarter is cut lower to avoid infringing on the lateral malleolus
  - High quarter-referred to as high top, offers mediolateral stability
- Tongue-strip of leather lying under the laces

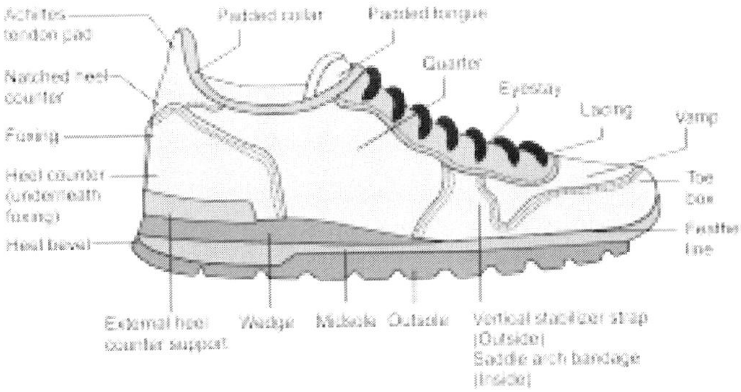

Fig. 7.35: Shoe Component

- Throat-opening at the base of the tongue, entrance to shoe
  - The more anteriorly the throat is located, the more room for internal modification (extra depth shoes also allow more room for shoe orthotics)
- Toe Box-anterior part of the vamp, protects toes from trauma

Sole-bottom part of the shoe; consists of three layers: insole, outsole and the filler between them

- Outsole-part that touches the ground; may be made of leather, rubber, crepe, plastic, wood, or other materials
- Insole-may be made of thin leather or man-made material; part closest to foot
- The filler is usually made of cork dust and latex
- Leather soles-indicated if shoe modifications are needed or attachment to metal AFO
- Rubber soles-modifications are more difficult
- Ball-widest part of sole, at the metatarsal heads

Can be modified internally or externally to help alleviate forefoot pain:

- Shank-narrowest part of sole, between heel and ball,
  - Usually reinforced with metal, leather, fiberboard, or other firm material (to provide additional support for the shoe in the region corresponding to the arch of the foot)
  - Can be reinforced with metal for attachment of metal Ankle Foot orthosis (AFO).

- External heel seat-the posterior part of sole to which heel is attached.

Heel-attached to Outer Sole

- The heel height varies from a negative heel that is lower than the forefoot position to 2-3 inches high.
- Purpose of heel:
  - Acts as a shock absorber and prevents shoe from wearing out
  - Shifts weight to the forefoot
- Materials-leather, wood, plastic, rubber, or metal
- Heel block-part attached to heel seat, made of firm material
- Breast-anterior part of heel; height of heel is measured in 1/8 inches at the breast
- Types of heels:
  - Flat heel-broad base, measures 0.75 to 1.25 inches in height
  - Thomas heel-flat with medial extension to support weak foot arch
  - Military heel-slightly narrower base, measures 1.25 to 1.375 inches
  - Cuban heel-still narrower base, higher heel
  - Spring heel-placed under outer sole, eliminates breast, only 0.125 inches.
- Many athletic shoes eliminate the heel because one can run faster this way
- Height may be a factor in clinical conditions
  - Shortening of gastrocnemius
  - Low back pain.
  - High heels make ankle and foot more unstable.
- Heel counter-reinforces the shoe, stabilizing the foot by supporting and controlling the calcaneus
  - Usually extends anteriorly to the heel breast
  - May extend further in specially made shoes.
- Collar-band of leather stitched to the top of the quarters
  - Sometimes used to reduce postioning
  - Can also prevent shoe from falling off.
- Lace Stay-portion containing the eyelets for laces
  - Usually part of the vamp
  - Can be part of the quarters

SHOE MODIFICATIONS

Internal Modifications

- **Heel cushion-relief/excavation:** is a soft pad with excavation under painful part of heel (e.g., a calcaneal spur)
- **Inner sole excavation/relief:** is a soft pad with excavation under one or more painful bony prominence (usually metatarsal heads). The excavation is usually filled with compressible material
- **Scaphoid pads/arch cookies/navicular pad (see Fig. 7.36) :** a rubber, cork, or plastic foam wedge used to provide medial longitudinal arch support.

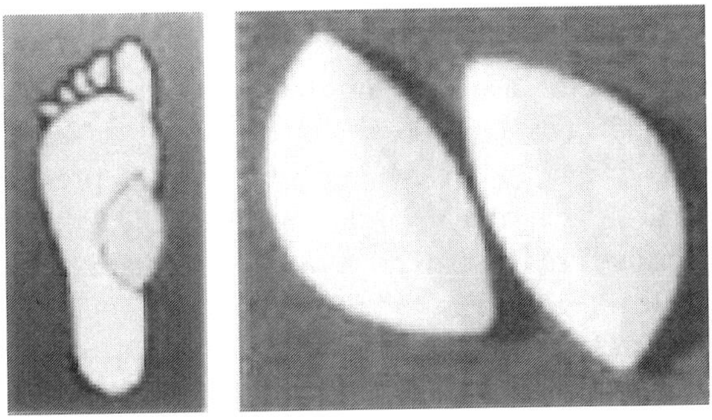

Fig. 7.36: Scaphoid pads

- Metatarsal pads: dome shaped pads glued to the inner sole with the apex under the metatarsal shafts. It relieves pressure from the metatarsal heads by transferring the load to the metatarsal shafts
- Internal heel wedges: can be applied medially and promote hind-foot inversion (e.g., in flexible pes planus) or laterally, and promote hindfoot eversion and relive pressure on the cuboid (e.g., in flexible pes varus.) It also increases total plantar-bearing area and can be used in fixed pes varus
- Toe crest: used to relieve pressure at the distal end and plantar surface of the toes (typically for hammer toes).

Foot Orthoses (inserts or inlays)

- **Univ. of California Biomechanics Lab orthosis (UCBL) (see Fig. 7.37):** custom-molded orthosis used to realign flexible flat foot; it

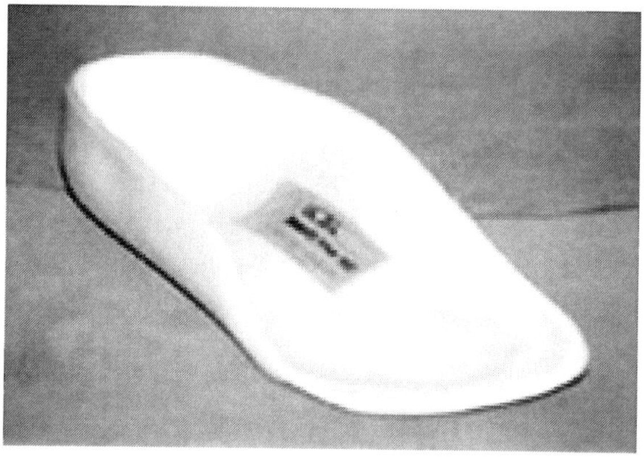

Fig. 7.37: UCBL

encompasses the heel and hindfoot, providing very effective longitudinal arch support.

- Heel cup: provides calcaneal support; used to prevent lateral calcaneal shift (calcaneal valgus) in the flexible flat foot.
- Longitudinal arch insert: can be applied medially or laterally.
- Plastazote full-contact insoles: custom molded, made of various densities and thickness. Accommodating many foot problems/ deformities, these insoles provide almost immediate comfort for plantar outgrowths.
- Other available foot orthoses include: sesamoid inserts, metatarsal inserts, Levy balancer, the Mayer, Morton's toe extension.

External Modifications

Sole Modifications

- **Rocker bar:** this is a convex strip placed across the sole just posterior to the metatarsal heads. It is longer than the metatarsal bar.
  - It can be used to relieve metatarsal pain (by relieving pressure), quicken the gait cycle (by assisting rollover during stance), assist dorsiflexion or decrease demand on weak plantar flexors (push off).
  - It can include entire heel and sole to become rocker-bottom shoe.

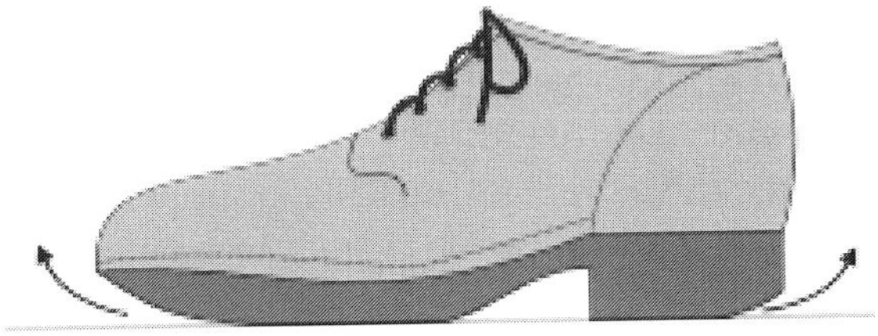

Fig. 7.38: Rocker bar

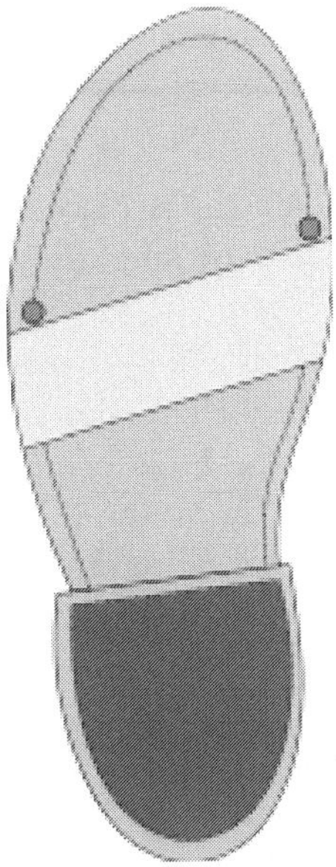

Fig. 7.39: Metatarsal Bar

- **Metatarsal bar (see Fig. 7.39):** This is a simple bar placed in the sole just posterior to the metatarsal heads; it relieves pressure from the metatarsal heads by transferring load to the metatarsal shafts during stance.
- **Sole wedge:** lateral sole wedge promotes forefoot eversion; medial wedge promotes forefoot inversion.
- **Toe wedge:** medial toe wedge is used to encourage toeing-in and is commonly used with a medial heel wedge. Lateral toe wedge (pigeon-toe wedge) is used to assist the foot to toe out.

- **Sole flare:** provides greater stability by widening the base of support of the shoe; a medial flare resists eversion, while a lateral flare resists inversion of the foot.
- **Shank filler:** can be applied medially to support medial longitudinal arch or it can be applied laterally to support lateral longitudinal arch.
- **Steel shank:** is inserted between the inner and outer soles to prevent motion of the anterior sole (bending of the sole) and thus reduce stress on metatarsals/phalanges. It is commonly used with the rocker bar to assist rollover.

Heel Modifications

- Heel wedge (see Fig. 7.40): can be placed either medially (to rotate hindfoot into inversion) or laterally (to rotate hindfoot into eversion).
- Heel flare: applied either medially (to resist hindfoot eversion) or laterally (to resist hind-foot inversion).
- Heel extension: can project anteriorly either medially (Thomas heel) or laterally (reverse Thomas heel). The Thomas heel provides support to the medial longitudinal arch; the reverse Thomas heel provides support to the lateral longitudinal arch.

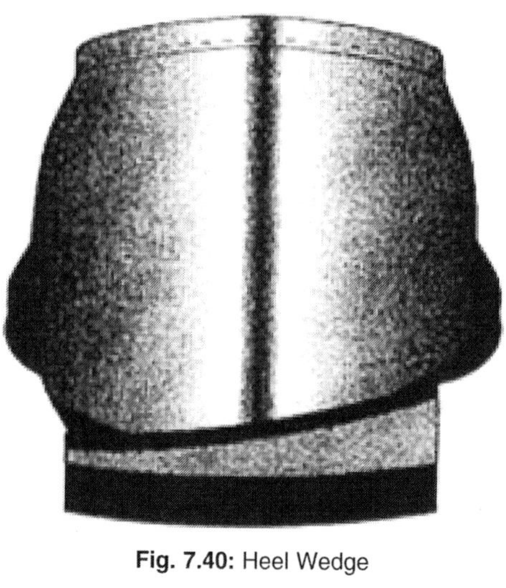

Fig. 7.40: Heel Wedge

- Cushioned Heel ("SACH" heel): is a heel with the posterior portion replaced by a rubberized, compressible material to absorb shock at heel (foot) strike. Cushioned heel with shift weight line (line of gravity) anterior to the knee joint at initial contact causing an extension moment of the knee (thus stabilizing knee).
- Heel lift: is used to compensate for fixed pes equinus deformity or for a leg length discrepancy of more than one fourth to one half inch (or if symptomatic).

SPLINTING

Splinting is a commonly used therapeutic procedure in the management of hand injuries. Splints can provide the essential therapeutic means of maintaining a position and holding it both statically and dynamically. The splint design follows specific principles with respect to the soft tissue trauma. Splinting is a combination of art and science and the creativeness of the therapist whose in-depth knowledge of anatomy and kinesiology is applied in the design and construction of custom-fabricated splints.

Splints are usually referred to as being either static or dynamic. The static splint is designed to support the hand, and the dynamic splint is designed to mobilize the hand.

Types of Splints

Static Splints

Splints are often classified as either static or dynamic. The static splint has no movable parts and is designed to support or limit joint activity. The rationale for static splints can be outlined as follows:

- Protects joint integrity by immobilization of the joint.
- Maintains correct joint alignment.
- Prevents developing contractures.
- Provides support for joint laxity or for a ligament injury.
- Maintains passive ROM gained with dynamic splinting or other therapeutic passive stretching techniques.
- Positions one joint to improve the function of another joint.

Dynamic Splints

Dynamic splinting is the application of a moving force compartment that remains approximately constant as the part moves. The use of carefully placed outriggers provides a direction of force for traction obtained by the pull of rubber bands and individual slings. More specifically, the outrigger serves as the fulcrum for the dynamic splint. These splints are applied when the inflammatory response is under control and when assistance is needed in gaining passive ROM, if the patient's ROM has started to plateau. The considerations for the design of a dynamic splint are as follows:

1. Provides resistance
2. Prolongs stretching
3. Substitution.

Indications

Temporary immobilization to improve pain and discomfort, decrease blood loss, reduce the risk for fat emboli and minimize the potential for further neurovascular injury associated with:

1. Fractures
2. Deep lacerations across joints
3. Painful joints associated with imflammatory disorders
4. Dislocated joint after reduction
5. Sprain: torn or stretched ligaments
6. Strain: torn or stretched muscles or tendons
7. Postoperative immobilization.

Contraindications

- Absolute: None.
- Relative: Injuries involving open wounds or infections need easily removable splints to allow soft tissue care.

Patient Education

- Instructions should be both verbal and written
- Explain and demonstrate the importance of elevation to minimize swelling and decrease pain

- Apply ice bags or cold packs (bags of frozen vegetables also work well) for at least 30 minutes at a time during the first 24-48 hours after injury to decrease swelling and pain
- Avoid getting the splint wet - some splints may be removable for bathing purposes, otherwise plastic bags may be placed over the splint to keep it dry while bathing
- Explain signs of infection and vascular compromise, instruct patient to seek help for any concerns
- Instruct patient to return for evaluation of damaged/broken or wet splint
- Discuss follow-up guidelines.

Mechanical Principles of Splint Design

- Increase the area of force application to disperse pressure
- Increase the mechanical advantage to reduce pressure and increase comfort
- Ensure three points of pressure (Three point rule of Jordan, F1=F2+F3) (see Fig. 7.41)
- Add strength through contouring
- Perpendicular traction for dynamic splinting
- Acceptable pressure for dynamic splinting.

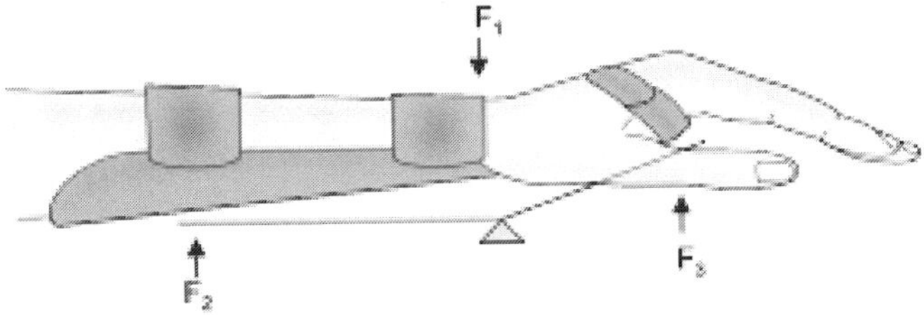

Fig. 7.41: Three point rule of Jordan, F1=F2+F3

Materials

- Plaster Rolls or sheets
  - Strips or rolls of various width made from crinoline-type, material impregnated with plaster which crystallizes or "sets" when water is added

- Prefabricated Splint Rolls (Ortho-Glass)
  - Layers of fiberglass between polypropylene padding
- Stockinette
- Cast padding
- Elastic bandages
- Adhesive tape
- Heavy scissors
- Bucket
- Protective sheets or pads to protect patient clothing
- Gloves.

UPPER EXTREMITY

Long Arm Posterior Splint (See Fig. 7.42)

Indications

- Elbow and forearm injuries
- Distal humerus fracture
- Both-bone forearm fracture
- Unstable proximal radius or ulna fracture (sugar-tong better).

Doesn't completely eliminate supination/pronation -either add an anterior splint or use a double sugar-tong if complex or unstable distal forearm fracture.

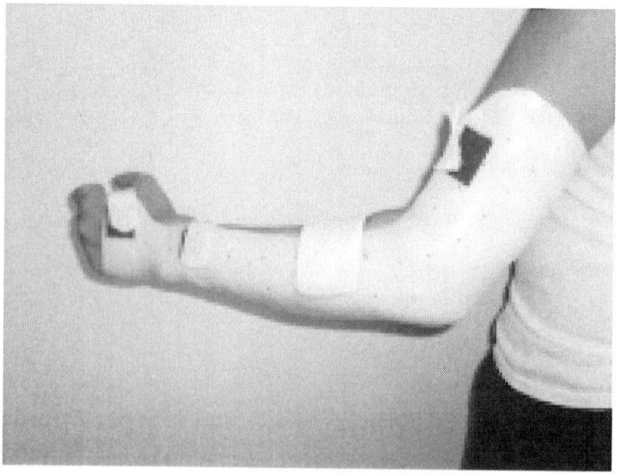

Fig. 7.42: Long Arm Posterior Splint

Double Sugar Tong

Indications

- Elbow and forearm fracture - prox/mid/distal radius and ulnar fracture.
- Better for most distal forearm and elbow fracture because limits flexion/extension and pronation/supination.

Forearm Volar Splint aka 'Cockup' Splint (see Fig. 7.43)

Indications

- The splint is of value because it corrects flexion deformity at the wrist, as well as maintaining dorsal flexion until muscle balance has been restored and there is no further need for its use.

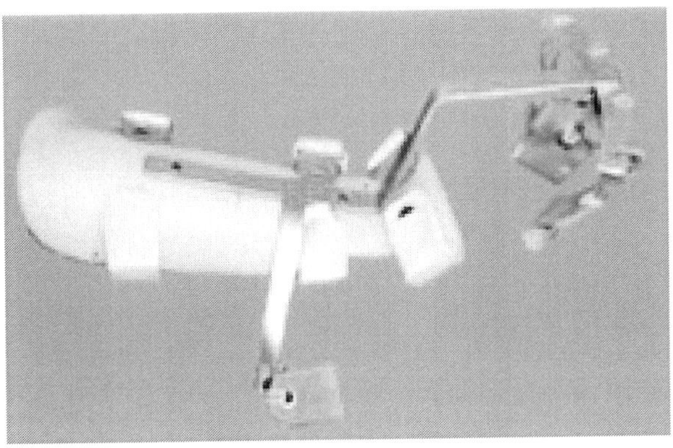

Fig. 7.43: Cockup Splint

- It is light in weight, easily applied and removed, so that any method of physiotherapy may be applied while it is in use.
- For the correction of flexion deformity at the wrist, it employs the principle of the screw. While any amount of power may be exerted by its use, the adjustment may be so fine as to cause the patient no discomfort.

Considerable pressure may be exerted on the dorsum of the wrist and to minimize this pressure effect, a piece of silence cloth or other material is interposed between the splint and the dorsal surface of the forearm.

Finger Splints (see Fig. 7.44)

- *Sprains* - dynamic splinting (buddy taping).
- *Dorsal/Volar finger splints* - phalangeal fracture, though gutter splints probably better for proximal fracture.

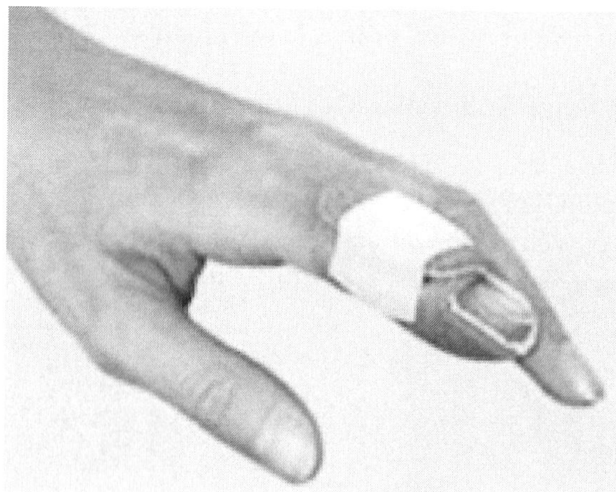

Fig. 7.44: Mallet Finger Splint

Posterior Ankle Splint (see Fig. 7.45)

- Indications
  - Distal tibia/fibula fracture

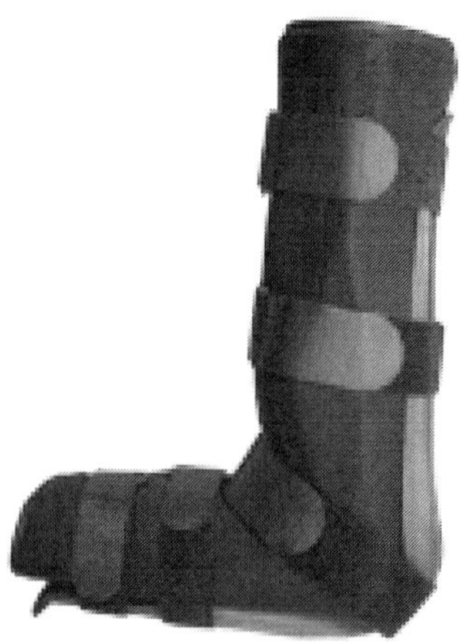

Fig 7.45: Posterior Ankle Splint

  - Reduced dislocations
  - Severe sprains
  - Tarsal/metatarsal fracture
- Use at least 12-15 layers of plaster.
- Adding a co-aptation splint (stirrup) to the posterior splint eliminates inversion/eversion - especially useful for unstable fracture and sprains.

COMPLICATIONS, PREVENTION AND MANAGEMENT

Compartment Syndrome

- Usually less common in splints than with circumferential casts
- May occur associated with splints from constricting webril (cast padding) or elastic bandages that cause increased pressure within a closed space on an extremity
- Increased pressure leads to inadequate tissue perfusion and loss of tissue (muscle, vascular and nerve) function within the compartment.
- *Presenting signs and symptoms:*
  (The "5 P's" are pathognomonic for ischemia: pain, pallor, paresthesias, paralysis, and pulselessness, but seldom all occur simultaneously, and when they do - indicate a late finding associated with poor prognosis).
  - Pain in the extremity
  - Tenderness over the involved compartment
  - Significant pain with passive stretching of ischemic muscle tissue
  - Diminished distal pulses and sensation
  - Delayed capillary refill, and pale cool skin.

Prevention

- Avoid wrapping bandages too tightly or making circumferential splints
- Elevate the extremity to decrease swelling
- Apply topical cold packs
- No weight bearing
- Early (24-48 hour) follow-up for high-risk injuries

Management

- Remove all constricting bandages and splint materials
- Consider compartment pressure monitoring
- Early consultation with orthopedist and/or vascular surgeon for possible fasciotomy.

Pressure Sores

- Uncommon with short term splinting
- Can result from stockinette wrinkles, irregular wadding of padding, insufficient padding over bony prominences or indentions in plaster form using fingers to mold splint
- If suspected, remove the splint materials and check the skin carefully, care for wounds and revise the splint if necessary.

Infection

- More common with open wounds, but may occur with intact skin
- Clean and debride wounds well prior to splint application
- Consider using a removable splint for periodic wound checks.

Joint Stiffness

- Expected to some extent after any immobilization of a joint
- Avoid prolonged immobilization if possible.

REFERENCES

1. Cerny, D, Waters R, Hislop H, Perry J. Walking and wheelchair energetics in persons with paraplegia. Phys Ther. 1980; 60(9): 1133-1139.[PubMed]
2. Gonzalez EG, Corcoran PJ, Reyes RL. Energy expenditure in below-knee amputees: correlation with stump length. Arch Phys Med Rehabil. 1974; 55: 111-119. [PubMed]
3. Huang CT, Jackson JR, Moore NB, Fine PR, Kuhlemeier KV, Traugh GH, Saunders PT. Amputation: energy cost of ambulation.Arch Phys Med Rehabil. 1979; 60(1): 18-24. [PubMed]
4. Kay HW, Newman JD. Relative medicine of new amputations: Statistical comparisons of 6,000 new amputees. Orthot Prosthet. 1975; 29: 3-16.

5. Saunders JB. Dec M, Inman, UT, and Eberhart, HD The major determinants of normal and pathological gait. J Bone Joint Surg. 1953; 35A: 543-58. [PubMed]
6. Seymour R. Prosthetics and Orthotics, Lower Limb and Spinal. Philadelphia: Lippincott, Williams and Wilkins; 2002.
7. Tan JC. Practical Manual of Physical Medicine and Rehabilitation: Diagnostics, Therapeutics, and Basic Problems. St. Louis: Mosby, 1998.
8. Traugh GH, Corcoran PJ, Reyes RL. Energy expenditure of ambulation in patients with above-knee amputations. Arch Phys Med Rehabil. 1975; 56: 67-71. [PubMed]
9. Jaipur foot journal, www.jaipurfoot.com
10. Berger N, Fishman S. (eds). Lower Limb Prosthetics. New York University Health Sciences Bookstore: New York, Prosthetics-Orthotics Publications, 1997.
11. Braddom, Randall L. Physical Medicine and Rehabilitation. Philadelphia: W.B. Saunders, 1996; 334-336, 1194-1196.
12. DeLisa JA, Gans BA. Rehabilitation Medicine: Principles and Practice, 3rd ed. Philadelphia: Lippincott-Raven, 1998; 167-187, 635-696.
13. DeLisa JA. Gait Analysis in the Science of Rehabilitation. Rehabilitation Research and Development Service. Department of Veterans Affairs-Veterans Health Administration. Monograph 002, 1998.
14. Downey JA, Myers SJ, Gonzalez EG, Lieberman JS. The Physiological basis of Rehabilitation Medicine. Boston: Butterworth-Heinemann, 1994.
15. Kottke FJ, Lehmann JF, eds. Krusen's Handbook of PM and R, 4th ed. Philadelphia: W. B. Saunders; 1990, 967-975.
16. O'Young B. Young MA, Stiens SA. Physical Medicine and Rehibilitation Secrets. Philadelphia: Hanley and Belfus, 1997.
17. New York University Medical Center Post-Graduate Medical School. Prosthetics and Orthotics: Upper Limb Prosthetics. New York: New York University Medical Center, 1986.
18. Reford JB (ed). Orthotics: Clinical Practice and Rehabilitation Technology. New York; Churchill Livingstone, 1995.

Eight

Disability Evaluation, Concession and Benefits for Disabled

Disability is defined as a physical, mental, or psychological condition that limits a person's activities.

In the past, this was interpreted according to a medical model. That is, disability was linked to various medical conditions, and was viewed as a problem residing solely in the affected individual. Disability was seen solely as the result of an individual's inability to function. Interventions usually included medical rehabilitation and the provision of social assistance.

This medical model has recently been replaced by the social model of disability, which conceptualizes disability as arising from the interaction of a person's functional status with the physical, cultural, and policy environments.

If the environment is designed for the full range of human functioning and incorporates appropriate accommodations and supports, then people with functional limitations would not be "disabled" in the sense that they would be able to fully participate in society. Interventions are thus not only at the individual level (e.g., medical rehabilitation) but also at the societal level, for example the introduction of universal design to make infrastructure more accessible, inclusive education systems, and community awareness programs to combat stigma.

According to the social model, disability is the outcome of the interaction of person and their environment and thus is neither person nor environment specific. The International Classification of Functioning, Disability and Health (ICF) developed by the World Health Organization are the starting point for recent developments in measuring functional capacity.

Based on a theoretical model that draws upon the social model of disability, disability in the ICF is not an "all or nothing" concept. People are not identified as having a disability based upon a medical condition, but rather are classified according to a detailed description of their functioning within various domains. The first of these domains - body structure and function - is the most closely related to the medical model as it refers to the physiological and psychological functions of body systems. Body structures are defined by the ICF as "anatomic parts of the body such as organs, limbs and their components." This domain relates to very specific capabilities, for example being able to lift one's arm over one's head or produce articulate speech sounds. Thus, it is not a "whole" person classification, as are the other domains – activities and participation.

Disability in the ICF arises out of Activity limitations and restrictions placed upon

Participation that grow out of the interaction between body structure and function limitations and an unaccommodating environment. These interactions are summarized in Figure 8.1.

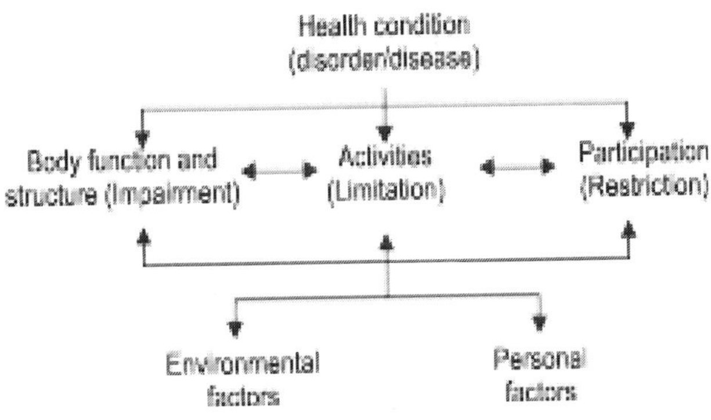

Fig. 8.1: The ICF Model

PREVENTION OF DISABLITIES

Prevention of disabling living conditions is a general societal concern and responsibility of all sectors. Health care has a specific role in the prevention of impairments that may lead to disabilities.

Prevention means actions aimed at preventing the occurrence of physical, intellectual or sensory impairment (primary prevention) or at preventing impairments from causing a permanent functional limitation or disability (secondary prevention).

Prevention includes: Provision of PHC services, prenatal and postnatal care, education, nutrition, immunization campaigns, measures to control endemic diseases, safety regulations, prevention of accidents (traffic safety, occupational safety), and environmental health.

The adequacy of prevention programs in the country context has to be analyzed within a wider framework than in the context of health sector interventions alone.

The following list contains some examples of prevention issues.

Prevention of Disabling Conditions

- Environmental health.
- Living conditions.
- Working conditions.
- Poverty reduction and alleviation.

DISABILITY EVALUATION

The Persons with Disabilities (PWD Act) (Equal Opportunities, Protection of Rights and Full Participation) Act, 1995" has come into enforcement on February 7,1996. This law is an important landmark and is a significant step in the direction to ensure equal opportunities for people with disabilities and their full participation in the nation building. The Act provides for both preventive and promotional aspects of rehabilitation like education, employment and vocational training, reservation, research and manpower development, creation of barrier free environment, rehabilitation of persons with disability, unemployment allowance for the disabled, special insurance scheme for the disabled employees and establishment of homes for persons with severe disability etc.

Main Provisions of the Act

- Prevention and Early Detection of Disabilities
- Education

- Employment
- Non-Discrimination
- Research and Manpower
- Affirmative Action
- Social Security
- Grievance Redressal.

Prevention and Early Detection of Disabilities

- Survey, Investigations and research shall be conducted to ascertain the cause of occurrence of disabilities.
- Various measures shall be taken to prevent disabilities. Staff at the Primary Health Centre shall be trained to assist in this work.
- All the children shall be screened once in a year of identifying "at-risk" cases.
- Awareness campaigns shall be launched and sponsored to disseminate information.
- Measures shall be taken for pre-natal, perinatal, and post-natal care of the mother and child.

Right to Free Education

- Every child with disability shall have the rights to free education till the age of 18 years in integrated schools or special schools.
- Appropriate transportation, removal of architectural barriers and restructuring of curriculum and modifications in the examination system shall be ensured for the benefit of children with disabilities.
- Children with disabilities shall have the right to free books, scholarships, uniform and other learning material.
- Special schools for children with disabilities shall be equipped with vocational training facilities.
- Non-formal education shall be promoted for children with disabilities.
- Teachers Training Institutions shall be established to develop requisite manpower.
- Parents may move to appropriate fora for the redressal of grievances regarding the placement of their children with disabilities.

Employment

- Three percent of vacancies in government employment shall be reserved for people with disabilities, 1% each for persons suffering from:
  - Blindness or Low Vision
  - Hearing Impairment
  - Locomotor Disability and Cerebral Palsy
- Suitable schemes shall be formulated for
  - The training and welfare of persons with disabilities
  - The relaxation of upper age limit
  - Regulating the employment
  - Health and safety measures and creation of non-handicapping environment in places where persons with disabilities are employed
- Government Educational Institutes and other Educational institutions receiving grant for Government shall reserve at least 3% seats for people with disabilities.
- All poverty allevation schemes shall reserve at least 3% for the benefit of people with disabilities.
- No employee can be sacked or demoted if they become disabled during service, although they can be moved to another post with the same pay and condition. No promotion can be denied because of impairment.

Affirmative Action

- Aids and appliances shall be made available to people with disabilities.
- Allotment of land shall be made at concessional rates to the people with disabilities for :
  - House
  - Business
  - Special Recreational Centres
  - Special Schools
  - Research Schools
  - Factories by Entrepreneurs with Disability

Non Discrimination

- Public buildings, rail compartments, buses, ships and air-crafts will be designed to give easy access to disabled people.
- In all public places and; in waiting rooms, toilets shall be wheel chair accessible. Braile and sound symbols are also to be provide in lifts.
- All the places of public utility shall be made barrier free by providing ramps.

Research and Manpower Development

- Research in the following areas shall be sponsored and promoted:
  - Prevention of Disability
  - Rehabilitation including CBR
  - Development of Assistive Devices
  - Job identification
  - On site Modifications of Offices and Factories.
- Financial assistance shall be made available to the universities, other institutions of higher learning, professional bodies and non-government research-units or institutions, for undertaking research for special education, rehabilitation and manpower development.

Social Security

- Financial assistance to non-government organizations for rehabilitation of persons with disabilities.
- Insurance coverage for the benefit of the government employees with disabilities.
- Unemployment allowance to people with disabilities registered with the special employment exchange for more than a year and who could not be placed in any gainful occupation.

Grievance Redressal

In case of violation of rights as prescribed in that act, people with disabilities may move an application to:

- Chief Commissioner for Persons with Disabilities in the Centre
- Commissioner for persons with Disabilities in the States

MAIN TYPES AND DEFINITIONS OF DISABILITIES

The P.W.D. Act, 1995 defines many aspects including various types of disabilities of handicap. They are:

I. Blindness

"Blindness" refers to a condition where a person suffers from any of the following conditions, namely:

- Total absence of sight; or
- Visual acuity not exceeding 6/60 or 20/200 (snellen) in the better eye with correcting lenses; or
- Limitation of the field of vision subtending an angle of 20 degree or worse.

II. Low Vision

"Person with low vision" means a person with impairment of visual functioning even after treatment or standard refractive correction but who uses or is potentially capable of using vision for the planning or execution of a task with appropriate assistive device.

III. Cerebral Palsy

"Cerebral palsy" means a group of non-progressive conditions of a person, characterized by abnormal motor control posture resulting from brain insult or injuries occurring in the pre-natal, peri-natal or infant period of development.

IV. Hearing Impairment

"Hearing impairment," means loss of sixty decibels or more in the better ear in the conversational range of frequencies.

V. Leprosy Cured

"Leprosy cured person," means any person who has been cured of leprosy but is suffering from:

- Loss of sensation in hands or feet as well as loss of sensation and paresis in the eye and eye-lid but with no manifest deformity

- Manifest deformity and paresis but having sufficient mobility in their hands and feet to enable them to engage in normal economic activity
- Extreme physical deformity as well as advanced age which prevent him from undertaking any gainful occupation, and the expression leprosy cured shall be construed accordingly.

VI. Locomotor

Locomotor disability means disability of the bones, joints or muscles leading to substantial restriction of the movement of the limbs or any form of cerebral palsy.

VII. Mental retardation

Mental retardation means a condition of arrested or incomplete development of mind of a person, which is specially characterized by subnormality of intelligence.

VIII. Mental illness

- Mental illness means any mental disorder other than mental retardation
- Person with disability means a person suffering from not less than forty per cent of any disability as certified by a medical authority.
- Medical authority means any hospital or institution specified for the purposes of this Act by notification by the appropriate Government.

There are five main types of Disabilities: ***(The Blind, The Deaf, The Orthopaedically Handicapped)***, The Negative Leprosy and The Mild Mentally Retarded. However, only the visually impaired, hearing impaired and locomotor disabled are covered for reservation in employment. Those afflicted by cured leprosy and cerebral palsy are covered under the group of locomotor disabled for training and employment purposes. The Mild Mentally Retarded with an IQ between 51 and 70 are served by the VRCs for evaluation and training in vocations.

The general guidelines for evaluation and assessment of various disabilities are issued by the Central ministry of welfare and various amendments from time to time are made. Accordingly Disability Certificate is to be issued by Medical Board constituted by Central and State Govt. consisting of at least three members. In pursuance of various notifications issued by the central and state Govt. it is mandatory that such certificate be granted free of cost and the medical board can avail the help and facility of private practitioners and institutions.

GUIDELINES FOR EVALUATION OF VARIOUS DISABILITIES

Locomotor Disability

Upper Limb

- The estimation of permanent impairment depends upon the measurement of functional impairment and is not expression of a personal opinion.
- The estimation and measurement must be made when the clinical condition is fixed and unchangeable.
- The upper extermity is divided into two component parts, the arm component and the hand component.
- Measurement of the loss of function of arm component consists of measuring the loss of motion, muscle strength and co-ordinated activities.
- Measurement of the loss of function of hand component consists of determining the Prehension, Sensation and Strength. For estimation of Prehension Opposition, lateral pinch, cylindrical grasp spherical grasp and hook grasp have to be assessed as shown in the column of "prehension component" in the proforma.
- The impairment of the entire extremity depends on the combination of the functional impairment of both components.

Arm Component

Total value of arm component is 90%.

Principles of evaluation of range of motion of joints :

- The value of maximum R.O.M. in the arm component is 90%
- Each of the three joints of the arm is weighed equally (30%).

Example

A fracture of the right shoulder joint may affect range of motion so that active abduction is 90%. The left shoulder exhibits a range of active abduction of 180%. Hence there is loss of 50% of abduction movement of the right shoulder. The percentage loss of arm component in the shoulder is 50 × 0.30 or 15 per cent loss of motion for the arm component.

If more than one joint is involved, same method is applied and the losses in each of the affected joints are added. Say:

- Loss of abduction of the shoulder = 60%
- Loss of extension of the wrist = 40%

Then, Loss of range of motion for the arm = (60 × 0.30) + (40 × 0.30) = 30%.

Principles of Evaluation of Strength of muscles

- Strength of muscles can be tested by manual testing like 0-5 grading.
- Manual muscle grading can be given percentages like:
  0. — 100 %
  1. — 80 %
  2. — 60 %
  3. — 40 %
  4. — 20 %
  5. — 0 %
- The mean percentage of muscle strength loss is multiplied by 0.30.
- If there has been a loss of muscle strength of more than one joint, the values are added as has been described for loss of range of motion.

Principles of Evaluation of Co-ordinated Activities

- The total value for co-ordinated activities is 90%.

- Ten different co-ordinated activates are to be tested as given in the Proforma.
- Each activity has a value of 9%.

Combining Value for the Arm Component

The value of loss of function of arm component is obtained by combining the value of range of movement, muscle strength and co-ordinated activities, using the combining formula:

$$a = \frac{b\,(90 - a)}{90}$$

Where a = higher value and b = lower value

Example:

Let us assume that an individual with a fracture of the right shoulder joint has in addition to 16.5% of motion his arm, 8.3% loss of strength of muscles, and 5% loss of coordination. We combine these values as:

Range of motion: 16.5%

Strength of Muscles: 8.3%

$$8.3\,(16.5 = \frac{8.3\,(90 - 16.5)}{90} = 3.3\%$$

Co-ordination : 5%

$$23.3 = \frac{5\,(90 - 23.5)}{90} = 27.0\%$$

So total value of arm component = 27.0%.

Hand Component

- Total value of hand component is 90%.
- The functional impairment of hand is expressed as loss of prehension, loss of sensation, loss of strength.
- Principles of evaluation of prehension
- Total value of prehension is 30%. It includes:
  - Opposition (8%): Tested against Index finger (2%), Middle finger (2%), Ring finger (2%) and Little finger (2%)
  - Lateral pinch (5%): Tested by asking the patient to hold a key.
  - Cylindrical raps (6%), tested for:

  - Large object of 4 inch size (3%)
  - Small object of 1 inch size (3%)
- Spherical Grasp (6%), tested for:
  - Large object 4 inch size (3%)
  - Small object 1 inch size (3%)
- Hook grasp (5%): Tested by asking the patient to lift a bag.

Principles of Evaluation of Sensations

Total value of sensation is 30%. It includes :

- Radial side of thumb (4.8%)
- Ulnar side of thumb (1.2%)
- Radial side of each finger (4.8%)
- Ulnar side of each finger (1.2%).

Principles of Evaluation of Strength

Total value of sensation is 30%. It includes :

- Grip strength (20%)
- Pinch strength (10%).

Strength will be tested with hand dynamo-meter or by clinical method (Grip Method).

10% additional weightage to be given to the following factors :

- Infection
- Deformity
- Malalignment
- Contractures
- Abnormal mobility
- Dominant extremity (4%).

Combining Value of the Hand Component

- The final value of loss of function of hand component is obtained by summing up values of loss of prehension, sensation and strength.
- Combining values for the extremity
- Values of impairment of arm component and impairment of hand component are combined by using the combining formula.

Example

- Impairment of the arm = 27.0%
- Impairment of the hand = 64%

$$64 = \frac{27\,(90 - 64)}{90} = 71.8\%$$

Guidelines for Evaluation of Permanent Physical Impairment in Lower Limbs

- The lower extremity is divided into two component and Stability component
- Mobility component.

Mobility Component

Total value of mobility component is 90 per cent. It includes range of movement and muscle strength.

Principles of Evaluation of Range of Movement

1. The value of maximum range of movement in the mobility component is 90 per cent.
2. Each of the three joints i.e. hip knee, foot-ankle component, is weighed equally - 0.30.

Example

- A fracture of the right hip joint may affect range of motion so that active abduction is 27 degree. The left hip exhibits a range of active abduction of 54 degree. Hence, there is loss of 50 per cent of abduction movement of the right hip. The percentage loss of mobility component in the hip is 50 X 0.30 or 15 per cent loss of motion for the mobility component.
- If more than one joint is involved, same method is applied and the losses in each of the affected joints are added. *For Example:*
  - Loss of abduction of the hip = 60%
  - Loss of extension of the knee = 40%
  - Loss of range of motion for mobility component (60 × 0.30) + 40 × 0.30) = 30%

Principles of Evaluation of Muscle Strength

- The value for maximum muscle strength in the leg is 90 per cent.
- Strength of muscles can be tested by manual testing like 0-5 grading.
- Manual muscle gradings can be given percentages like

  Grade 0 = 100 %

  Grade 1 = 80 %

  Grade 2 = 60 %

  Grade 3 = 40 %

  Grade 4 = 20 %

  Grade 5 = 0 %
- Mean percentage of muscle strength loss is multiplied by 0.30.
- If there has been a loss of muscle strength of more than one joint, the values are added as has been described for loss of range of motion.

Combining Values for the Mobility Component

Let us assume that the individual with a fracture of the right hip joint has in addition to 16 per cent loss of motion, 8 per cent loss of strength of muscles.

Combining Values

Motion 16%

Strength 8%

$$16 + \frac{8\,(90 - 16)}{90} = 22.6\%$$

Where a = higher value b = lower value

Stability Component

1. Total value of stability component is 90 per cent.
2. It is tested by 2 methods.
   i. Based on scale method
   ii. Based on clinical method.
   - Three different readings (in kilograms) are taken measuring the total body weight (W). Scale 'A' reading and scale 'B' read.

- Guidelines for Evaluation of Permanent Physical Impairment of Trunk (Spine)
- The local effects of lesions of spine can be divided into traumatic and non-traumatic lesions.

Traumatic Lesions

Cervical Spine Fracture	*Percent Whole Body Permanent Physical Impairment and Loss of Physical function to whole Body*
A. Vertebral compression 25 per cent, one or two vertebral adjacent bodies, no fragmentation, no involvement of posterior elements, no nerve root involvement, moderate neck rigidity and persistent soreness.	20
B. Posterior elements with X-ray evidence of moderate partial dislocation.	
• No nerve root involvement, healed	15
• with persistent pain, with mild motor and sensory manifestations	25
• With fusion, healed, no permanent motor or sensory changes.	20
C. Severe dislocation, fair to good reduction with surgical fusion.	
• No residual motor or sensory changes	25
• Poor reduction with fusion, persistent radicular pain, motor involvement only slight weakness and numbness	35
• Same as (b) with partial paralysis, determine additional rating for loss of use of extremities and sphincters.	

Contd...

Contd...

Cervical Intervertebral Disc	
1. Operative, successful removal of disc, with relief of acute pain, no fusion, no neurologic residual.	10
2. Same as above with neurological manifestations, persistent pain, numbness, weakness in fingers	20
Thoracic and Dorsolumbar Spine Fracture	
	Percent whole body Permanent Physical Impairment and Loss of Physical Function to whole body
• Compression 25 per cent, involving one or two vertebral bodies, mild, no fragmentation, healed, no neurological manifestations.	10
• Compression 50 per cent, with involvement posterior elements, healed, no neurologic manifestations, persistent pain, fusion, indicated.	20
• Same as above with fusion, pain only on heavy use of back.	20
• Total paraplegia	100
• Posterior elements, partial paralysis with or without fusion, should be rated for loss of use of extremities and sphincters.	

Contd...

Contd...

Low Lumbar

1. Fracture

• Vertebral compression 25 per cent one or two adjacent vertebral bodies little or fragmentation, no definite pattern or neurologic changes.	15
• Compression with fragmentation posterior elements, persistent pain, weakness and stiffness, healed, no fusion, no lifting over 25 pounds	40
• Same as above, healed with fusion, mild pain	25
•. Same as above, nerve root involvement to lower extremities, determine additional rating for loss of industrial, function to extremities.	
• Same as above, with fragmentation of posterior elements, with persistent pain after fusion, no neurologic findings.	35
• Same as above, with nerve root involvement to lower extremities, rate with functional loss to extremities.	
• Total paraplegia.	100
•. Posterior elements, partial paralysis with or without fusion, should be rated for loss of use of extremities and sphincters.	

2. Neurogenic Low Back Pain-Disc Injury

• Periodic acute episodes with acute pain and persistent body list, test, tests for sciatic pain positive, temporary recovery 5 to 8 weeks.	5
• Surgical excision of disc, no fusion, good results, no persistent sciatic pain.	10
• Surgical excision of disc, no fusion, moderate persistent pain and stiffness aggravated by heavy lifting with necessary modification of activities.	20

Contd...

Contd...

D. Surgical excision of disc with fusion, activities of lifting moderately modified.	15
E. Surgical excision of disc with fusion, persistent pain and stiffness aggravated by heavy lifting, necessitating modification of all activities requiring heavy lifting	25

Non-Traumatic Lesions

Scoliosis

The whole Spine has been given rating of 100 per cent and region wise the following percentages are given :

- Dorsal Spine - 50 per cent
- Lumbar Spine - 30 sper cent
- Cervical Spine - 20 per cent

Kobb's method for measurement of angle of curve in standing position is to be used. The curves have been divided into three sub groups (see Table 8.1).

Table 8.1

	Cervical Spine	*Thoracic Spine*	*Lumbar Spine*
Less than 30° (Mild)	20%	5%	5%
1° - 60° (Moderate)	3%	15%	12%
Above 60° (Severe)	5%	25%	33%

In the curves ranging above 60 degree, cardio-pulmonary complications are to be graded separately. The junctional curves are to be given that rating depending upon level of apex of curve. For example, if apex of dorso-lumbar curve falls in the dorsal spine the curve can be taken as a dorsal curve. When the scoliosis is adequately compensated, 5 per cent reduction is to be given from final rating (for all assessment primary curves are considered for rating).

Kyphosis

The same total rating (100 per cent) as that suggested for scoliosis is to be given for kyphosis. Region-wise percentages of physical impairment are:

- Dorsal 50 per cent
- Cervical Spine 30 per cent
- Lumbar Spine 20 per cent.

For dorsal spine the following further grading are:

- Less than 20 degree 10 per cent
- 21 degree - 40 degree 15 per cent
- 41 degree - 60 degree 20 per cent
- Above 60 degree 25 per cent.

For kyphosis of lumbar and cervical spine 5 per cent and 7 per cent respectively have been allocated.

Paralysis of flexors and extensors of dorsal and lumbar spine.

The motor power of these muscles to be grouped as follows:

- Normal
- Weak - 5 per cent
- Paralysed - 10 per cent

Paralysis of Muscles of Cervical Spine

For cervical spine the rating of motor power is as follows (see Table 8.2):

Table 8.2

	Normal	*Weak*	*Paralysed*
Flexors	0	5%	10%
Extensors	0	5%	10%
Rotators	0	5%	10%
Side bending	0	5%	10%

Miscellaneous

Those condition of the spine which cause stiffness and pain, etc. are rated as follows (see Table 8.3):

Table 8.3

	% physicalimpairment
A. Subjective symptoms of pain. No involuntary muscle spasm. Not substantiated by demonstrable structural pathology.	0%
B. Pain, Persisent muscle spasm and stiffness of spine, substantiated by demonstrable mild radiological changes.	10%
C. Same as B, with moderate radiological changes	15%
D. Same as B, with severe radiological changes involving and one of the region of spine (cervical, dorsal or lumbar)	20%
E. Same as D, involving whole spine	30%

In kypho-scoliosis, both curves to be assessed separately and then percentage of disability to be summed.

Guidelines for Evaluation of Permanent Physical Impairment in Amputees

Basic Guidelines

1. In case of multiple amputees (see Tables 8.3, Table 8.4 and Table 8.5), if the total sum of percentage permanent physical impairment is above 100 per cent, it should be taken as 100 per cent.
2. Amputation at any level with uncorrectable inability to wear and use prosthesis, should be given 100 per cent permanent physical impairment.
3. In case of amputation in more than one limb percentage of each limb is counted and another 10 per cent will be added, but when only toes or fingers are involved, only another 5 per cent will be added.
4. Any complication in the form of stiffness, neuroma, infection etc. has to be given a total of 10 per cent additional weightage.
5. Dominant upper limb has been given 4 per cent extra percentage.

Table 8.4

	Upper Limb Amputations	Per cent Permanent Physical Impairment and loss of physical function of each limb
1.	Fore-quarter amputation	100 per cent
2.	Shoulder Disarticulation	90 per cent
3.	Above Elbow upto upper 1/3 of arm	85 per cent
4.	Above Elbow upto lower 1/3 of arm	80 per cent
5.	Elbow disarticulation	75 per cent
6.	Below Elbow upto upper 1/3 of forearm	70 per cent
7.	Below Elbow upto lower 1/3 of forearm	65 per cent
8.	Wrist disarticulation	60 per cent
9.	Hand through carpal bones	55 per cent
10.	Thumb through C.M. or through 1st MC Joint	30 per cent
11.	Thumb disarticulation through metacarpo-phalangeal Joint or through proximal phalanx	25 per cent
12.	Thumb disarticulation through inter phalanageal Joint or through distal phalanx.	15 per cent

Table 8.5

		Index Finger (15%)	Middle Finger (5%)	Ring Finger (3%)	Lit Fin (2%)
1.	Amputation through promimal phalanx or disarticulation through MP joint	15%	5%	3%	2%
2.	Amputation through middle phalanx or disarticulation through PIP joint	10%	4%	2%	1%
3.	Amputation through distal phalanx or disarticulation through DIP joint	5%	2%	1%	1%

Table 8.6

Lower Limb Amputations

1.	Hind quarter	100 per cent
2.	Hip disarticulation	90 per cent
3.	Above knee upto upper 1/3 of thigh	85 per cent
4.	Above knee upto lower 1/3 of thigh	80 per cent
5.	Through knee	75 per cent
6.	B.K. upto 8 cm	70 per cent
7.	B.K. upto lower 1/3 of leg	60 per cent
8.	Through Ankle	55 per cent
9.	Syme's	50 per cent
10.	Upto mid-foot	40 per cent
11.	Upto fore-foot	30 per cent
12.	All toes	20 per cent
13.	Loss of first toe	10 per cent
14.	Loss of second toe	5 per cent
15.	Loss of third toe	4 per cent
16.	Loss of fourth toe	3 per cent
17.	Loss of fifth toe	2 per cent

Guidelines for Assessment of Physical Impairment in Neurological Conditions

- Assessment in neurological conditions (See Tables 8.6, 8.7 and 8.8) is not the assessment of disease but it is the assessment of the effects. i.e. clinical manifestations.
- Any neurological assessment has to be done after six months of onset.
- These guidelines will only be used for Central and upper motor neurone lesions.
- Proforma A and B will be utilized for assessment of lower motor neurone lesions, muscular disorders and other locomotor conditions.
- Total percentage of physical impairment in neurological conditions will not exceeds 100 per cent.
- In the mixed cases the highest score will be taken into consideration. The lower score will be added to it and calculations will be done by the formula :

$$a + \frac{b\,(100 - a)}{100}$$

- Additional rating of 4 per cent will be given for dominant upper extremity.
- Additional 10 per cent has been given for sensation in each extremity, but the maxi -mum total physical impairment will not exceed 100 per cent.

Table 8.7: Motor System Disability

	Disability Rate
Monoparesis	25 per cent
Monoplegia / Hemiparesis	50 per cent
Paraparesis	75 per cent
Paraplegia	100 per cent
Hemiplegia / Quadriparesis	75 per cent
Quadriplegia	100 per cent

Table 8.8: Sensory System Disability

	Disability Rate
Anaesthesia/Rypoaesthesia/ Paraesthesia Each Limb	10 per cent
FOR INVOLVEMENT	
For involvement of hand/hands foot/feet	25 per cent

Table 8.9: Speech disability

	Disability Rate
Mild	25 per cent
Moderate	50 per cent
Severe	75 per cent
Very Severe	100 per cent

Tested by a 100 word text. Ability to read (in educated), comprehend when read out, answer question on text clearly and ability to write a synopsis (in educated).

Guidelines for Evaluation of Physical Impairment due to Cardio Pulmonary Diseases

Basic Guidelines

- Modified New York Heart Association subjective classification should be utilised to assess the functional disability.
- The physician should be alert to the fact that patients who come for disability claims are likely to exaggerate their symptoms. In case of any doubt, patients should be referred for detailed physiological evaluation.
- Disability evaluation of cardiopulmonary patients should be done after full medical, surgical and rehabilitative treatment available, because most of these diseases are potentially treatable.
- Assessment of a cardiopulmonary impairment should also be done in diseases which might have associated cardiopulmonary problems, e.g. amputees, myopathies etc.

The proposed modified classification is as follows:

- Group 0 : A patient with cardiopulmonary disease who is a symptomatic (i.e. has no symptoms of breathlessness palpitation, fatigue or chest pain).
- Group 1 : A patient with cardiopulmonary disease who becomes symptomatic during his ordinary physical activity but has mild restriction (25 per cent) of his ordinary physical activities.
- Group 2 : A patient with cardiopulmonary disease who becomes symptomatic during his ordinary physical activity and has 25 - 50 per cent restriction of his ordinary physical activity.

Mental Disorders

Source: Glossary and guide to their classification A Publication by W.H.O.

Mental Retardation: A condition of arrested or incomplete development of mind which is especially characterized by subnormality of intelligence. The coding should be made on the individual's current level of functioning without regard to its nature of causation - such as psychosis, cultural deprivation. Down's syndrome etc, where there is a specific cognitive handicap - such as in speech - the four digit coding should be based on assessments of cognition outside the area of specific handicap. The assessment of intellectual level should be based on whatever information is available, including clinical evidence, adaptive behaviour and psychometric findings. The IQ levels given are based on a test with a mean of 100 and a standard deviation of 15 - such as the Wechsle scales. They are provided only as a guide and should not be applied rigidly. Mental retardation often involves psychiatric disturbances and may often develop as a result of some physical disease or injury. In these cases, an additional code or codes should be used to identify and associated condition, psychiatric or physical. The impairment and handicap codes should also be consulted.

Mild Mental Retardation

Feeble - minded — Moron
High Grade defect — IQ 50 - 70
Mild mental subnormality

Other Specified Mental Retardation

- Moderate mental retardation Imbecile IQ 35 - 49 - Moderate mental subnormality
- Severe mental retardation IQ 20 -34 - Severe mental subnormality
- Profound mental retardation Idiocy IQ under 20 - Profound mental subnormality.

Unspecified Mental Retardation

Mental deficiency NOS Mental subnormality NOS.

CONCESSIONS OFFERED BY THE CENTRAL GOVERNMENT TO THE PERSONS WITH DISABILITIES

1. Travel Concessions For The Disabled

a. By Train

As per the order of Ministry of Railways, Government of India, the following concessions are available for the disabled:

(i) Blind Person

The blind person travelling alone or with an escort, on production of a certificate from Government doctor or a registered medical practitioner, is eligible to get the concession as below (See Table 8.10):

Table 8.10: Element of Concession

Class	*First Class*	*Second Class*	*Sleeper Class*	*Season First Class*	*Ticket Second Class*
Percentage of Concession	75	75	75	0	50

(ii) Orthopaedically Handicapped Person

The orthopaedically handicapped person travelling with an escort, on production of a certificate from a Government doctor to the effect that the person concerned is orthopaedically handicapped and cannot travel without the assistance of an escort, is eligible for getting concession (see Fig. 8.11).

Table 8.11: Element of Concession

Class	*First Class*	*Second Class*	*Sleeper Class*	*Season First Class*	*Ticket Second Class*
Percentage of Concession	75	75	75	50	50

(iii) Deaf and Dumb Person

A Deaf and Dumb person travelling alone (both afflictions together in the same person) on production of a certificate from a government doctor is eligible for the concession.

Table 8.12: Element of Concession

Class	*First Class*	*Second Class*	*Sleeper Class*	*Season First Class*	*Ticket Second Class*
Percentage of Concession	75	75	75	50	50

Notes

- A deaf person is allowed 50% concession in railway fare both in first and second class, but concession is not available for the escort.
- A deaf and dumb person is permitted to travel by 2-tier A.C. Sleeper on payment of concessional fare for first class and full surcharge for 2-tier A.C. Sleeper).

(IV) Mentally Retarded Person

A Mentally Retarded person, accompanied by an escort, on production of a certificate in the prescribed form, from a government doctor, is eligible to get the concession.

Note

Mentally Retarded person is permitted to travel by 2-tier A.C. Sleeper on payment of concessional fare for first class and full surcharge for 2-tier A.C. Sleeper.

(b) By Air

(i) Blind Persons

The Indian Airlines Corporation allows 50 percent concessional fare to blind persons on single journey or single fare round trip journey on all domestic flights.

(ii) Locomotor Disability

Locomotor Disabled persons (80% and above) are allowed following concessions in Indian Airlines :

- Fifty percent of Normal Economy Class INR Fare or Point to Point Fare. Full Inland Air Travel Tax and Passenger Service Fee applicable.
- Fifty percent of INR fare applicable to foreigners resident in India for travel on Domestic Sectors. Full Inland Air Travel Tax and Passenger Service Fee applicable.
- By Bus. In state transport the seats are reserved for disabled person.

COMMUNICATION

(a) Postage

Payment of postage, both inland and foreign, for transmission by post of Blind Literature packets is exempted if sent by surface route only. If packets are to be sent by air, prescribed air mail charges should be paid.

The relevant rule from the Post Office Guide is reproduced below:

Exemption from Postal Fees

- Blind Literature packets are exempted from the payment of postage and also for (i) registration fee,
  - fee for acknowledgement, and
  - fee for the attested copy of the receipt
- Postage free 'Blind Literature' packets will be transmitted by surface route only, and if they are to be sent by air, the air mail charge as prescribed for packets has to be paid.

(b) Telecommuncation

- Concessional Telephone Connection to Blind Persons
- It has been decided to provide telephone facility to blind persons on concession and priority basis on the following terms:
  - Rental Rebate-50 percent of the normal rental.
  - Advance Rental-50 percent of the annual advance rental and bimonthly rental as applicable to a private subscriber. This facility is available in Non-OYT (S) category only.

(c) Preference in Allotment of STD/PCO to Handicapped Persons

- Educated unemployed persons are eligible for allotment of STD/ PCOs.
- The educational qualification for the applicant is:
  - VIIIth or Middle School Pass for rural areas.
  - Atleast Matriculation or High School for urban areas.

CUSTOMS CONCESSIONS

Individuals

(Notification No. 105/86 dated 17.2.86 Annexure Issued by the Deptt. of Revenue, Ministry of Finance)

The Central Government exempts goods specified below, when imported into India by a handicapped or disabled person for his personal use, from the whole of the duty of customs and the additional duty.

- Braille writers and Braille writing equipment
- Hand writing equipment, Braille Frames, Slates, writing guides, Braille
  - Erasers, Script writing guides.
- Canes, Electronic aids like the Sonic Guide
- Optical, Environmental Sensors
- Arithmetic Aids like the Taylor Frame (Arithmetic and Algebra Types)
  - Cubarythm, Speaking or Braille Calculator
- Geometrical Aids like Combined Graph and Mathematical Demonstration Board, Braille Protractors, Scales Compasses and Spar Wheels
- Electronic measuring equipment, such as calipers, micrometers, comparators, gauges, blocks levels, and yard sticks
- Drafting drawing aids, tactile displays
- Specially adapted clocks and watches
- Orthopaedic appliances falling under Heading 90.21 of the First Schedule to the said Tariff Act
- Wheel Chairs falling under Heading No. 87.13 of the said First Schedule
- Artificial electronic Larynx and Spares there of.

Institutions

The Institutions for the Blind and the Deaf are permitted to import equipment and apparatus as below, being bonafide gifts to, as purchased out of donations received in foreign exchange.

- All tangible appliances for the blind

- Hearing aids and other audio-visual aids for the education of the deaf
- Vocational aids for the blind and the deaf
- Articles including instruments, apparatus, appliances, machinery and spares or component parts of accessories thereof required by such institution for the purpose of giving training or imparting instructions to the blind and the deaf.

Exemption for Braille Paper

Import of Audio Cassettes

CONVEYANCE ALLOWANCE

In accordance with the revised Orders No.F.19029/2/86-E.IV and F. 19029/1/ 89-E.IV dated 16.5.87 and 12.9.89 respectively, issued by the Ministry of Finance, Department of Expenditure, the Central Government employees who are on regular establishment (including work charged staff) and who are blind or orthopaedically handicapped (with disability of upper or lower extremities) are to be granted conveyance allowance at 5 percent of basic pay subject to a maximum of Rs. 100 p.m. subject to the following conditions:

- An orthopaedically handicapped employee will be eligible for conveyance allowance only if he/she has a minimum 40 percent permanent/partial disability of either upper or lower limbs or 50 percent permanent/partial disability of both upper and lower limbs together.
- Conveyance allowance will be admissible to the orthopaedically handicapped employee on the recommendation of the head of Orthopaedic Department of a Government Civil Hospital.
- In the case of a blind employee the allowance will be admissible on the recommendation of the head of Opthalmological Department of a Government Civil Hospital.
- Conveyance allowance is also applied to Central Government employees suffering from spinal deformity (generally known as hunch back disability) at the same rate as available to other Physically Handicapped persons.

The allowance will not be admissible during leave (except casual level), joining time or suspension.

CHILDREN'S EDUCATIONAL ALLOWANCE

As per Office Memorandum No.21011/21/88-Estt(Allowances) dated 17.10.88, issued by the Ministry of Personnel Grievances and Pensions (Department of Personnel and Training), grant of children educational allowance, reimbursement of tuition fee, etc., to Central Govt. employees will be governed by the Central Civil Services (Educational Assistance) Orders, 1988.

Under this order, the reimbursement of tuition fee in respect of physically handicapped and mentally retarded children of the Central Govt. employee has been enhanced to Rs. 100 p.m. (from class I to XII) in comparison with general category where it restricts only to Rs. 40 p.m. The disabled children will however, get other assistance under this scheme as per rates prescribed for the other children.

SCHEME OF INTEGRATED EDUCATION FOR THE DISABLED CHILDREN

Under the scheme, handicapped children are sought to be integrated in the normal school system. Hundred per cent assistance is provided to the States/UTs for education of the children suffering from certain mild handicaps in common schools with the help of necessary aids, incentives and specially trained teachers.

The following types of disabled children are covered under this scheme:

- Children with locomotor handicaps (O.H.)
- Mildly and moderately hearing impaired
- Partially sighted children
- Mentally handicapped-educable group (IQ 50-70)
- Children with multiple handicaps (blind and orthopaedic, hearing impaired and orthopaedic, educable mentally retarded and orthopaedic, visual impaired and mild hearing handicap).
- Children with learning disabilities.

1. The handicapped children are provided the following allowances and facilities under this scheme:
   - Books and stationery allowance of Rs. 400 per annum
   - Uniform allowance of Rs. 50 per annum
   - Transport allowance of Rs. 50 per month (if a disabled child admitted under the scheme resides in a hostel of the school within the school premises, no transportation charges would be admissible)
   - Reader allowance of Rs. 50 per month in case of blind children after class V
   - Escort allowance for severely handicapped children with lower extermity disabilities @ Rs. 75 per month
   - Actual cost of equipment subject to a maximum of Rs. 2,000 per student for a period of five years.
2. In the case of severly orthopaedically handicapped children, it may be necessary to allow one attendant for 10 children in a school. The attendant may be given the standard scale of pay prescribed for Group 'D' employees in the States/U.Ts concerned.
3. Disabled children residing in school hostels within the same institution where they are studying may also be paid boarding and lodging charges as admissible under the State Govt. rules/schemes. Where there is no State Scheme of Scholarships to hostelers, the disabled children, whose parents income does not exceed Rs. 3,000 per month, may be paid actual boarding and lodging charges subject to a maximum of Rs. 200 p.m.
4. Severely orthopaedically handicapped children residing in school hostels may need the help of a helper or an ayah, a special pay or Rs. 50 p.m. is admissible to any employee of the hostel willing to extend such help to children in addition to his/her duties.
5. In a school in rural areas where at least 10 handicapped children are enrolled, capital cost for purchase of school rickshaw for free use of these children and expenses for Rickshaw Puller Rs. 300 p.m. will be provided under the scheme. In such cases, no transport allowance will be payable to the students.

INCOME TAX CONCESSIONS

Relief For The Handicapped

Section 80 DD: Section 80 DD provides for a deduction in respect of the expenditure incurred by an individual or HUF resident in India on the medical treatment (including nursing) training and rehabilitation, etc., of handicapped dependants. For officiating the increased cost of such maintenance, the limit of the deduction has been raised to Rs. 41,000.

Section 80 V: A new Section 80 V has been introduced to ensure that the parent in whose hands, income of a disabled minor has been clubbed under Section 64, is allowed to claim a deduction upto Rs. 40,000 in case of an individual who is suffering from a permanent disability (including blindness) or is subject to mental retardation.

Section 88 B: This Section provides for an additional rebate from net tax payable by a resident individual who has attained the age of 65 years, has been amended and a tax rebate of Rs. 10,000 has been allowed.

In his budget speech on 15th March, 1995, Sh. Manmohan Singh, Finance Minister, Govt. of India made the following anouncements: Deductions from the total income of handicapped persons under Section 80 V of the Income Tax Act has been raised from Rs. 20,000 to Rs. 40,000.

AWARD OF DEALERSHIPS/AGENCIES BY OIL COMPANIES

Award of Retail Outlet , 2/3 Wheeler Outlet, Kerosene-LDO Dealerships and LPG Distributorships

Ministry of Petroleum and Natural Gas has reserved 7½ percent of all types of dealership agencies of the public sector oil companies for Physically Handicapped/Government personnel (other than Defence personnel) disabled on duty/widows of Government personnel (other than Defence personnel who die in the course of duty).

The oil industry appoints its dealers/distributors through an advertisement in one english daily and one regional daily newspaper having maximum circulation in the district in which the dealership/ distributorship is to be located.

RESERVATION OF JOBS AND OTHER FACILITIES FOR THE DISABLED PERSONS

(i) Three Percent Reservations in Grade 'C' and 'D' Posts

As per the order of Government of India reservation of 3 percent in jobs have been made in Grade 'C' and Grade 'D' posts for the PH persons. The category of andicapped persons benfitted are the blind, the deaf and the Orthopaedically Handicapped (O.H.) Persons, as given below:

Category of Handicapped Percent of Reservation

1. The Blind 1
2. The Deaf 1
3. The O.H. 1

For effective implementation of the reservation it has been advised to maintain a roaster of vacancies arising in Grade 'C' and Grade 'D' posts from year to year. The 34th vacancy may be earmarked for the blind. Similary the 67th vacancy and 100th vacancy would be reserved for the Deaf and the O.H. respectively in a cycle of 100 vacancies.

(ii) Definitions of Disabled for the Purpose of Reservation

1. The Blind: The blind are those who suffer from either of the following conditions:
   a. Total absence of sight.
   b. Visual acuity not exceeding 6/60 or 20/200 (Snellen) in the better eye with correcting lenses.
   c. Limitation of the field of vision subtending an angle of 20 degree or worse.
2. The Deaf: The Deaf are those in whom the sense of hearing is nonfunctional for ordinary purposes of life. They do not hear and understand sounds at all events with amplified speech. The

cases included in this category will be those having hearing loss more than 90 decibles in the better ear (profound impairment) or total loss of hearing in both ears.

3. The Orthopaedically Handicapped: The orthopaedically handicapped are those who have a physical defect or deformity which causes an interference with the normal functioning of the bones, muscles and joints.

(iii) Identification of Jobs

In order to implement these reservations, without loss of productivity some posts are identified disability wise. To ensure sufficient recruitment of blind persons, separate list has been identified for the blind and partially blind persons.

(iv) Posting of Handicapped Candidates

As per the decision of Government of India Grade 'C' and Grade 'D' posts recruited on regional basis and who are physically handicapped may be given posting as far as possible near to their native place within the region subject to administrative constraints. PH employees may be given preference in transfer case near to their native place.

(v) Relaxation of Ban Order on Recruitment to Vacancies Earmarked for PH Persons

As per the Government order regarding ban on filling up of non-operational vacant posts will not be applicable in case of reserve vacancies to be filled up for PH person.

(vi) Carry Forward of Vacant Posts Under Reserve Category

As per the Government order if a reserve category of person is not available or the nature vacancy in an office is such that the given category of person cannot be employed then the post may be carried forward for a period of three subsequent years.

(vii) Appointment of VI Persons as Caner in Government Department

As per the decision of Government of India it has been instructed that recaning of chairs in Government Offices should be done by blind persons as far as possible when the volume of work require a full time chair caner then a suitable post may be created in consultation with the Finance Department.

For the purpose of recaning the chairs in Government offices Vocational Rehabilitation Centres and Special Employment Exchange for the PH persons may be contacted.

(viii) Instruction to Appointing Authority for Intimating Vacancies Reserved for Handicap

As per the existing instruction of the Government all the vacancies in Grade 'C' and 'D' irrespesctive of their nature and duration are to be notified to the Employment Exchange and also to be filled through the agency unless filled through UPSC/SSC. It has also been decided that all the appointee should send their request to Employment Exchange/Special Employment Exchange/nearest Vocational Rehabilitation Centre for P.H. for nominating suitable handicapped persons.

(ix) Grant of Age Concession to PH Persons

As per the Government order it has been decided to extend the age concession of 10 years in favour of handicap persons to recruitment to posts filled through the SSC and through Employment Exchange in Grade 'C' and Grade 'D' posts.

(x) Relaxations in Typing Qualifications

As per the order, PH persons who are otherwise eligible for appointment to posts of LDC but cannot be so appointed for being unable to satisfy the typing qualifications due to their disability may be exempted from the typing qualification for appointment.

(xi) Consideration for Confirmation in Job for Blind Persons

It has been instructed to all the Ministries/Departments of Government of India that there should not be any delay in confirmation of officers including blind persons on account of administrative delay. Ministry/Department should ensure, especially in which blind persons are employed that confirmation is made without delay and at appropriate time.

(xii) Reservation for PH Persons in Posts Filled by Promotion

As per the order handicapped persons may be promoted to Grade 'C' from 'D' and within Grade 'C' against the identified post if they are capable of being filled/held by the appropriate category of PH.

(xiii) Exemptions from Payment of Examinations Fee

As per the order PH persons recruited to Grade 'B' and Grade 'C' posts advertised by the UPSC and SSC will be exempted from the payment of applications and examination fee as prescribed by UPSC/SSC.

SPONSORSHIP POWER TO NATIONAL INSTITUTIONS

The Ministry of Labour in consultation with the Ministry of Social Justice and Empowerment and Department of Personnel and Training has decided to grant co-sponsoring power to the National Level rehabilitation institutes as given below:

1. National Instt. for the Visually Handicapped, Dehradun.
2. National Instt. for the Mentally Retarded, Secunderabad.
3. Ali Yavar Jung National Instt. for the Hearing Handicapped, Mumbai
4. Naional Institute for the Orthopaedically Handicapped, Kolkata
5. Naional Institute for Rehabilitation Training and Research, Cuttack.
6. The Institute for the Physically Handicapped, Delhi.

ECONOMIC ASSISTANCE

Public Sector Banks

Under the Scheme of Public Sector Banks for Orphanages, Women's Homes and Physically Handicapped Persons the benefits of the differential rate of interest are available to physically handicapped persons as well as institutions working for the welfare of the handicapped.

Keeping in view the social objective the interest will uniformly be charged @ 3 percent per annum, Physically handicapped persons including blind eligible under DRI Scheme are also given loans for purchasing of artificial limbs, hearing aids, wheel chair, etc., subject to maximum of Rs. 2,500 per borrower provided such assistance is given along with the advances for productive activities and self-employment ventures and all other requirements under DRI scheme are fulfilled.

Under the scheme of 'Financing Small Scale Industries' a special provision has been made to allow concession of 1/2 percent in the rate of interest to the physically handicapped availing working capital limit above Rs. 25,000 and upto Rs. 2 lakhs.

Subsidy to Handicapped Under the Integrated Rural Development Programme (IRDP)

Under the IRDP, 3 percent quota is earmarked for the Physically Handicapped persons. The Government has now decided that per family subsidy limit under the IRDP be raised from:

- Rs. 3,000 to Rs. 4,000 in normal areas.
- Rs. 4,000 to Rs. 5,000 in drought prone areas and desert development programme areas.
- Rs. 5,000 to Rs. 6,000 for Physically Handicapped beneficiaries.

Nine

Aerobic Fitness

Aerobic simply means in the presence of oxygen. Aerobic refers to those types of exercises that require oxygen to burn fat stores for energy.

Aerobic exercise uses the same large muscle groups, rhythmically, for a period of 15 to 20 minutes or longer while maintaining 60-80% of your maximum heart rate.

Fitness - Ability to perform physical work

- Physical work requires
  - > Cardio respiratory functioning
  - > Muscular strength and endurance
  - > Musculoskeletal flexibility.

Physical fitness is to the human body what fine tuning is to an engine. It enables us to perform up to our potential. Fitness can be described as a condition that helps us look, feel and do our best. More specifically, it is:

"The ability to perform daily tasks vigorously and alertly, with energy left over for enjoying leisure time activities and meeting emergency demands. It is the ability to endure, to bear up, to withstand stress, to carry on in circumstances where an unfit person could not continue, and is a major basis for good health and well-being."

Physical fitness is most easily understood by examining its components, or parts. There is widespread agreement that these four components are basic:

Cardiorespiratory Endurance: the ability to deliver oxygen and nutrients to tissues, and to remove wastes, over sustained periods of time. Long runs and swims are among the methods employed in measuring this component.

Muscular Strength: the ability of a muscle to exert force for a brief period of time. Upper-body strength, for example, can be measured by various weight-lifting exercises.

Muscular Endurance: the ability of a muscle, or a group of muscles, to sustain repeated contractions or to continue applying force against a fixed object. Pushups are often used to test endurance of arm and shoulder muscles.

Flexibility: the ability to move joints and use muscles through their full range of motion. The sit-and reach test is a good measure of flexibility of the lower back and backs of the upper legs.

Body Composition is often considered a component of fitness. It refers to the makeup of the body in terms of lean mass (muscle, bone, vital tissue and organs) and fat mass. An optimal ratio of fat to lean mass is an indication of fitness, and the right types of exercises will help you decrease body fat and increase or maintain muscle mass.

Warmup: 5-10 minutes of exercise such as walking, slow jogging, knee lifts, arm circles or trunk rotations. Low intensity movements that simulate movements to be used in the activity can also be included in the warmup.

Muscular Strength: a minimum of 2– 20-minute sessions per week that include exercises for all the major muscle groups. Lifting weights is the most effective way to increase strength.

Muscular Endurance: at least 3–30-minute sessions each week that include exercises such as calisthenics, pushups, situps, pullups, and weight training for all the major muscle groups.

Cardiorespiratory Endurance: at least 3–20-minute bouts of continuous aerobic (activity requiring oxygen) rhythmic exercise each week. Popular aerobic conditioning activities include brisk walking, jogging, swimming, cycling, rope-jumping, rowing, cross-country skiing, and some continuous action games like racquetball and handball.

FLEXIBILITY: 10-12 minutes of daily stretching exercises performed slowly, without a bouncing motion. This can be included after a warmup or during a cooldown.

COOL DOWN: a minimum of 5-10 minutes of slow walking, low-level exercise, combined with stretching.

BASAL METABOLIC RATE (BMR)

Energy Requirement at Rest

- BMR - liters of O2 consumed per minute
- MET - Multiple of the resting metabolic rate
- 1 MET - Resting oxygen consumption
- 1 MET - 3.5 ml O2/kg-1/ min.
- Men - 2700 × 3000 kcal/ day
- Women - 2000 × 2100 kcal/day
- Light Work - 3 times of resting MET.
- Heavy Work - 6 to 8 times of resting MET.
- Maximal - 9 times of resting MET.

  For, e.g. - Sitting < 20 mins - 1-2 METS
  - Walking for 5-10 mins - 2-2.5 METS
  - Stair case climbing–3-3.5 METS
- METS is linearly related to the heart rate.

Principles of Training

Overload

- The body and its systems must be stimulated at a greater level than normal to enhance the physiological activity.
- Progressive overload allows the body to function more efficiently
- It can be achieved by manipulating combination of training frequency, duration, mode and intensity.
- Overload means that to improve any aspect of physical fitness, the individual must continually increase the demands placed on the appropriate body systems. For example, to develop strength, progressively heavier objects must be lifted. Overload in running programs is achieved by running longer distances or by increasing the speed.

Specificity

- The effects of training are specific to those parts and systems of the body are overloaded.
- As an example of wt.—lifting exercises. Produces muscle hypertrophy where as distance running produces cardiovascular endurance.

The principle of specificity derives from the observation that the adaptation of the body or change in physical fitness is specific to the type of training undertaken. Quite simply this means that if a fitness objective is to increase flexibility, then flexibility training must be used. If one desires to develop strength, resistance or strengthening exercises must be employed. This principle is indeed simple; however, it is frequently ignored. Many fraudulent claims for an exercise product or system promise overall physical fitness from one simple training technique. A person should be suspicious of such claims and should consider whether or not the exercise training recommended is the type that will produce the specific changes desired.

Reversibility

- The effects of training are transient and reversible. Detraining occurs when person stops exercising. After 2 wks of detraining, there is significant reduction in both metabolic and working capacity.

Maintenance

Necessary to avoid effects of detraining.

Progression

Individuals frequently make the mistake of attempting too rapid a fitness change. A classic example is that of the middle-aged man or woman who has done no exercise for 20 years and suddenly begins a vigorous training program. The result of such activity is frequently an injury or, at the least, stiffness and soreness. There are no hard-and-fast rules on how rapidly one should progress to a higher level of activity. The individual's subjective impression of whether or not the body seems to be able to tolerate increased training serves as a good guide. In general it might be reasonable not to progress to higher levels of activity more often than every one or two weeks.

Basic components of Exercise Programme

- Frequency-The inactive person should exercise. one to three times per week, gradually can be increase to 3 to 4 times per week and then every day.
- Duration- For cardiorespiratory endurance, exercise. Session should last for 20 to 30 mins, gradually increasing to 40 to 60 mins
- The total pragramme consist of 3 phases
  - Warm up- 5 to 10 mins
  - Conditioning - 15 to 30 mins
  - Cool down-- 5 to 10 mins

Intensity

- Low intensity with longer duration for Endurance.
- High intensity with shorter duration for Strengh.

A frequency of about every other day or three days per week appears minimally sufficient. Many individuals exercise more frequently than this, and, of course, such additional exercise is acceptable provided that one does not become overtrained and suffer illness or injury.

The intensity of exercise required to produce benefits has been the subject of much study. Many people have the impression that exercise is not doing any good unless it hurts. This is simply not true. Regular exercise at 45 to 50 percent of one's maximal capacity is adequate to improve one's physiological functioning and overall health. This level of intensity is generally comfortable for most individuals. A reliable way to gauge exercise intensity is to measure the heart rate during exercise. An exercise heart rate that is 65 percent of a person's maximal heart rate corresponds to approximately 50 percent of his maximal capacity. Maximal heart rate can be estimated by subtracting one's age in years from 220 (or, in the case of active males, by subtracting half of one's age from 205). Thus, a sedentary 40-year-old man has an estimated maximal heart rate of 180 beats per minute. Sixty-five percent of this maximal rate is 117 beats per minute; thus by exercising at 117 beats per minute, this individual is working at about 50 percent of his maximal capacity. To determine exercising heart rate, a person should exercise for several minutes, to allow the heart rate to adjust. The exerciser should then stop exercising, quickly find the pulse, and count the number of beats for 15 seconds. Multiplying this by four gives the rate in beats per minute. The pulse must be taken immediately after stopping exercise, since the heart rate rapidly begins to return to the resting level after work has been stopped. As noted above, exercising at the 50 percent level of intensity will improve physiologic functioning and provide health benefits. This level of exercise will not produce the maximum fitness needed for competitive athletics.

The physiological response to exercise is dependent on the intensity, duration and frequency of the exercise as well as the environmental conditions. During physical exercise, requirements for oxygen and substrate in skeletal muscle are increased, as are the removal of metabolites and carbon dioxide. Chemical, mechanical and thermal stimuli affect alterations in metabolic, cardiovascular and ventilator function in order to meet these increased demands.

Testing as a Basis for Exercise Program

- Fitness testing of healthy subjects
- Field test running (1.5 miles) or distance run for 12 minutes
- Multistage test measure of vo_2 max (treadmill with 6 stages with 3-6 mins per stage)

STRESS TESTING

- Should have Percent efficiency first, monitored by ECG, be observed at rest, during exercise, during recovery
- Percent efficiency = useful work output × 100 energy expended or work input
- (Treadmill) WORK = weight of the subject × vertical distance the subject is raised walking up the incline of the treadmill)

- (Ergometer bike) WORK = distance (circumference of the flywheel times the number of revolutions) x the bicycle resistance.

Principles of Stress Testing

- Changing the workload by increasing the speed (treadmill) resistance (ergo meter)
- An initial workload that is low in terms of the individual's anticipated aerobic threshold
- Maintenance of each workload
- Termination of the test at the onset of symptoms or abnormality in the ECG
- When available, measurement of the individual's maximal oxygen consumption.

Purpose of Stress Testing

- Helps establish a diagnosis of overt or latent heart disease
- Evaluates cardiovascular functional capacity as a means of clearing individuals with strenuous work
- Determines the physical work capacity (METS)
- Evaluates responses to exercise training and/or preventive programs
- Assists in the selection and evaluation of appropriate modes of treatment programs
- Increases the patient's motivation for entering and adhering to exercise programs
- Used clinically to evaluate patient with chest sensations or history of chest pain.

Preparation for Stress Testing

- Have had a physical examination
- Be monitored by ECG, closely observed at rest and during recovery
- Sign a consent form,

Precautions for Stress Testing

- Monitor the pulse

- BP increases with exercise 7-10 mm of mercury per MET of physical activity (Systolic pressure not exceed 220 to 240mmHg; Diastolic >120 mm Hg)
- Rate and depth and respiration (respiration should not be labored and no SOB)
- Increase in blood flow while Exercising Termination of Stress Testing
- Progressive angina
- Significant drop in systolic pressure in response to an increasing load
- Lightheadedness, confusion, pallor, cyanosis, nausea, or peripheral circulatory insufficiency
- Abnormal ECG responses including ST segment depression greater than 4 mm
- Excessive rise in BP
- Subject wishes to stop.

GENERAL GUIDELINES FOR AN AEROBIC TRAINING PROGRAM

- Establish the target heart rate
- Warm-up for 5 to 10 minutes gradually increasing (speed and effort)
- Increase the pace of activity
- Cool down for 5 to 10 minutes
- Aerobic activity (3-5x/week)
- Use appropriate equipment, correct footwear.
- To avoid overuse syndromes, proper warm-up and stretching
- Individualize the program of exercise

Physiological effects of Exercises

I. **Musculoskeletal System**
   - Increase muscle tone - proper shape and ideal posture.
   - To reduce the fat.
   - Increase strength and flexibility of the muscle.
   - Bone becomes stronger and dense under exercises.

II. **Cardiovascular System**
- Decrease in resting heart rate.
- Heart size - the weight and volume of the heart increases.
- Increase in stroke volume.
- Increase in cardiac output.
- Decrease in blood pressure.

III. Respiratory System
- Increase in tidal volume and force vital capacity.
- Increase minute ventilation.
- Ventilation and perfusion increases.
- Respiratory muscles become stronger and flexible.

IV. Digestive System
- Increase in appetite.
- Increase in speed of peristalsis activity - decrease constipation.
- Liver and pancreas - improves their function and size.

V. Overall increase co-ordination, skill and flexibility.

VI. Relaxation - Physical and Mental.

Normal Respiratory and Cardiovascular Responses to Exercises

Respiratory

- Increase in respiratory rate
  Respiratory mechanism can be stimulated by many physiology changes occurs during ex. such as :
  - Decrease in venous O2 saturation
  - Increase in PCO2 and H+
  - Increase in body temperature
  - An increased stimulation of receptors of the joints and muscles.
- Increase in alveolar ventilation and diffusion of gases.
- Minute ventilation increases.

Cardiovascular Responses

- Cardiovascular phase
  - Mild increase in heart rate, cardiac output and Systolic BP.
  - Increase in venous tone throughout the body.
  - Therefore blood volume shifts to centre from the periphery.

- Initial phase
  - Intense rise in sympathetic nervous system.
  - Increase heart rate
  - Increase myocardial contractility
  - Increase systolic BP and constant or fall in diastolic BP
- Steady State - Hemodynamic parameters are sustained.
- Cardiovascular drift

  As exercise. Continues
  - Progressive fall in VR, SV and BP.
  - Progressive redistribution of blood flow.
  - Blood volume and flow is directed to the skin, Splanchnic and non working muscle

Benefits of Aerobic Exercise

- Increased resistance to fatigue
- Extra energy and stamina
- Toned muscles and increased lean body mass
- Decreased tension and stress
- Improved quality of sleep
- Psychological benefits - exercise improves mood, reduces depression and anxiety
- Social - exercise is fun and can be shared with friends and partners.
- Control of body fat - aerobic exercise in conjunction with strength training and a proper diet will reduce body fat
- Decreased risk of diseases - hypertension, diabetes, osteoporosis (weight-bearing activities), various cancers, and heart disease.

Warm-up

Any period of activity should ideally begin with a warm-up. The importance of warming up is based on sound physiological principles. During the warm-up the temperature of the large muscle groups is increased, which allows increased force and velocity of muscular contraction as well as increased blood and oxygen supply to the fibers. Chemical reactions within the muscle tissue are increased and energy from muscle contraction is increased. Finally the warm-up helps prevent tears and damage to connective tissue and thereby prevents joint injury. Warm-up for a beginner should be at least 10 min and should consist of extremely light large muscle group activity, such as walking, swinging the arms, easy jogging and gentle movements.

If warm-up is too short or omitted within the first few minutes of starting the main exercise session, the exerciser will feel discomfort, rapid heart rate, heavy breathing and muscular fatigue due to the body's inability to use its aerobic system and its dependence on the anaerobic system.

Flexibility Exercises

Once warm-up is completed, the beginner exerciser is advised to engage in some flexibility practice of the large muscle groups. Modern stretching techniques are designed to produce slow and gradual lengthening of the muscles, with the full stretch being held for 15-30 see. Muscles stretched in this way are also relaxed.

There are many different kinds of stretching exercises.

Aerobic Exercise

Essential aerobic activity is rhythmic, repetitive and causes the muscles to work at a level where they require oxygen for the release of energy. There is a wide selection of activities suitable for the aerobic component of an exercise or physical activity programme. It is best to select those which are appropriate to the individual's needs and which are enjoyable. If, for example, the beginning exerciser is overweight, she or he may feel very uncomfortable performing high impact or jarring activities, such as jogging or work with a skipping rope. He or she may also feel ill-at-ease in a class situation where skimpy and tight clothing is the norm. However, the same individual may feel relaxed and comfortable using a bicycle or rowing machine or walking briskly. A regular exerciser may choose a mixture of swimming, playing football, canoeing or running sports for his programme. Examples of aerobic exercises include brisk walking, cycling, cross country skiing, hill walking, canoeing, rowing, jogging, swimming and any running game. As muscles, including the heart muscle, become conditioned to activity, it is possible and desirable to work for longer or to increase the intensity over a period of weeks or months.

The intensity of exercise for a training effect can be calculated from the heart rate: '220 - the age' will give an estimate of maximum heart rate in beats per minute. In order for fitness to be improved, the pulse rate should between 65 and 85 per cent maximum heart rate. It is wise to calculate what the heart rate should be for a 10 or 15 s count, as this is easy to take during the exercise session. For example, a 45-year-old woman, who enjoys cycling, has decided to enter a cycle marathon. She would like to target her training programme towards becoming fitter. Using the calculation to find her estimated maximum heart rate (220 - 45 ¼ 175 beats per minute), she can work out that, in order to be training hard enough, she will need to cycle so that her heart rate is raised to between 65 and 85 per cent of 175; that is between 114 and 149 beats per minute. If gaining fitness is not as important as gaining health benefits, then the target heart rate may be only between 50 and 60 per cent of the maximum heart rate.

Muscular Endurance

Muscular endurance activities also play an important part in the complete exercise or physical activity programme. Without a degree of muscular endurance, simple tasks such as gardening, housework or changing a car tyre can become difficult and may result in injury or muscle strain. There are several training principles that should be understood before embarking on the muscular endurance part of the training programme.

In order to improve muscular endurance, the principle of progressive overload must be applied. The beginning exerciser will be unfamiliar with the load values which he/she is capable of lifting. So it is best to start with fairly light weights. The number of repetitions performed (that is, how many times the same exercise is repeated) is normally around 12 to induce endurance. At the correct load, the individual will find repetitions 10, 11 and 12 hard to complete, but still manageable.

At the beginning of an exercise programme, it is best to limit the number of sets of repetitions to one or two to avoid muscle soreness. As the exerciser becomes more able, and muscles become used to endurance, another set of 12 repetitions can be added to the programme. Eventually a full three sets can be performed regularly.

A complete muscle endurance programme will include a wider variety of different types of exercises so that a balance is achieved. Often a person's own body weight serves well as the load in the exercise. Muscular endurance improves in those muscles that are specifically being trained. These have been chosen because no special equipment is required and they can be done anywhere. Exercises can be made progressively more difficult by increasing the level or be increasing the repetitions.

It is important to work all of the large muscle groups in any one programme.

Cooling Down and Post-exercise Effects

Once the physical activity session is completed, it is necessary to spend a few minutes cooling down. If the body goes from a state of pumping blood at a much increased rate to stopping suddenly, dizziness, nausea or light-headedness might be experienced. The working muscles push blood back to the heart, but when they stop suddenly, without a period of cooling down, the blood pools in the muscles instead of being forced back to the heart. A transition period is required for transferring from hard muscular work to light muscular work. Cooling down is as important as warming up.

Planning

Choosing how to fit exercise or periods of physical activity into an already busy life does take a great deal of thought and planning. In order to gain either health or fitness benefits, exercise or physical activity must be performed on a regular basis. It may be easier for people with diabetes to achieve a better blood glucose balance when each day's energy expenditure is relatively stable, but the sedentary individual who decides to aim for health benefits by taking short periods of physical activity, such as walking to work or cycling to the shops, adding up to 30 min per day, should remember that a complete programme includes muscular endurance, aerobic and flexibility components. It is likely that the short bursts of physical activity throughout the day will be largely aerobic in nature and provision needs to be made to include some muscular endurance and flexibility components at other times during the week. One of the most difficult problems in exercise and physical activity programmes is to find ways to change behaviour and to 'stay with' physical activity that is to increase long-term compliance.

Define - Special Population

A special population may be defined in terms of exercise on a group with a special medical condition who may require expertise and supervision to overcome that medical situation. Other special populations may just need to improve their skill level and knowledge or increase awareness and social interaction of conditioning by participating in a regular physical activity.

Example

Diabetes, hypertension, arthritis older Adults etc.

Benefits of Exercise for Individual with Diabetes

- Has shown improvement in glucose tolerance and overall metabolism.
- Improvement in overall blood glucose control, cholesterol and strength.
- Exercise like aerobic or strength training has insulin like affect on glucose uptake into cells.

Benefits of PACE Program

PACE: (People with Arthritis can exercise)
- Maintaining range of motion for all of its participants.
- Clearing waste products that accumulate in joints through muscle toning.
- ROM (Range of Motion) exercise participant can perform there three times or more during a given day.

- Increasing muscle tone through resistance training with external work loads and minimum the fibromyalgia component and some of the suffering.
- Using exercise as a social interaction to guard against depression, which is one of the major reasons arthritis patients deteriorate in health.

Two Types of Arthritis

- *Osteoarthritis* : is a non-systematic disease and usually attacks on joint in the body.
- *Rheumatoid Arthritis:* is a systemic disease that like type 1 diabetes, has an autoimmune etiology.

Three Categories of Seniors

1. **50-65 years old:** May participate in most moderate weight training routines with only slight modifications (joint problem, decreased range of motion, any cardiovascular abnormalities)
2. **65-80 years old:** For thin group modified programs should be modified and based on medical recommendation, ROM limitations, and signs of fatigue, initial muscle tone and joint pain.
3. **80 years old and up:** For this age level, low exertion level should be monitored and emphasis placed on individual muscle group strength, overall posture and strength enhancement to avoid injury.

Three Types of Hypertension

a. **Stage 1:** Patients may use low intensity training to keep their blood pressure level in check on opposed to the use of medication.
b. **Stage 2:** Patients may have some organ damage due to increased pressure over time including left ventricular hypertrophy. For these patients an exercise program should consists of aerobics but no heavy straining or lifting.
c. **Stage 3:** For patients with advance blood pressure and heavier organ and heart damage exercise itself is contraindicated.

Type of Exercise Program for an Individual with Arthritis

- The most common exercise program is the PACE exercise routine, And I also believe in this, because this is the safest exercise program for Arthritis individuals.
- Suggest the individual according to PACE program that aerobic activities (low impact or without impact) 2-Days a week, and followed by the Body conditioning with moderate weight, incorporating range of motion (ROM) 2 days a week.
- And also will put him/her in light flexibility five to ten minutes before and after each session.
- According to the condition of the client the program can be modified more and also can give them the same exercises for 5 to 6 days also.

Cystic Fibrosis

- This is a common fatal genetic disease. It is characterized by the following traits : an increase in electrolytes suggesting a defect in cellular transport mechanisms and pancreatic insufficiency. This impairs growth and reduces absorption of nutrients and in the major cause of morbidity (which is impaired pulmonary mucous clearance) and subsequent infections of the respiratory tract.
- Cystic fibrosis is an insidious disease. Its affects on women are greater than that of men, showing a 2:1 mortality ratio in comparison.
- Exercise would be beneficial for individuals with cystic fibrosis disease:
- **Warm up:** Diaphragmatic breathing (abdominal breathing) minimum of 10 to 15 slow breaths for approx. 2 minutes. Low intensity cardiovascular works (treadmill, cycle or rowing machine), 5 to 8 minutes.
- Weights Exercise (Basic) for all the body parts:
  = 2-3 sets each part
  = 8-10 reps each set
- **Cool down:** A recommended program is more cardiovascular exercise (5-8 minutes) coupled with stretching and flexibility

work and 10-15 repetitions of rhythmic diaphragmatic breathing exercise.

- Exercise is not a cure for clients that suffer from Cystic fibrosis. It is only the means to help CF patients improve their lung function and heighten their awareness about the benefits of fitness.
- Important precautionary measures to consider concerning exercise and children :
  - Make sure medical clearance has been obtained.
  - Determine the appropriate level of participation.
  - Insure appropriate shoes are worn.
  - Instruct children how to breathe properly during exercise.
  - Give class orientation, describe the day's activities and teach a healthy message.
  - Have children hydrate before, during and after exercise.

Immediate Benefits of Exercise for Children

- Improved ability to meet the demands of daily physical activity.
- Improved results in Physical Performance tests.
- Improved motor skills.
- Reduced Injuries
- Fewer chronic health conditions and a lower risk for developing chronic health problems than sedentary children introducing fitness for preschool years.

Contraindications to Exercise for (5-12 years) Children

- Training at too high level of intensity and for long duration.
- Training in hotter and more humid environment as thermo regulatory mechanisms in the child's body are not fully developed.
- Sports injuries are problematic in this group.

Contraindications to Exercise for Pregnant Woman

a. Pregnancy induced hypertension.
b. Pre-term rupture of membranes
c.. Pre-term labor during a prior or current pregnancy or both.
d. Incompetent cervix or a cerclage.
e. Persistent second or third trimester bleeding.
f. Intrauterine growth retardation.

ASTHMA

- Exercise may cause airways to tighten, swell and fill with mucous
- Asthma attacks often occurs 5-15 minutes after initiating strenuous exercise
- No Cure. Manage symptoms by taking medication before exercising
- Air pollution and certain medications (like beta blockers) can make attacks worse.

Triggers

- Upper respiratory infections
- Pollen from flowers, trees or grasses
- Molds or dust
- Smoking
- Emotional distress
- Exercise
- Cold air
- Dry air
- Air pollution.

Medications

- Rescue - Theophyline (short acting), adrenaline -used in hospital ER, and Beta-antagonist inhalers (albuteral, ventolin or proventil) preventive
- Prophylactic - Theophyline (long acting), Cromolyn sodium, Leukotriene inhibitors, cortocosteriods.

Pre-exercise assessment

- Pulmonary function testing: FVC (forced vital capacity), FEV1 (forced expiratory volume in one sec), PEFR (peak expiratory flow rate)
- Exercise tolerance testing using Borg or Dyspnea scale rating.

Helpful tips

- Begin with activities least likely to trigger asthma (kayaking, swimming, walking)

- Progress as tolerated to cycling, treadmill running, outdoor running
- Prolong warm up to at least 15 minutes
- Always have rescue medication available
- Maintain hydration
- Use diaphragmatic breathing
- Monitor for signs of an asthma attack,

F-I-T-T

- F - 3-5 days a week
- I - Based on pulmonary function and triggers, generally 50-60% MHR
- T - CV 20-30 min. goal
- T - Strength training high volume low intensity 2 × 15 min, or 1 × 30 min, 4-5 days per week.

Exercise Program for a Client with Asthma

- Warm up - Deep breathing exercise, abdominal breathing, breathing through the nose 5 minutes stretching, and range of motion exercise.
- Resistance Training Program:

  Body Parts 2 sets of 10 Reps each exercise

Chest	Bench press/
Shoulders	Shoulder press/overhead
Back	Lat pulls, reverse flys, shrugs
Abdominal	Machine crunches
Biceps	Dumbbell biceps curls
Triceps	Triceps kickback
Hips/Adductors	Total hip or abductor/adductor
	Middle Back Rows

Cool Down: More respiratory work, plus walk recovery and flexibility.

Supervision

- Ensure adequate hydration
- Verify preventive medications are taken prior to exercise session and rescue medications ready

- Use dyspnea scale to measure potential for attack, avoid sudden intense exercise
- Have client use peak-flow meter readings regularly to monitor effectiveness
- Consult with HCP on monitoring, treatment plan and breathing exercises.

HYPERTENSION

- Cause of primary HTN is unknown in 90-95% of cases
- Two resting BP readings greater than 140/90mm Hg on two different days
- Uncontrolled HTN can lead to blood vessel and organ failure - the silent killer
- Physical activity/aerobic fitness markedly reduce mortality for HTN patient
- Medication and lifestyle modification are effective in improving outcome
- 52% of people with HTN are not taking medication
- 21% receive inadequate medical therapy to lower their elevated BP
- Smoking, obesity, poor diet, and sedentary lifestyle increase risk.

Classifications of Cardiac Exercise Programs

Stage - 1: Programs denote patients who have just had surgery and are using exercise for first time. Aerobics instructors will probably not be working with this group, as they are physician assisted, and therein with use of heart monitors which record EKG response to training.

Stage - 2: Patients are past the initial stage of medical intervention, and some that are a symptomatic may participate in outpatients programs. Some will wear 24 hours monitors and heart rate strips that are then checked by phone hook-up to a physician's office.

Stage - 4: Patients are basically self-paced with their exercise and schedule regular visits with their exercise and cardiology team.

Assessment Considerations

- Preferred test: Physician supervised 12 lead exercise stress test, with noted BP response to increasing workloads determining upper limits of intensity.
- Is BP well controlled?
- Which lifestyle modifications are being followed?
- Type of medications regularly used and effect on HR and BP?
- Affect of additional clinical conditions?

Contraindications of individual with hypertension

- Training contraindications include systolic BP>175 mm Hg. Training should be postponed until this number is lowered to below 140 mm Hg.
- Exercising without consent of physician is also contraindicated.
- All persons training in a health club who have hypertension should be under the care of a physician. Instructor should be aware of all physical limitations (perceived exertion orthopedic etc.) before working with any hypertensive patient.

F - I - T - T

- F – 5-6 days per week
- I – 40-70% MHR (40-70% Vo2)
- T – 30-60 min. per session
- T – Emphasize aerobic activities
- ST Circuit weight training best to reduce blood pressure

Precautions

- Avoid isometric exercises to lessen impact of sodium and potassium retention on kidneys
- For HTNs on diuretics, monitor hydration levels when exercising, especially on high heat index days
- Avoid high intensity exercise and highly competitive activities

DIABETES

- Insulin (hormone) is secreted by the pancreas and converts glucose so it can enter muscle cells and produce energy

- With limited or no insulin production, blood glucose rises, depriving the body of energy and causing serious complications for all organ systems.

Types of Diabetes

Type I

- Insulin dependant
- Affects children and young adults
- Daily doses of insulin are required to keep blood glucose levels controlled.

Type II

- Non-insulin dependant
- Primarily affects mostly > 40 yrs old and overweight
- Achieving optimal glucose control (ideal body weight, exercise, oral medications) can reduce complications

Precautions

- Glucose levels over 250 mg/dl are a contraindication for exercise
- Neuropathy decreases ability to feel pain and increases risk for abnormal heart rate, abnormal BP and overheating
- Proliferative retinopathy increases risk for hemorrhages and retinal detachment
- Type 1 diabetics should avoid vigorous or prolonged exercise if hypoglycemic or fasting plasma glucose exceeds 250-350 mg/dl.
- Avoid exercise in climatic extremes
- Check feet daily for cuts and blisters, especially after exercise

F-I-T-T IDDM/NIDDM

- F- 3-5 days per week / 5-6 days per week
- I - 55-75% VO_2 Max or 3-5 RPE / 40-70% , 2-5 RPE
- T- 30 min. aerobic / 20-30 min for glucose control 40-60 min. per session

- T- Aerobic and aerobic interval, low impact
- ST- 2-3 days per week 40-60% 1RM, 2-3 sets per exercise.
- Warm up and cool down 5-10 min.

OSTEOPOROSIS

- 40% of Americans over 50 will experience a fracture due to bone loss
- 1 in 4 women over 40 have osteoporosis
- Prevention: Adequate calcium intake, exercise, decrease ETOH, smoking and caffeine
- Hip and spine fractures cause disability and death.

Assessment

- Medical history and physical examination including DEXA - often monitored yearly
- Medications and effect on HR and BP
- Functional fitness testing
- Balance, flexibility and walking skills.

Women at High Risk for Osteoporosis

- Menopause earlier than 45
- High volume aerobic athletes: Distance runners, swimmers, gymnasts, dancers
- Low calcium intake
- Smokers
- Competitive or high intensity activities that predispose individual to fractures.

Training Guidelines

- Weight bearing activity is essential
- Becoming physically active helps prevent more bone loss
- Exercise and hormone therapy may be necessary to prevent further bone loss
- Goals: Improve strength, flexibility, and balance to reduce falls and fractures.

F-I-T-T for Clients with Osteoporosis

- F - 3-7 days per week
- I - Age appropriate, generally 60-80% MHR
- T - 20-60 minutes per session
- T - Weight bearing aerobics, strength training, functional exercises, balance
- ST - 75% 1RM, progress to 3 set/10 to 15 rep program.

Supervision

- Lower body exercises in sitting position
- Light dumb bell work standing
- Monitor overhead exercises carefully
- Avoid abdominal curls and sit and reach
- Provide stable, non-slippery floor and lifting surfaces
- Know medications and side effects especially those causing dizziness.

ARTHRITIS

- Rheumatoid and Osteoarthritis are the most common of 100 arthritic conditions
- OA is most common, affects hips, knees and spine, usually only one joint is affected
- RA is progressive, symmetrical, cartilage destroying, can fuse and scar joints < ROM
- Arthritis is the most common cause of disability in America.

Treatment Goals

- Reduce pain
- Decrease inflammation
- Improve function
- Decrease joint damage
- Manage through lifestyle changes, weight reduction, medication, heat/cold, and joint protection strategies.

Assessment

- Isokinetic machines for muscle strength and endurance - 60-90 E/second major muscle
- 6 min, or 1 mile walk test
- Goniometry for ROM and symmetry
- Gait analysis and balance assessment
- Functional capacity - assess ability to walk, sit, stand several times.

Training Guidelines for Clients with Arthritis

- Preserve or restore motion and flexibility around affected joint
- Increase muscle strength and endurance
- Increase aerobic conditioning to enhance mood, maintain function and overall health
- Revise training as new symptoms present.

F - I - T - T

- F - Progress to 3-5 days per week
- I - 50-75%
- T - Slowly increase to 30 min. sessions
- T - Light weight bearing, non-weight bearing, Tai Chi and aquatic exercise is best
- ST - Stretching, ROM, isometric then progressive resistance isotonic exercises - 3 second contraction, 6 second hold.

PACE: (People with Arthritis can exercise)

- Maintaining range of motion for all of its participants.
- Clearing waste products that accumulate in joints through muscle toning.
- ROM (Range of Motion) exercise participant can perform their three times or more during a given day.
- Increasing muscle tone through resistance training with external workloads decreases to a minimum the fibromyalgia component and some of the suffering.

- Using exercise as a social interaction to guard against depression, which is one of the major reasons arthritis patients deteriorate in health.

Precautions/Arthritis

- If pain increased after exercise for more than two hours reduce level of exercise
- Pain, stiffness and biomechanical inefficiency increase metabolic cost 50%
- Progress training gradually
- Ensure joint safety, adapt plan to joints
- Refer new or worsening joint pain to HCP and adjust training.

Cardiovascular Disease

- Atherosclerosis causes 1.5 million AMIs every year, 1/3 will die from their AMI
- When coronary arteries are affected it is called coronary artery disease (CAD), devoid of symptoms it is a silent killer
- Risk factors: Smoking, HTN, high cholesterol and physical inactivity
- Prevention: Increase activity, decrease body weight, decrease HTN.

Assessment

- Obtain physician signed referral
- Document risk factors and changes
- Understand cardiac medications, actions and effect on HR and BP
- Consider age, sex, clinical status, related medical conditions, habitual practices and MS limitations
- 12 lead ECG is mandatory for functional capacity, diagnostic and prognostic value.

Training Guidelines for CAD

- Uncomplicated hospital course
- No resting or exercise induced ischemia
- Functional capacity 6 METs, 3 wks post event

- Normal ventricular ejection fraction > 55%
- No significant resting or exercise induced ventricular arrhythmias.

F - I - T - T

- F - 3-5 days per week
- I - 60-85% MHR
- T - 20-60 min. sessions
- T - Any type aerobic activity, modify for medical limitations
- ST - 2-3 X/week, up to 60% 1RM, 10-15 reps/2-3 sets slow progression, limit lower intensity isometrics.

Supervision

- Obtain physician signed referral noting exercise capacity, limitations, risk factors and medications
- Monitor exercise intensity carefully
- Understand cardiac medications, actions, treatment plans
- Maintain CPR certification
- Give feedback to physician, share concerns

Stroke (CVA)

- Decreased oxygen and blood flow to brain cells caused by atherosclerotic plaque, blood clot or hemorrhage
- Results in motor, sensory and/or communication skill impairment
- Can occur at any age and during exercise sx confusion, dizziness, severe HAs, slurred speech and transient ischemic attacks (TIAs)
- Prompt recognition and treatment can prevent sharp declines in function
- Receiving clot busting drugs within the first three hours can rescue neurons
- 50% of brain cells die in the first hour; 90% die by three hours
- Rehab goals: OT, PT, independent functioning, gain strength, coordination and balance, disability adaptations

Training Guidelines

- Perform ROM below pain threshold, some restriction is a protective limitation
- Low intensity resistance work
- Have therapist check proprioception, static and dynamic balance to reduce fall risk
- Utilize client feedback to monitor progress
- Apraxia - mind willing, body won't respond. Be patient and assist when necessary
- Dynamic balance compromised - place equipment on good side, give step-by-step directions
- New tasks may precipitate resistance. Offer support and encouragement. Repetition will make the task easier

F-I-T-T

- F - Aerobically progress as tolerated to 3-5 days per week. ROM daily, initially with assistance. Goal: volitional/unassisted
- I - 50-70% MHR
- T - Short intervals progress to 30 min
- T - Aquatic exercise preferred. Initially use a, stationary bike for balance deficits
- ST - Seated position initially, low intensity, keep HR and BP from rising too high.

Children

- TV viewing is up, weight is up, physical activity is down, signs of early CVD are increasingly evident in children and adolescents
- Children's aerobic capacity increases before anaerobic capacity
- Due to high metabolic rate, children tire quickly.

Assessment

- At 12 years of age basic field tests safely establish training guidelines
- Aerobic - 1.5 mile run/12 min. walk
- Anaerobic - 30-60 meter sprint (power), 200 meter sprint (capacity).

Precautions for Training Children

- Due to high metabolic rate children's muscles fatigue quickly
- Body fat has significantly greater effect on endurance runs than body mass
- First priority: secure energy for healthy growth and development. Monitor load to rest ratio.
- Be alert for overtraining: excessive fatigue, weakness or decreased attention span
- Sequence of load increases is critical development stimulus
  - **1st -** increase frequency of workouts
  - **2nd -** increase the duration of workouts,
  - **3rd -** increase the intensity of exercises without increasing duration
- Base workouts on child's training and biological age NOT chronological age

F - I - T- T

- **F - Hrs/wk**

6-10 yrs.	4 hrs.
11-14 yrs.	4 - 6 hrs.
15-19 yrs.	6 - 8 hrs.

- **I and T**

6-10 yrs.	emphasize play and flexibility
11-14 yrs.	team games, in to long easy intervals
15-19 yrs.	moderate length and short intervals, regular training at anaerobic threshold

- **ST -3 days/wk**

6-10 yrs.	own body weight	15 min.
11-14 yrs.	12-20 reps strength / endurance	30 min.
15-19 yrs.	10-12 reps strength/power	45 min.

Training Guidelines

- Target heart rate restrictions unnecessary
- < 2 hours of TV or video games per day

- Create more opportunities for fun physical activity. Involve friends and peers. Encourage confidence in sports
- Encourage family, teachers and adults to model active lifestyle.

Strength Training Guidelines

- Obtain medical check-ups before training
- ST just one part of varied fitness program
- Use calisthenics to build muscle endurance and strength
- Use variety of training methods
- Proper technique first, low resistance
- Progress from low resistance/high reps to higher resistance/fewer reps
- Limit ST to 3X/week, avoid negative or eccentric exercises, use full ROM
- Circuit system maximizes CV fitness
- Warm up before, flexibility after training
- Provide constant experienced adult supervision
- Head pain as a warning, seek medical advice

OBESITY

Obesity: Obesity (see Fig. 9.1) is defined as a condition of excessive amount of body fat.

The WHO itself describes an escalating global epidemic of overweight and obesity- "globesity"-that is taking over many parts of the world.

"Obesity is an abnormal accumulation of fat, usually 20% or more over an individuals ideal body weight and is a heterogeneous disorder in which energy intake chronically exceeds energy expenditure."

- *Overweight:* a body weight that exceeds some average for stature, and perhaps age.
- *Overfat:* condition whereby body fat exceeds an age- and/or gender appropriate average by some predetermined amount.
- *Obesity:* overfat condition that accompanies comorbidities that include one or more components of the obese syndrome.

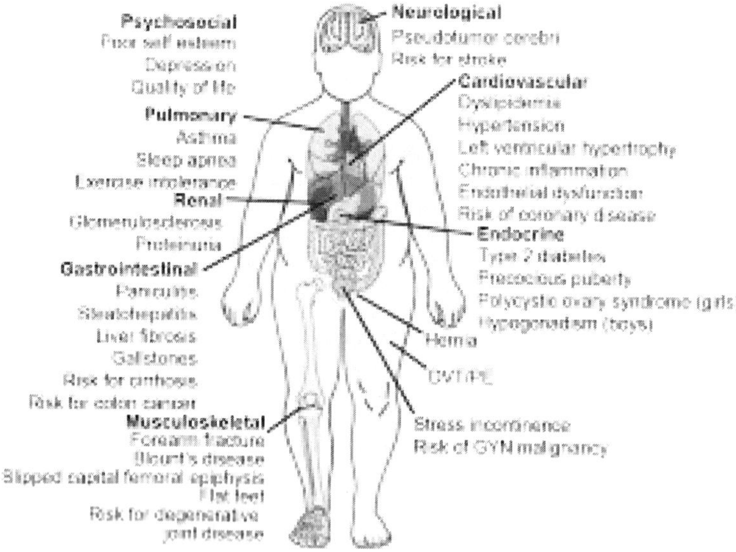

Fig. 9.1: Obese

Obese Syndrome Components

- Glucose intolerance
- Insulin resistance
- Dyslipidemia
- Type 2 diabetes
- Hypertenision
- Elevated plasma leptin concentration
- Increased visceral adipose tissue
- Increased risk of CHD and some cancers

Causes of Obesity

- **Age:** As you grow older, your metabolic rate slows down and you do not require as many calories to maintain weight. Ages 25-44 yrs are dangerous time for development of excessive fatness by adult.
- **Gender:**

  Males — lean body mass — Resting metabolic rate

  Females — due to menopause — Resting metabolic rate [25 - 44]

- **Physical inactivity:** It is the main reason for increase in obesity among people in affluent societies.
  - Physical activity decreases appetite in obese individuals and increases body's ability to metabolize fat as an energy source.
- **Hereditary factors:** If biological mother is obese as an adult, there is approx. 75% chance of her children to be obese and vice versa.
- **No. of fat cells:** People who are obese in childhood are more likely to be obese in adulthood because of more no. of fat cells. Number of fat cells can't be decreased, weight can only be lost by decreasing size of fat cells.
- **Pregnancy:** Gaining weight in pregnancy is necessary . However for some, pregnancy is beginning of weight problems.
- **Menopause:** After menopause hormonal changes causes fat to be redistributed in body and accumulate around waist.
  - It increases health risk. Also reduces physical activity.
- **Hormonal disorders:** Rare cause of obesity is excess production of cortisol by adrenal glands. In this fat accumulates only in trunk while arms and legs remain thin.
  - Polycystic ovary syndrome causes increased level of insulin in blood which can cause obesity.
- **Drugs:** Antidepressants, antipsychotic, antihypertensive, corticosteroids, insulin therapy, OC pills. Stopping smoking usually results in weight gain. Nicotin appetite and metabolic rate.
- **Psychological aspect :** Depression
- **Behavioral influences :**
  - Physically inactive people
  - High fat diet/faulty eating habits
  - Snacking intermittently
  - Having energy dense food and drinks
  - Alcohol consumption
  - Irregular exercise.
- **Genetics plays a role**
  - How much variation in weight gain among individuals can be accounted for by genetic factors?
  - Largest transmissible variation is cultural.

- **A Mutant Gene**
- **What is leptin?** *[ob protien]*
  - A satiety hormone that influences the appetite control in the hypothalamus.
  - Describe the role of the mutant "obese" gene in obesity development.
- Second genetic defect is affected body's response to the "signal" leptin provided.

Health Risks of Excessive Body Fat

Obesity is the second leading cause of preventable death in America:

- Impaired cardiac function from increased mechanical work and autonomic and left ventricular dysfunction
- Hypertension, stroke and DVT
- Increased insulin resistance in children and adults and type II diabetes
- Renal disease
- Sleep apnea, Mechanical ventilatory constraints and pulmonary disease
- Problems receiving anesthetics during surgery
- OA, degenerative joint disease and gout
- Endometrial, breast, prostate and colon cancers
- Abnormal plasma lipid and lipoprotein levels
- Menstrual irregularities
- Gall bladder disease
- Enormous psychological burden and social stigmatization and discrimination
- Skin disorders : Heat burns.

Evaluation of Obese Patient

- Medical history
- Assessment of the degree of obesity
- Exercise and obesity history
- Assessment of obesity-related comorbidities
- Contraindications to exercise
- Nutritional habits

- Exercise testing
- Treatment modalities.

Obesity History

- Family history
- Age of onset
- Pounds/years overweight
- Landmark medical weight
- Lowest weight maintained 2 years
- Loss/regain history
- Social support
- Coping skills
- Control eating.

Exercise History

- Types of activities
- Time of day
- Planned vs. incidental
- Social component
- Clothing/shoes
- Perception of intensity/duration
- Frequency/consistency
- Typical interruptions
- Long term patterns
- Seasonal patterns.

Assessment for Overweight and Obesity

- Determine BMI
- Body fat measurements/Body composition assessment
- Determine fat distribution
- Assess risk factors and presence of obesity related diseases

Body Mass Index: Body Mass Index is the ratio of the body weight in kilograms to the height in meters squared. This is the Quetelet Index-kg/(mt.)^2

Table 9.1

Classification	*BMI (kg/m²)*	*Risk of co-morbidities*
Underweight	<18.5	Low (but risk of other clinical problems increased)
Normal range	18.5–24.9	Average
Overweight	25.0–29.9	Mildly increased
Obese	**> 30.0**	
Class I	30.0–34.9	Moderate
Class II	35.0–39.9	Severe
Class III severe (for 'morbid obesity' or 'super' obesity)	> 40.0	Very severe

BMI Limitations (see Table 9.1)

- BMI does not provide actual information on body composition.
- High BMI may be due to excessive lean body mass
- Use clinical judgment
- Elevated BMI without other risk factors may indicate a healthy weight
- Assess other risk factors
- It should not be used for :
  - Children
  - Adolescents
  - Pregnant and Lactating women
  - People with large body frame
  - Highly muscular individuals
  - Human body composition.
- J. Matiega described a Four component model consisting of :
  - Weight of the skeleton (S) Skin
  - Subcutaneous tissue (Sk+St)
  - Skeletal muscle (M)
  - Remainder (R).
- So, Total body mass = S + [Sk = St] + M + R
- Two distinct compartments:
  - Fat free body mass
  - Fat mass

- Essential fat:
  - Fat in Heart, Lungs, Liver, Spleen, Kidneys, Intestines, Muscles and lipid rich tissues of CNS and bone marrow.
  - In reference men : 3% of body mass
  - In reference women : Sex-specific essential fat
- Storage fat:
  - Includes fat primarily in adipose tissue, Adipose tissue energy reserve contains approx. 83% pure fat, 2% protein, 15 % water within its supporting structures.
  - In men : 12% of body mass
  - In women: 15% of body mass
- Lean body mass: contains small % of non sex specific essential fat i.e.3% of body mass
- Fat free body mass [FFM] : Body mass devoid of all extractable fat [FFM = body mass - fat mass].

Common Techniques to Asses Body Composition

- **Direct measurements :** Chemical analysis of the animal carcass or human cadaver
- **Indirect measurements :** *Laboratory methods*

– Hydrostatic weighing	– Lung analyser Bod Pod
– Isotope dilution	– Dual energy X-ray absorptiometry
	– MRI, CT, Near infrared interactane and ultrasound

- **Field methods**
  - Bioelectrical impedance analysis
  - Skin fold and girth measurements
  - Anthropometry.
- Waist Hip Ratio: Waist Hip Ratio is defined as the ratio of the circumference of the waist to the circumference of the hip (see Fig. 9.1).
- Waist to Hip Ratio
  - W/H ratio
- Upper Body Obesity when W/H is:
  - > 0.8 females
  - > 0.9 males

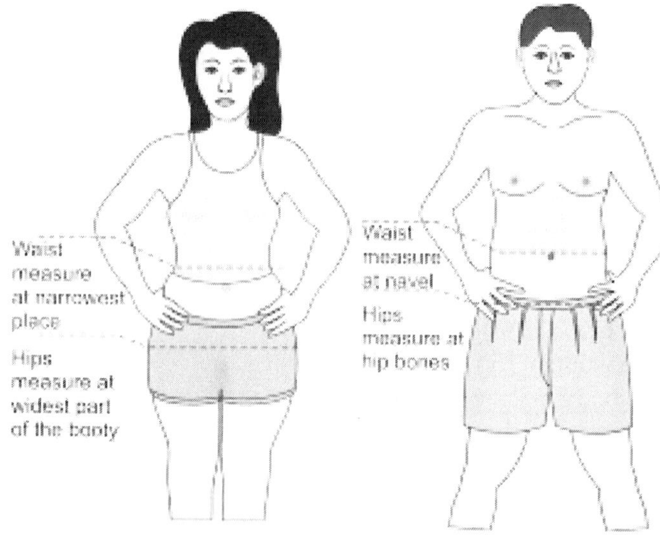

Fig. 9.1: Measurement of waist Hip ratio

Skin fold Measurement: The skin fold was measured on the right side of the body. Skin fold was firmly grasped by the thumb and index finger of the left hand and was pulled away from the body. Then the caliper was held in the right hand perpendicular to the skin fold and with the caliper dial facing up and easily readable. The caliper hands were placed 1/2-1/4th of an inch away from the fingers holding the skin fold. The data was read approximately four seconds after the pressure from the hand was released on the lever arm of the caliper jaw. The skin fold measurement was taken from the following sites:

Thigh: The subject was standing with the body weight shifted to the other foot. The knee of the leg being tested was slightly flexed and the foot was on the ground. The skin fold measurement was taken from a vertical fold on the anterior aspect of the thigh midway between the hip (inguinal crease) and the nearest border of the patella.

Triceps: The arm was hanging loosely by the side. A vertical fold on the rear midline of the upper arm half way between the lateral projection of the acromion process and the inferior part of the olecranon process with elbow flexed at 90 degrees was measured.

Suprailiac: The person was standing erect with feet together. A diagonal fold above the crest on the ilium at the spot where an imaginary line would come down from the midaxillary line was measured.

The treatment of obesity includes

- Education
- Exercise
- Diet
- Medication
- Surgery

Education and behavior therapy are considered important parts of treatment. It is important to make the patient aware of the hazards of obesity. Behavioral modification plays an essential role in controlling weight gain. Various diets have been formulated keeping in mind severity and amount of weight loss desired.

Medications like appetite suppressants and lipid-lowering drugs are prescribed for moderate obesity. Surgeries like gastric reduction and liposuction are considered in cases of moderate to severe obesity.

Aerobic Exercises

Aerobic exercises utilize oxygen to generate the energy required for the activity. The substrate used is preferentially fat to prevent depletion of the carbohydrate stores. Low-intensity, long-duration exercises are aerobic exercises. With adaptation there is an earlier onset of fat mobilization.

Mechanism

Prolonged exercise can result in lowering of fasting plasma triglyceride (TG) concentration. Repeated exercise on successive days can bring about a progressive decline in elevated TG levels. It is not known whether the lowering of TG is attributable to a specific effect of exercise on lipid metabolism, or to a decreased availability of substrate for TG synthesis secondary to the increased energy expenditure.

Exercise training brings about a decrease in body weight. It alters the blood lipid profile favorably i.e. increases HDL and decreases total cholesterol, triglycerol and LDL. Exercise training increases the levels of HDL more systematically than dietary change or weight loss. The content of HDL is increased due to stimulation of lipoprotein lipase activity in adipose tissue.

The endurance exercise is prescribed to an obese individual considering four parameters:

1. Mode of exercise
2. Duration of exercise
3. Intensity of exercise
4. Frequency of exercise.

Mode

- Exercise training must include only high energy cost activities i.e. 5-7 times more energy expenditure as compared to resting energy expenditure.
- Walking and jogging are such activities.

Duration

Prolonged, low intensity, dynamic and continuous activities that emphasize endurance tend to be aerobic and hence utilize more free fatty acids. Long duration and low intensity exercises yield better results. A minimum session of 20 minutes with a 5-minute warm and 5 minute cool down is required.

Frequency

The minimum frequency of exercise to produce health and fitness benefits is thrice a week.

Intensity

The intensity prescribed should be demanding to produce both cardiovascular conditioning and lipid mobilization. The target can be set by:

Target HR = 0.6(HR max - HR rest) + HR rest

The patient can be taught to monitor his own heart rate and can increase the intensity gradually. This is particularly important when planning the home program (see Table 9.2).

Table 9.2q

Location	*Environmental Factors*	*Potential Impact on Energy Balance*
Home	• Reduce time spent watching television and in other sedentary behaviors • Build physical activity into regular routines	• Increases daily and leisure time physical activity • Increases calories used
Schools	• Ensure that the school breakfast and lunch programs meet nutrition standards • Provide food options that are low in fat, calories, and added sugars • Provide all children, from prekindergarten through grade 12, with quality daily physical education	• Decreases excessive calorie consumption • Increases daily physical activity
Work	• Create more opportunities forphysical activity at work sites	• Increases daily physical activity Increases calories used
Community	• Promote healthier choices including at least 5 serving of fruits and vegetables a day, and reasonable portion sizes • Encourage the food industry to provide reasonable food and beverage portion sizes • Encourage food outlets to increase the availability of low-calorie, nutritious food items • Create opportunities for physical activity in communities	• Decreases in excessive calorie consumption • Increases leisure time physical activity

OSTEOPOROSIS

Definition

- A reduction in bone density and a change in bone structures
- The rate of bone resorption is greater than the rate on bone formation
- Bones become previously porous, brittle and fragile
- Bones fracture easily under stresses that would not break in normal bone

Incidence: The prevalence of osteoporosis in women older than 80 years old of age is 84%. The average 75 years-old woman has lost 25% of her cortical bone and 40% of her trabecular bone.

Predisposing and Risk Factors

Predisposing Factors

- Caucasian or Asian
- Females
- Family history
- Small frame.

Risk Factors

Age

- Post-menopause
- Advance age
- Low testosterone in men
- Decreased calcitonin.

Nutrition

- Low calcium intake
- Low vitamin D
- High phosphate intake
- Inadequate calories.

Physical exercise

- Sedentary

- Lack of weight-bearing exercise
- Low weight and body mass index.

Lifestyle Choices

- Caffeine
- Alcohol
- Smoking
- Lack of exposure to sunlight.

Medications

- Corticosteroids
- Antiseizure medications
- Heparin
- Thyroid Hormone.

Manifestation

In the early stages of osteoporosis, you probably will not have symptoms. As the disease progresses, you may have symptoms related to weakened bones, including:

- Back pain
- Loss of height and stooped posture
- A curved upper back (dowager's hump)
- Broken bones (fractures) that might occur with a minor injury, especially in the hip, spine, and wrist
- Compression fractures in the spine that may cause severe back pain. But sometimes these fractures cause only minor symptoms or no symptoms at all.

Types of Osteoporosis

Primary Osteoporosis: Occurs in women after menopause (usually after 45 and 55 years) and later in life in men, but it is not merely a consequence of aging. Failure to develop optimal one peak bone mass during childhood, adolescence, and young adult contributes to the development of osteoporosis without resultant bone loss.

Secondary Osteoporosis: result of medications or other conditions and disease that affect bone metabolism. Specific disease states (eg.

celiac disease, hypogonadism) and medications (e.g. corticosteroids, antiseizure medications) that place patients at risk need to be identified and therapies instituted to reverse the development of osteoporosis.

Pathophysiology Diagnostic Studies

1. **Dual-energy X-ray Absorptiometry (DEXA):** analyzed and reported as T-scores (the number of standard deviations above or below the average BMD value for young, healthy woman. A normal BMD is less than 1 SD below the young adult mean value.
   - The WHO defines the osteoporosis as being present when the T-score is at least 2.5 SD below the young adult mean value. Ostopenia is diagnosed when the BMD T-score is between 1 and 2.5 SD below the young adult mean value.
2. **Quantitative ultrasound studies (QUS):** use to diagnose osteoporosis and to predict the risk of hip and nonvertebral fracture.

Management

Medical Management

1. Hormone replacement therapy (HRT) - the mainstay of therapy to retard bone loss and prevent occurrence of fractures. Estrogen replacement.

Genetics

- Caucasian or Asian
- Females
- Family history
- Small frame.

Age

- Post-menopause
- Advance age
- Low testosterone in men
- Decreased calcitonin.

Nutrition

- Low calcium intake
- Low vitamin D
- High phosphate intake
- Inadequate calories.

Physical Exercise

- Sedentary
- Lack of weightbearing exercise
- Low weight and body mass index.

Lifestyle Choices

- Caffeine
- Alcohol
- Smoking
- Lack of exposure to sunlight.

Medications

- Corticosteroids
- Antiseizure medications
- Heparin
- Thyroid Hormone
  - Bones needed stress for bone maintenance
  - Affects calcium absorption and metabolism
  - Reduces osteogenesis in bone remodeling
  - Reduces nutrients needed for the bone remodeling
  - Predisposes to low bone mass.

Hormones (estrogen, calcitonin, and testosterone) inhibit bone loss. Decreases bone resorption and increases bone mass, reducing the incidence of osteoporotic fractures.

2. **Raloxifene (Evista):** reduce the risk for osteoporosis by preserving bone mineral density without estrogenic effects on the uterus. They are indicated for both prevention and treatment of osteoporosis.
3. **Bisphosphonates:** reduce spine and hip fractures associated with osteoporosis

4. **Alendronate:** offers an alternative to HRT and produces increase bone mass inhibiting osteoclast function and decrease bone loss.
5. **Calcitonin:** primarily suppresses bone loss through direct action on osteoclast and reduced one turnover. It is effective in increasing BMD. It is administered by nasal spray or by subcutaneous or intramuscular injections.

Rehabilitative interventions

1. **Promoting and Understanding of Osteoporosis and the Treatment Regimen**
   - Adequate dietary or supplemental calcium (1200-1500 mg/day) and vitamin D
   - Regular weight-bearing exercise
   - Modification of lifestyle like cessation of smoking, reduce the use of caffeine and alcohol
   - Help to maintain bone mass
   - Instruct to take the calcium supplements with meals
   - Teach patient to drink adequate fluids to reduce the risk of renal calculi
   - For Alendronate users, it must be taken on an empty stomach with water and the patient must not consume foods or liquids for 30-60 minutes.
2. **Relieving Pain**
   - Rest in bed in a supine position or side-lying position several times a day. The mattress should be firm and non-sagging.
   - Intermittent local heat and back rubs promote muscle tension.
   - Instruct to move the trunk as a unit and avoid twisting.

Ten

Ergonomics

Ergonomics is a science concerned with the 'fit' between people and their work. It puts people first, taking account of their capabilities and limitations. Ergonomics aims to make sure that tasks, equipment, information and the environment suit each worker.

The term *Ergonomics* first introduced 125 years ago by Wojciech Jastrzebowski (a Professor of Natural Sciences) at the Agronomical Institute in Warsaw Poland.

The word "Ergonomics" comes from two Greek words: "ergon" meaning work, and "nomos" meaning laws. Today, however, the word is used to describe the science of *"designing the job to fit the worker, not forcing the worker to fit the job."* Ergonomics covers all aspects of a job, from the **physical stresses** it places on joints, muscles, nerves, tendons, bones and the like, to **environmental factors** which can affect hearing, vision, and general comfort and health.

Ergonomics is the study of how to improve the fit between the physical demands of the workplace and the employees who perform the work. That means considering the variability in human capabilities when selecting, designing, or modifying equipment, tools, work tasks, and the work environment. Employee's abilities to perform physical tasks may vary because of differences in age, physical condition, strength, gender, stature, and other factors.

If work is performed in awkward postures or with excessive effort, fatigue and discomfort may result. Under these conditions, muscles, tendons, ligaments, nerves, and blood vessels can be damaged. Injuries of this type are known as musculoskeletal disorders. MSDs can increase the cost of doing business both directly and indirectly. Direct costs may include medical services and higher worker's compensation premiums. Indirect costs from increased employee turnover, absenteeism, and retraining may also occur. Productivity, product quality, and employee morale may also suffer.

Purpose of Ergonomics

The improvement of human health, safety, and performance through the application of sound people and workplace principles.

Principles of Ergonomics

1. Keep everything in easy reach
2. Work at proper heights
3. Reduce excessive forces
4. Work in good postures
5. Reduce excessive repetition
6. Minimize fatigue
7. Minimize direct pressure
8. Provide adjustability and change of posture
9. Provide clearance and access
10. Maintain a comfortable environment
11. Enhance clarity and understanding
12. Improve work organization,.

Benefits of Ergonomics

- Improved health and safety for workers
- Higher morale
- Improved quality
- Improved productivity and competitiveness
- Lower absenteeism and turnover
- Fewer workplace injuries and health problems
- Reduced workman's compensation rates

Ergonomics in the Workplace

Jobs are made up of tasks. Tasks are the *things* employees must do to accomplish their jobs. Put simply, tasks are the parts of a job. Some jobs may contain only a single task, but many jobs are made up of multiple tasks. Below are some examples:

Job Tasks

Cabinet shop worker	Retrieving wood, feeding saw, stacking cut wood
Custodial worker	Emptying trash, dusting, vacuuming
Jewelry manufacturer	Waxing, cutting, finishing
Metal fabricator	Shaping bar stock, cutting, threading
Supermarket clerk	Stocking shelves, checking out groceries
Warehouse worker	Filling containers, shrink-wrapping, loading trucks

Contributing Factor

Contributing factors are aspects of work tasks that can lead to fatigue, musculoskeletal disorder (MSD) symptoms and injuries, or other types of problems. These factors may be present in one or more of the tasks employees must perform to accomplish their jobs. The contributing factors both employers and employees should be aware of include:

- Work environment
- Awkward postures
- Visual effort
- Repetitive motions
- Forceful exertion
- Pressure points (e.g., local contact stress)
- Vibration

Work Environment

There are also environmental factors associated with the workplace that can cause problems.

- Extreme high temperatures can increase the rate at which the body will fatigue. Alternatively, exposure of the hands and feet to cold temperatures can decrease blood flow, muscle strength, and manual dexterity. These conditions can also cause excessive grip force to be applied to tool handles or objects. Another problem may be caused by tools or equipment that exhaust cold or hot air directly onto the operator.

- The lighting in a workplace may be too dark or too bright for the work task. This may result in employees assuming awkward postures to accomplish work tasks and a loss of product quality.
- An employer should be aware of the amount of time in a workday that employees spend performing physically demanding or repetitive tasks (i.e., the duration of tasks). Both the total time per work shift and the length of uninterrupted periods of work can be significant in contributing to problems. As repetitive motions, forceful exertions, and other contributing factors increase in work tasks, so does the recovery time (i.e., the length and frequency of muscle relaxation breaks) needed to help reduce fatigue and prevent injury.

It is very important to uncover why (i.e., the reasons or root causes) the contributing factors are occurring in work tasks because it allows employers to fully understand the nature of the problem and eventually to come up with effective improvement options.

Awkward Postures

Posture affects muscle groups which are active during physical activity. Awkward postures can make work tasks more physically demanding by increasing the exertion required from smaller muscle groups and preventing the stronger, larger muscle groups from working at maximum efficiency. The increased exertion from the weaker, smaller muscle groups impairs blood flow and increases the rate of fatigue. Awkward postures typically include repeated or prolonged reaching, twisting, bending, working overhead, kneeling, squatting, and holding fixed positions or pinch grips. They may affect various areas of the body such as the hands, wrists, arms, shoulders, neck, back, and knees. The effects of awkward postures are worse if work tasks also involve repetitive motions or forceful exertions. Awkward postures may be caused by poorly designed or arranged workstations, tools, and equipment and by poor work practices.

Visual Effort

Sometimes employees assume awkward postures or experience eyestrain and fatigue because it is hard for them to see their work.

For example, when the lighting is bad, the work is too far away, or materials are blocking the field of vision, employees may have to bend, reach, twist, or hold fixed positions. Similarly, handling or assembling very small parts and materials or performing extremely precise tasks may contribute to eyestrain and awkward postures.

Repetitive Motions

In repetitive work, the same types of motions are performed over and over again using the same muscles, tendons, or joints. The amount of repetition can be affected by the pace of work, the recovery time provided (i.e., number and length of muscle relaxation breaks), and the amount of variety in work tasks. The pace of work may be controlled by the employee performing the task, machines, other employees, or administrative procedures. Examples of jobs involving machine-controlled pace include working on assembly, packaging, or quality-control lines. Work tasks linked to performance or incentives are examples of administratively controlled pace.

The risk of injury is greater when repetitious jobs involve awkward posture or forceful exertions. Injuries may also develop when highly repetitive jobs are combined with low-force exertions, such as in light assembly tasks involving the hands, wrists, elbows, and shoulders. An example could be, having to grip a cutting or trimming tool throughout the entire work task without being able to set it down momentarily to rest the hand.

Forceful Exertions

Force is the amount of muscular effort expended to perform work. Exerting large amounts of force can result in fatigue and physical damage to the body. The amount of force exerted when moving or handling materials, tools, or objects depends on a combination of factors, including:

- Load shape, weight, dimensions, and bulkiness
- Grip type, position, and friction characteristics
- Amount of effort required to start and stop the load when moving it (i.e., how physically demanding it is to accelerate or decelerate the load)

- Length of time *continuous force* is applied by the muscles (e.g., the amount of time the load or object is held, carried, or handled without a muscle-relaxation break)
- Number of times the load is handled per hour or work shift
- Amount of associated vibration
- Body posture used
- Resistance associated with moving the load (e.g., over rough flooring or with poorly maintained equipment)
- Duration of the task over the work shift
- Environmental temperature
- Amount of rotational force (e.g., torque from tools or equipment).

Pressure Points (Local Contact Stress)

Pressure points result from the body pressing against hard or sharp surfaces. Certain areas of the body are more susceptible because nerves, tendons, and blood vessels are close to the skin and underlying bones. These areas include the sides of the fingers, palms, wrists and forearms, elbows, and the knees.

Vibration

Vibration exposure is of concern when it is continuous or of very high intensity. Using vibrating tools such as sanders, grinders, chippers, routers, impact guns, drills, chain saws, and circular saws can cause exposure to hand-arm vibration. Tools that are not properly maintained or are inappropriate for the task may increase the amount of hand-arm vibration. These exposures may result in fatigue, pain, numbness, tingling, increased sensitivity to cold, and decreased sensitivity to touch in the fingers, hands, and arms.

Whole-body vibration commonly results from sitting or standing on work surfaces that vibrate. Examples of such surfaces include vibrating vehicles, equipment, and platforms. Whole-body vibration may be associated with general discomfort and lower back pain.

Ergonomics Job-Analysis Methods

There are many different types of ergonomics job-analysis methods. These methods consist of various techniques for taking a systematic look at jobs and work tasks. They help decide which jobs and specific tasks may contribute to problems. Once it is known where the problems exist, it is easier to come up with ideas for making improvements.

Some methods are relatively simple, and others require detailed analysis and sophisticated equipment. Checklists are generally a simpler, less comprehensive type of ergonomics job-analysis method. More comprehensive methods break jobs down into specific movements (e.g., reach, grasp, place) or use other complicated techniques.

Ergonomics job-analysis methods also vary according to what types of work activities they address. Some focus on workstation design. Others are more specific to certain types of work (e.g., manual materials handling or the office environment) or focus on the work environment (e.g., lighting, cold exposures).

Work Site Analysis

- Hazard Prevention and Control
- Engineering Controls
- Work Practice Controls
- Personal Protective Equipment
- Administrative Controls

Training and Education

- General Training
- Job-specific Training
- Training for Supervisors
- Training for Managers
- Training for Engineers and Maintenance Personnel

Site Analysis

- Gathering information from available sources (injury reports, employees, worker modifications to workstations, personal observations, etc.)
- Conducting screening surveys
- Performing ergonomic Job Hazard Analysis
- Conducting periodic surveys and follow-ups.

Informational Sources

- Perform records analysis and tracking to identify ergonomic hazards
- Medical, Safety, or Insurance Records
- Employee surveys

Incidence Rates

- $IR = \frac{\textit{New Cases/yr (200,000 hrs)}}{\text{Hours Worked/yr}}$
- Note: Per Facility
- Why 200,000 hours? Average worker puts in 2000 hours (work) per year – The IR considers the hours of 100 workers in its determination

Worksite Analysis

- Checklists (chairs, workstations, job requirements, etc.)
- Ergonomic Risk Factors
- Cumulative Trauma Disorder Risk Factors
- Back Disorder Risk Factors
- Multiple Risk Factors
- Lifting Hazards
- Videotaped Analysis
- Periodic Ergonomic Surveys
- Employee Feedback and Follow-up
- Trend Analysis.

Hazard Prevention and Control

- **Purpose:** Make the job fit the person *and to not* make the person fit the job
- **Activities:**
  - Workstation design
  - Design of work methods
  - Tool design and handles
  - Understand your workplace population (Age, heights, etc.)

Workstation Design (see Fig. 10.1)

- Designed for the individuals who actually use them

- Not sufficient to design it for the "average" person (aim is 90% of workforce population)
- Should be designed large enough to allow for a full range of required movements.

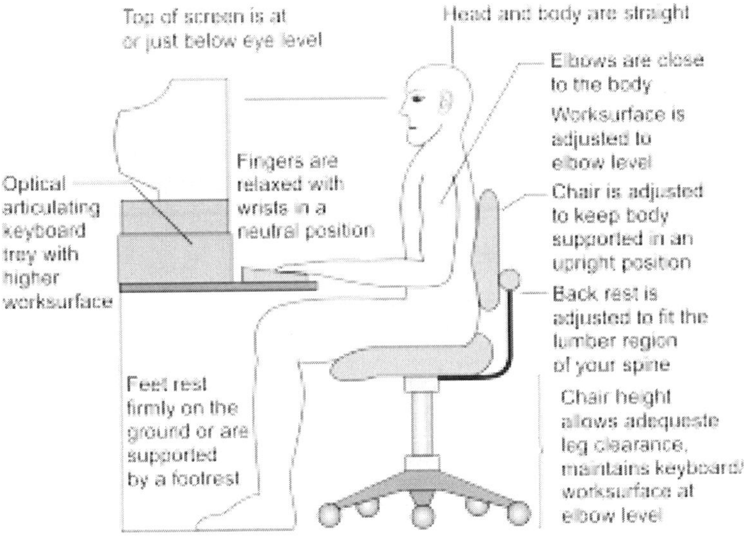

Fig. 10.1: Work Station Design

Design of Work Methods

- Traditionally considers static postures and repetition rates
- Should also look at force levels required
- Hand and arm postures involved
- Alter tasks to alleviate CTD causing stresses
- Identify light-duty as well as high-risk jobs.

Tool Design and Handles

- Design for both left and right handed
- Triggers that depress easily, activated by one or two fingers
- Grips should distribute pressure over the fleshy part of the palm, and not dig into it
- Design should incorporate minimum weight to be handled, counterbalancing provided if required
- Minimum vibration and proper maintenance

Medical Management

Purpose: To aid in the early identification, evaluation, and treatment of signs and symptoms and to prevent their occurrence and aid in their prevention

- Employee Training and Education.
- Encourage Early Report of Symptoms.
- Protocols for Health-Care Providers.
- Evaluation, Treatment and Follow-up.
- OSHA Record-Keeping Forms.
- Monitor Trends.

Components of Medical Management

- Medical Personnel trained in treatment of Cumulative Trauma Disorders
- Periodic Workplace Walk-through
- Symptoms Survey Review (measures the extent in each area of the workplace)
- Employee Symptoms Survey.

Common Indicators of Problems

- Apparent trends in accidents and injuries
- Incidence of CTD's
- Absenteeism and high turnover
- Employee complaints and *informal* modifications made to work stations
- Poor quality output with high amounts of manual material handling.

Identifying Ergonomic Problems

- General Observation
- Questionnaires and Interviews
- Videotaping and Photography
- Drawing or Sketching
- Measurements of the work environment
- Understanding the ergonomic aspects of aging (along with diverse workforce populations).

Ergonomics of Aging

- About the age of 45: Nerve conduction, hand-grip strength, muscle mass, range of motion, and flexibility diminish
- Height diminishes, beginning about age 30
- Lower back pain is much more common
- Visual acuity at close range diminishes
- Weight and mass increases.

Strategies for Ergonomic Problem Solving

- Seated Repetitive Work with Light Parts
- Seated Work with Larger Parts
- Seated Control Work/Standing Work
- Standing for Heavy lifting and Carrying
- Work requirements with hands above the chest
- Hand Tools.

Economics of Ergonomics

- Highly debated : A cost-benefit analysis for ergonomics (injuries occur over time, hard to pin down causation factor)
- Hard to perform with a cause/effect analysis
- Requires a high commitment of time and money
- Requires extensive follow-up evaluations
- Industry apprehensive of costs to be incurred.

Repetitive Strain Injuries (RSIs)

- An umbrella term that covers a number of cumulative trauma disorders (CTDs) caused by forceful or awkward movements repeated frequently over time
- Factors involved: Improper workstation design, poor posture, and job stress

Prevention of Repetitive Strain Injuries (RSI's)

- Employee training
- Exercise (see Fig. 10.2)
- Select tools wisely
- Medical monitoring

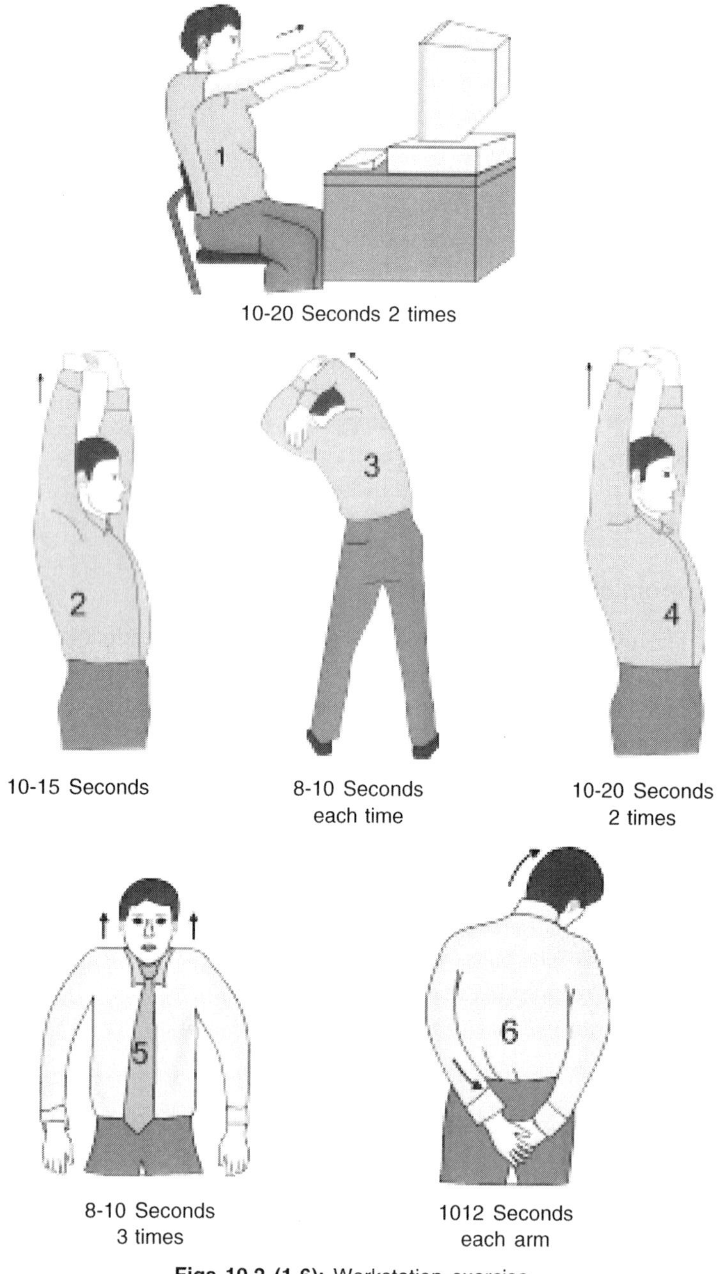

Figs 10.2 (1-6): Workstation exercise

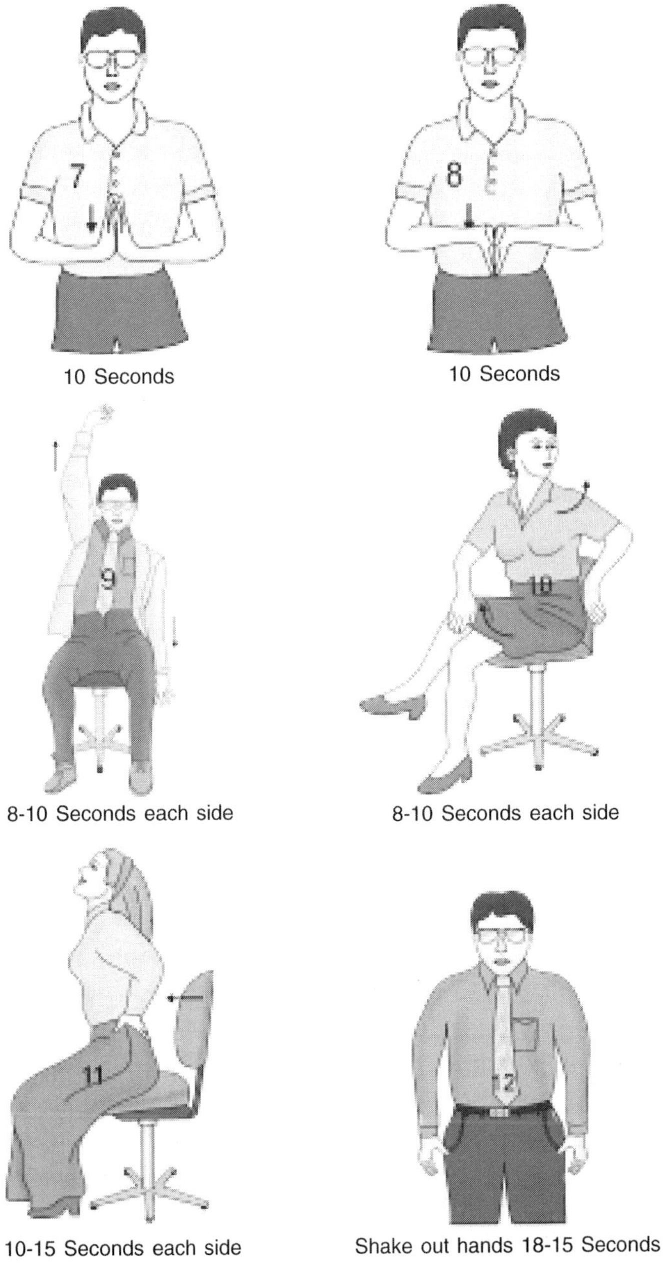

Figs 10.2 (7-12): Workstation exercise

Ergonomic Improvements

Ergonomic improvements are changes that can be made to improve the "fit" between a job and the capabilities of the employees performing it. They are commonly grouped into three categories:

1. ***Engineering Improvements:*** Engineering improvements include rearranging, modifying, redesigning, or replacing tools, equipment, workstations, packaging, parts, or products. These improvements can be very effective because they may reduce or eliminate contributing factors. The best time to select engineering improvements is when new facilities, processes, or work procedures are being planned. Some engineering improvement options:
   a. Raise or lower the work surface or the employee — reduces bending, reaching, and awkward postures.
   b. Use cutout work surfaces — allows employees to get closer to their work, reducing visual effort and awkward postures.
   c. Reposition the work — reduces bending and reaching.
   d. Reconfigure the workstation — sliding and rolling replaces lifting and carrying.
   e. Use adjustable equipment — allows comfortable, upright working posture.
   f. Provide close, convenient storage for frequently used materials, parts, or tools — reduces reaching and awkward postures.
   g. Provide comfort.
   h. Be innovative.
   i. Lifting aids reduce force, repetition, and awkward postures in lifting or handling tasks.
   j. Mechanical aids reduce force, repetition, and awkward postures in transporting materials and products around the workplace.
   k. Provide adequate, well-lit storage with easy access for employees — reduces repetitive reaching, bending, twisting, and forceful exertions.
   l. Increase the efficient use of storage space by grouping stored items by container size or shape.

m. Good design and proper maintenance can help reduce pressure points on the hands, awkward postures (e.g., bent wrists), forceful exertions, and other contributing factors.

n. Find ways to reduce hand-arm and whole-body vibration through:
   - Routine maintenance
   - Vibration-dampening wraps on handles
   - Isolating the tool from the operator
   - Properly fitting vibration-dampening gloves
   - Good design of an alternate or low-vibration tool
   - Suspending or supporting tools (e.g., by a fixture)
   - Providing vibration isolators (e.g., springs or pads) for seated work tasks
   - Providing cushioned floor mats for standing work tasks
   - Mounting equipment and work platforms on vibration-dampening pads or springs
   - Altering the speed or motion of tools and equipment.

2. ***Administrative Improvements***: Administrative improvements include changing work practices or the way work is organized. They may not address the reasons for the contributing factors or other problems. Administrative improvements usually require continual management and employee feedback to ensure that the new practices and policies are effective. Some administrative improvements options:

   a. *Providing variety in jobs:* Job rotation and job enlargement strategies could be used to increase variety in jobs. *Job rotation* means rotating employees through different jobs. *Job enlargement* means increasing the variety by combining two or more jobs or adding tasks to a particular job. To be effective, both of these improvements rely on rotating through or combining jobs and tasks which differ in the following ways:
      - Muscles or body parts used
      - Working postures
      - Amount of repetition
      - Pace of work
      - Amount of physical exertion required
      - Visual and mental demands
      - Environmental conditions

b. *Adjusting work schedules and work pace:* Try to limit the amount of time any employee has to spend performing a "problem job." If you have new employees or employees returning from long absences, introduce them to a normal work pace and workload gradually, like athletes in spring training.

c. *Providing minibreaks:* Work should be broken up with frequent, short recovery periods or minibreaks. These short breaks (5–10 min every hour) can help prevent the accumulation of fatigue and injury to muscles and their associated structures. Even breaks as short as a few seconds on a regular basis are helpful.

d. *Modifying work practices:* Pay close attention to how the work is being performed. Our bodies are stronger, more efficient, and less injury prone when we work in midrange postures. Maintaining midrange working postures simply means sitting or standing upright and not bending the joints into extreme positions. This can be done by trying to keep the neck, back, arms, and wrists within a range of neutral positions. Employees should be encouraged to be comfortable, to change positions, and to stretch when working. Other work-practice improvements for work tasks involving manual handling include encouraging employees to do the following:
   - Minimize carry, push, or pull distances.
   - Try to carry roughly equal amounts of weight in each hand.
   - Turn or pivot the entire body instead of twisting at the waist.
   - Avoid jerking by using smooth, even motions.
   - Use their legs to do the work, not the upper body or back.
   - Plan by making sure paths are clear, even-surfaced, and free of obstructions.
   - Organize their work to provide gradual increases in exertion or pace.
   - Make sure their shoes have the appropriate soles for the surfaces in the workplace.

Tags can be used to identify loads that may be unstable and heavy. Before moving or handling loads you have tagged, consider:

- Testing for stability
- Reconfiguring or repackaging
- Using mechanical or other alternate means to move or handle them.

e. *Regular housekeeping and maintenance:* Ensure regular housekeeping and maintenance of work spaces, tools, and equipment. Regular housekeeping to eliminate clutter can reduce reaching, bending, or twisting when handling materials, tools, or objects. Floor surfaces kept dry and free of obstructions help eliminate slipping and tripping hazards. Regular maintenance of tools and equipment can help reduce or prevent problems in work tasks. For example, keeping cutting or drilling tools sharpened and in good condition, can reduce the amount of force and repetition required when using the tools. Fixing broken handles or replacing worn padding can help reduce vibration and awkward postures, when performing work tasks. Making sure that carts and other equipment are in good working condition can reduce the amount of force required to move materials.

a. *Encouraging exercise:* Long-term, sensible exercise has many benefits, which may include better health and reduced injuries. Individuals in good physical condition are generally more productive and less injury prone. Regular exercise can increase an individual's energy level, alertness, and coordination. The range of motion of joints and the circulation may also improve with regular exercise. Remember to encourage your employees to warm up, perform gentle stretching (e.g., without bouncing), and increase their physical exertion gradually. New, returning, or injured employees should gradually increase their physical activity.

3. ***Personal Protective Equipment:*** Personal protective equipment (PPE) includes gloves, knee and elbow pads, footwear, and other items that employees wear.
   - Gloves can protect hands from cold or injury. However, gloves may decrease manual dexterity and make it harder to grip, if they do not fit correctly.

- Proper footwear and antifatigue soles can prevent employees from slipping and prevent fatigue from long hours of standing on hard surfaces.
- Knee and elbow pads can protect the body from pressure points, when pressing against hard or sharp surfaces.
- Back belts are not typically considered to be personal protective equipment. They may help maintain the proper curvature of the spine during lifting or physical exertion and may also provide comfort and confidence while performing work tasks but it has not been proven that they are effective in reducing back injuries.

Training

An important part of an effective ergonomics program is training and education. For improvements to be effective, employees need to be trained thoroughly and given opportunities for hands-on practice with any new tools, equipment, or work procedures. The goals for training should include a mix of the knowledge and the skills needed to work safely. Employees should always be informed of any workplace changes.

A training program should include the following individuals:
- All affected employees
- Engineers and maintenance personnel
- Supervisors
- Managers
- Health care providers

The program should be designed and implemented by qualified persons. Appropriate special training should be provided for personnel responsible for administering the program. The program should be presented in a language and at a level of understanding appropriate for the individuals being trained. It should provide an overview of the potential risk of illnesses and injuries, their causes and early symptoms, the means of prevention, and treatment.

The program should also include a means for adequately evaluating its effectiveness. This might be achieved by using employee interviews, testing, and observing work practices, to determine if those who received training understand the material and the work practices to be followed.

Training for affected employees should consist of both general and specific job training:

1. ***General Training:*** Employees who are potentially exposed to ergonomic hazards should be given formal instruction on the hazards associated with their jobs and with their equipment. This includes information on the varieties of CTDs, what risk factors cause or contribute to them, how to recognize and report symptoms, and how to prevent these disorders. This instruction should be repeated for each employee as necessary or at least annually.
2. ***Job Specific Training:*** New employees and reassigned employees should receive an initial orientation and hands on training prior to starting their duties. Each new hire should receive a demonstration of the proper use of and procedures for all tools and equipment. The initial training program should include the following:
   - Care, use, and handling techniques for tools and equipment they might use as part of their job
   - Use of special tools and equipment associated with individual work stations
   - Use of appropriate guards and safety equipment, including personal protective equipment
   - Use of proper lifting techniques and devices.

   On the job training should emphasize employee development and use of safe and efficient techniques.
3. ***Training for Supervisors:*** Supervisors are responsible for ensuring that employees follow safe work practices and receive appropriate training to enable them to do so. Supervisors therefore should undergo training comparable to that of the employees, and such additional training as will enable them to recognize early signs and symptoms of CTDs, to recognize hazardous work practices, to correct such practices, and to reinforce the employer's ergonomic program, especially through ergonomic training of employees as may be needed.

4. ***Training for Managers:*** Managers should be aware of their safety and health responsibilities and should receive sufficient training pertaining to ergonomic issues at each work station and at the organizational level as a whole so that they can effectively carry out their responsibilities.
5. ***Training for Engineers and Maintenance Personnel:*** Plant engineers and maintenance personnel should be trained in the prevention and correction of ergonomic hazards through job and work station design and proper maintenance, both in general and as applied to the specific conditions of the facility.

To assess the fit between a person and their work, ergonomists have to consider many aspects.

These include

- The job being done and the demands on the worker
- The equipment used (its size, shape, and how appropriate it is for the task)
- The information used (how it is presented, accessed, and changed)
- The physical environment (temperature, humidity, lighting, noise, vibration)
- The social environment (such as teamwork and supportive management).

Ergonomists consider all the physical aspects of a person, such as:

- Body size and shape
- Fitness and strength
- Posture
- The senses, especially vision, hearing and touch
- The stresses and strains on muscles, joints, nerves.

Ergonomists also consider the psychological aspects of a person, such as:

- Mental abilities
- Personality
- Knowledge
- Experience.

Benefits of ergonomics to the workplace:

- Reduces the potential for accidents
- Reduces the potential for injury and ill health
- Improves performance and productivity.

COMPUTER WORKSTATION EVALUATION CHECKLIST

This checklist is designed to help you adapt/adjust your computer workstation and your video display terminal (VDT) to help prevent common stresses and injuries associated with VDT usage.

Chair

A well-designed and adjusted chair improves circulation and posture and prevents back strains and fatigue. Check the following:

- Chair height (up/down) and backrest tension/angle are easily adjustable
- Chair is equipped with a padded seat and back cushion
- Front edge of seat pan is rounded and seamless
- Seat is at least 18" wide × 15" long
- Chair has non-slippery upholstery with porous "breathable" fabric
- Backrest has height adjustable lower back support
- Backrest is at least 18" tall × 14" wide
- Seat tilts back only slightly as the backrest tilts back
- Chair swivels easily on casters
- Chair is supported with five legs for stability
- Base of chair is at least 24" around
- Height and width adjustable arm rests provided if needed.

Foot/Leg Positions

The proper foot and leg positions help prevent stress in your neck and shoulders plus prevent cramping and stiffness in your legs. Check the following:

- Feet are flat on the floor or on a footrest
- 3" - 6" of leg room between legs and workstation
- Thighs are parallel to floor
- Knees are at 90-110 degree angle.

Keyboard/Arm and Wrist Positions

Proper positioning of your keyboard and your arms and wrists will improve comfort and avoid injury. Check the following:

- Keyboard is detachable and slightly sloped at about 10-15 degrees
- Keyboard is prevented from slipping
- Wrists are relaxed and straight (neutral)
- Wrist rest or parallel support arm rests used if needed
- Arms are close to body with elbows at 90-degree angle
- Wrist/forearms are parallel to floor
- Mouse is at same level as keyboard and within easy reach

Workstation

A well-designed and arranged workstation encourages good posture and provides less stress on the body. Check the following:

- Table height is adjustable if needed
- Table surface is 25" - 27" above the floor and 30" deep
- Adequate space to adjust height/location of monitor
- Front edge of table is rounded
- Materials used most often are arranged within easy reach
- Document holder is at same height and distance as the display screen
- Telephone headset or speakerphone used if needed
- Storage drawers located under desk/table do not restrict knee clearance

Display Screen/Monitor

Adjusting the viewing distance, height, angle and clarity of the display screen can reduce eye and neck strain. Check the following:

- Display screen is 18"- 30" away from your eyes
- Top line of display (print) is slightly below eye level
- Display is tilted slightly to reduce reflections and glare
- Display screen is clean and free of flickering
- Brightness and contrast controls are adjusted for viewing comfort.

Lighting/Glare Reduction

Proper lighting and glare reduction will reduce the strain on your eyes. Check the following:

- Indirect or shielded lighting used to reduce reflections and glare
- Window blinds or drapes are adjusted or closed when needed
- Lighting levels are adjusted (where possible) throughout the day
- Face of display screen is at right (90 degree) angles to windows
- Ceiling lights are located to the side of the screen (not directly overhead)
- Anti-glare screen/filter used if necessary
- Task lighting or desk lamp adjusted to avoid glare and reflections.

Equipment to Consider

- Adjustable document holder
- Wrist/mouse rest
- Keyboard extension for wrist rest
- Anti-glare screen/filter
- Task light/desk lamp
- Lumbar support
- Footrest
- Telephone headset or speakerphone.

Work Task Evaluation

Name of Employee ---

Job Title --

Tasks in this job are:

For *each task* you have noted for this job, ask the employee(s) performing the work the following questions:

How hard is this task? Score	Score How often is this task done? Score
Very easy 1	Seasonally (a few times a year) 1
Easy 2	Occasionally (a few times a shift or week) 2
Somewhat hard 3	Frequently (up to 4 hours per shift) 3
Hard 4	Constantly (more than 4 hours per shift) 4
Very hard 5	Extended hours (more than 8 hours per shift) 5

Total the scores for *each task* and multiply the totals for the two questions to get a total for the task.

Tasks	Score for "how hard"	×	Score for "how often"	=	Total for the task

ERGONOMICS AWARENESS CHECKLIST

Job title ____________________ Job location ______________

Name of employee ________________________________

Name of observer ____________ Date: __________________

Contributing Factor Descriptions

- *Awkward postures:* Repeated or prolonged reaching, twisting, bending, working overhead, kneeling, squatting, holding fixed position, or pinch grips
- *Repetition:* Performing the same types of motions over and over again using the same muscles, tendons, or joints
- *Forceful exertion:* The amount of muscular effort expended to perform work
- *Pressure points (local contact stress):* The body pressing against hard or sharp surfaces
- *Vibration:* Continuous or high-intensity hand–arm or whole-body vibration
- *Other factors:* Extreme high or low temperatures; lighting too dark or too bright

For each task list, the contributing factor(s) you observe and the reasons for them.

Contributing Factor (CF)	Reason for CF	Comments
Task 1		**Total Score**
______________		______________
______________		______________
______________		______________
______________		______________
______________		______________
______________		______________

Contd...

Contd...

Contributing Factor (CF)	Reason for CF	Comments
Task 2		Total Score
Task 3		Total Score
Task 4		Total Score

Table 10.5: Checklist for Risk Factors

Things to look for:	*Possible solutions, depending on further analysis:*
Prolonged hunched or elevated shoulder while holding the phone	• Telephone headset • Speakerphone
Elbows splayed out (shoulder abduction)	• Lower work surface • Lower chair armrests • Bring chair armrests in closer • Awareness and habit training
Raised or tensed shoulders	• Habit or tension training • Lower worksurface or keyboard • Lower chair armrests • Raise chair, if foot contact with the floor can be maintained
Twisting the head to the side	Bring viewed item closer to centerline of view
Elbow flexed for long periods using the telephone	• Telephone headset • Speakerphone
Elbow or forearm resting for long periods on hard or sharp worksurface, chair armrests	• Pad or round surfaces, corners, and armrests • Replace armrests • Telephone headset • Habit training
Wrists bent to the sides when using side keys	• Habit training • Keyboard with more accessible keys or split keyboard design
Wrists bent back (extended) or forward (flexed) for prolonged periods	• Habit training • Palm rest • Lower, raise, or change slope of the keyboard
Wrists or palms resting for long periods on hard or sharp keyboard or work surfaces	• Habit training • Palm rest • Padded or rounded surfaces, corners
Hands held actively over the keyboard during keying pauses	• Habit training • Palm or forearm rest

Contd...

Contd...

Things to look for:	*Possible solutions, depending on further analysis:*
Rapid, sustained, or prolonged keying	• Greater work variety • Aggressive break schedule • Reduce overtime
Forceful keying, key pounding	• Habit training • Light-touch keyboard
Significant amounts of hand stapling, punching, lifting, opening mail, or other forceful exertions, especially combined with awkward postures	• Mechanical aids, such as electric stapler or punch • Reduce size of lifted loads • Bring heavy loads close to the body, at a medium height • Substitute sliding (worksurface) or wheeling (floor) • Sharpen letter openers
Prolonged mouse use	• Greater work variety • Aggressive break schedule • Alternate hands • Alternative pointing devices • Arm support, including small table • Mouse close to body (extended keyboard tray) • Learn keystroke substitutes for menus
Prolonged sitting, especially in only one posture	• Greater work variety • Aggressive break schedule • Chair that supports posture change, through movement, size, or easy adjustability • Habit training • Move phone and printer to the other side of the office to force standing, or suggest standing when on phone • Check chair fit • Monitor in-out mechanism • Sit-stand worksurface

Contd...

Contd...

Things to look for:	***Possible solutions, depending on further analysis:***
Lumbar back area not supported	• Lumbar cushion • Backrest height and tilt • Check chair fit, especially backrest/lumbar height
Feet dangling, not well supported, or a posture which seems to put pressure on the backs of the thighs	• Lower chair • Lower worksurface • Habit training • Foot rest (last resort)
Chair backrest not used for long periods	• Check chair fit, especially seat pan depth and height • Check leg room • Check monitor distance and character height • Habit training
Twisted torso	• Rearrange work • Provide more knee space • U-shaped worksurface layout • Swivel chair
Frequent or prolonged leaning or reaching	• Rearrange work • Mouse pad, palm or forearm rest • Bring mouse and keyboard closer to body
Working with one or both arms "reaching" toward a mouse or keyboard	• Bring keyboard closer to body • Mouse pad, palm or forearm rest • Bring mouse closer to keyboard
Light sources that can be seen by the worker	• Cover or shield light sources • Rearrange work arena • Lower other viewed objects to lower field of view
Reflected glare on the screen	• Shield light sources • Shade screen • Glare screen • Move monitor so light enter from side angle, not back Do NOT tip monitor down • Lower light levels • Move light sources

Contd...

Contd...

Things to look for:	***Possible solutions, depending on further analysis:***
Too much contrast between screen and surroundings or document; worker feels relief when bright areas are shielded	• Lower ambient light levels • Turn off, reposition, or dim task lights • Block offending light sources • Change screen polarity to black on white
Very bright ambient lighting (above 500 lux or 50 fc) or shadowed areas caused by over-illumination	Lower ambient light levels to 200-500 lux (20-50 fc) and use task lights
Monitor closer than approximately 65 cm (25")	• Push monitor back (enlarge font size) • Habit training for reclining • Computer glasses • Bring keyboard forward, possibly with a keyboard tray
Different viewed objects (screen, documents) at different distances from the eyes	Use document stand or otherwise equalize distances to within about 10 cm (4") if rapid viewing changes are required
Screen or documents not oriented perpendicular to the line of sight (tipped back slightly is even better)	Change monitor, document stand angle
Prolonged near focusing throughout the day with few far-focusing opportunities	• Move monitor back as far as possible • Habit training • Rearrange space to provide view • Introduce glazing
Monitor image dim, fuzzy, flickery, small, or otherwise difficult to read	• Upgrade monitor • Use software toenlarge image
Shiny, low-contrast, or small-print documents	Improve lighting on documents if documents cannot be changed

Contd...

Contd...

Things to look for:	*Possible solutions, depending on further analysis:*
Forward head posture (peering) or squinting	• Lower monitor • Tilt monitor back • Check for monitor image quality problems, character height or monitor distance • Suggest consultation with vision specialist
Eyestrain complaints	• Check all aspects of visual environment • Suggest consultation with vision specialist
Neck extended backwards, head tilted back, even slightly	• Remove CPU from under monitor • Remove tilt-swivel base from monitor (leave ventilation space) • Check for bifocals and suggest full-frame "computer glasses" prescription
Neck severely flexed (downward)	• Tilt face of monitor back • Tilt document - do not lay flat on work surface • Raise document or monitor to a comfortable height • Adjust posture • Habit retraining • Check glasses for proper prescription.

THINGS YOU SHOULD KNOW ABOUT EYESTRAIN

1. Eyestrain means different things to different people. It can be experienced as burning, tightness, sharp pains, dull pains, watering, blurring, double vision, headaches, and other sensations, depending on the person. If you have any eye discomfort caused by viewing something, you can call it eyestrain.
2. 2. In VDT workstations, the principal factors affecting the ability to see well are:

- Glare
- The luminance (brightness) difference between what is being Looked at and its immediate environment
- The amount of light
- The distance between the eye and the screen and document
- The readability of the screen and document
- The worker's vision and his or her corrective lenses.

3. Watch out for direct glare. Direct glare involves a light source shining directly into the eyes — ceiling lights, task lights, or bright windows. To determine the degree of direct glare, you can temporarily shield your eyes with a hand and notice whether you feel immediate relief.
4. Reflected glare, such as on computer screens, sometimes causes eyestrain. But its worst effect may be causing you to change your posture to an uncomfortable one, in order to see well.
5. The most overlooked cause of eyestrain in offices is contrast — usually, a dark screen surrounded by a bright background such as a window or a lit wall. The best solution is to find a way to darken the area around the screen. This problem occurs mainly on screens with light letters on a black background.
6. How much light is right? It depends on your age, the quality of the print you are reading, and other factors. There should be plenty of light for easy reading, but too much can, depending on the person, cause eyestrain.
7. Eyes are strained more by close viewing than by distant viewing. The "right" distance for computer monitors and documents depends entirely on how clearly they can be read at a given distance. The general rule is to keep viewed material as far away as possible, provided it can be read easily.
8. If you gaze at something too long, your eyes can tire. Eyes need to focus at different distances from time to time. It's a good idea to follow the "20/20 rule" — every twenty minutes, look twenty feet away for twenty seconds.
9. If two objects are only a couple of inches different in their distance from the eyes, the eyes actually do NOT have to refocus to look from one to another. Greater distance differences, however, can overwork the eyes if you have to look from one object to another

frequently — as when typing from printed copy and looking at the screen. In general, keep viewed objects at about the same distance if you have to look back and forth a lot.

10. Can computer work cause nearsightedness? Rarely, according to optometrists. It's more likely that computer work makes you realize that you need glasses.
11. Sometimes eyestrain is just a case of dry eyes. Lowering the monitor can help. Looking downward means more of the eye surface is covered by the eyelid, and two other things happen: the eyes unconsciously blink more, and they produce more lubrication. People who need bifocals should consider other options besides bifocals. Two good ones are:
    - Computer glasses that focus at the right distance for the computer screen.
    - Wearing contact lenses — corrected for computer or reading distance in one eye, and for far distance (if needed) in the other eye.
12. Bifocal wearers often experience sore necks and shoulders because they have to tip their heads back to see the computer screen.
    - Lower the screen as much as possible — if it sits on the CPU, move the CPU.
    - If necessary, remove the monitor's tilt-swivel base (consult a computer hardware person first) to gain a couple additional inches.
    - Lower the work surface that the monitor sits on.

ABOUT BACK PAIN

1. Back pain is as mystifying today as it was decades ago. Despite excellent tests and procedures, modern back specialists admit that up to eighty percent of all cases have no clear physiological cause. In fact, many pain-free people show bulging or herniated discs in x-rays.
2. Also, despite everything we know about back pain, ninety percent of us are going to have a disabling episode at some point in our lives.

3. It is difficult to predict which individual person will develop back pain. Strength, fitness, and back x-rays are not good predictors. One major study concluded that the only predictors were 1) whether the person has had back pain before, and 2) whether the person smokes cigarettes.
4. On the other hand, job characteristics are predictors of back pain. Jobs with heavy or frequent lifting are high risk, as are jobs involving prolonged standing or sitting.
5. There is little agreement on how to do lifting with little risk. Lifting with the legs is easy on the back, but hard on the legs and muscles. Lifting with the back puts strain on the disks but is less fatiguing.
6. So-called 'back belts' have not been proven to strengthen backs or prevent back problems. On one hand, they may help remind wearers to lift carefully. On the other hand, they may give wearers a false sense of greater strength, encouraging them to lift more than they should.
7. People who sit for long periods are at risk for back disorders. The two greatest problems seem to be 1) sitting upright or forward, and 2) not changing position.
8. An upright posture with a ninety-degree hip position is actually unhealthy, from the perspective of the intervertebral discs. For a number of reasons, the discs experience more pressure—and the pressure is more lopsided—than while standing. So it's a good idea to sit with the hip joints somewhat straightened. Yes, this resembles a slouch, with your rear end forward in the seat. A supported slouch may be healthy in the long run. Forward-tilt chairs support this posture, but so do chairs with level seats and reclined backrests.
9. Even if the hip joints aren't somewhat straightened, sitting in a reclined posture is healthier than sitting upright. This is because reclined sitting puts more of your weight onto the chair's backrest. If the chair backrest holds-up more weight, the discs in the lower back hold up *less* weight. (Well-designed armrests also take some of the upper body weight from the discs). And reclined sitting lets the back muscles relax.

10. All sitters should move around. In addition to helping the muscles relax and recover, this alternately squeezes and unsqueezes the intervertebral discs, which results in better filtration of fluids into and out of the cores of the discs. Discs stay plumper and, in the long run, healthier. One implication: chairs should follow the sitter as he/she changes posture.
11. The most important chair adjustments are
    - Seat height from the floor — the feet should be able to rest flat on the floor. (however, this doesn't mean the feet should always be flat on the floor). Legs should be free to stay in different positions.
    - Depth from the front of the seat to the backrest — sitters should be able to use the backrest without any pressure behind the knees.
    - Lumbar support height — every person is shaped differently.
12. The 'proper' chair adjustments and chair posture are greatly influenced by the rest of the work area. In particular, the eyes can affect posture, especially if the work material is too far, low, or high. Hand positions (especially working far from the body) can also affect body position, particularly the posture of the upper back and neck.
13. Upper back and neck discomfort is often related to upward viewing angles (for example, monitors above eye height) or leaning, twisting, or reaching (for example, looking down and sideways at a document on the desk, or reaching for a mouse).
14. For people with existing, chronic, difficult back pain: all the above rules are optional, because each back pain case is different. Rules for prevention of back pain or treatment of medium- level cases may be completely inappropriate for individual cases of severe back pain. Before accepting any advice, trust the "advice" of your own body's discomfort reactions.

HAND AND WRIST PAIN (CUMULATIVE TRAUMA DISORDERS OR CTDS)

1. There are many kinds of CTD medical conditions that have ergonomic causes among office workers, including carpal tunnel

syndrome and various kinds of tendon inflammation. Some other disorders, such as myofascial pain syndrome, fibromyalgia, thoracic outlet syndrome, and reflexive sympathetic dystrophy are believed to be the results of cumulative trauma in some cases.

- Because of the complexity and subtle differences between disorders, physicians don't always diagnose CTD's correctly or easily. The most knowledgeable medical specialists for CTD's are generally considered to be physiatrists, or physical medicine specialists.

2. CTDs can happen when there is very little repetitious work. Besides repetition, other possible causes include:
   - Holding one position: Muscles that hold a body part in position for long periods are more prone to fatigue than muscles that move a body part around.
   - Non-neutral postures: In this context, "posture" is the position of an individual joint, not overall body posture. Any posture significantly different from "neutral" is considered to be at risk for musculoskeletal distress. "Neutral" is considered to be the position about halfway through the available range of motion for the joint.
   - Localized pressure: Direct pressure on nerves or tendons can cause damage in the long run. The wrist is one location of concern. The elbow (the funny bone or crazy-bone nerve) is another.
   - Use of force: Even small exertions can cause stress if small muscles are involved. Sudden, fast motions involving a jerk or snap.
   - Cold temperatures.
   - Vibration, as with hand-held power tools or whole-body vibration as caused by driving heavy equipment.
3. Keeping these causes in mind, some of the rules of thumb for preventing CTD's are:
   - Break up repetitious work.
   - Relax: Don't use your muscles to hold your hands or shoulders in a particular position. Keep your limbs and shoulders limp as much as possible, even during short pauses.

- Use moderate postures for individual joints. Stay away from positions near the extremes of your joints' range of motion — the most neutral joint position is about halfway.
- Minimize contact with hard or sharp surfaces. This is especially important at the wrists and elbows.
- Don't use too much force. Notice any exertions you have to make and see if they can be eliminated. "Exertions" don't have to involve breaking into a sweat. They can be subtle, such as pulling a hard-to-reach drawer or lifting a heavy file.
- Move with an even motion. Avoid snapping the wrist or jerking against outside forces.
- Keep your hands and fingers warm. Consider gloves or even fingerless gloves.
- Break up exposures to vibration.

4. "Fitting the physical workspace to the worker" is often touted as the best way to prevent CTD. This is an incomplete view. Although physical workstation design, physical tool design, and adjustability are important, there are many other work-related factors. Three less tangible but extremely important factors are job design, stress control, and individual workstyle.
   - Examples of job design are infrequent or inflexible breaks, low activity variety, and fast pace. Examples of stressors are deadlines, monitoring, and bad management. Examples of harmful workstyles (in the context of computer work, for instance) are how hard the individuals hits keys, how the individual holds his/her wrists, and where the individual places the mouse.
5. Most CTD's are preventable and curable if caught early. The key is to notice trouble when it starts — and do something about it. Early signs may include persistent pain, tingling, numbness, burning, or aching. The signs may be constant or may occur mostly after certain activities. The drastic cures — such as surgery, are not reliable and should be a last resort. Nevertheless, a health professional should be consulted when you are concerned about possible early signs.
6. Some people get CTD's because their bodies are vulnerable to them. For example, carpal tunnel syndrome seems to be related

to diabetes, overweight, thyroid conditions, hormone conditions such as those caused by hysterectomy or removal of both ovaries, rheumatoid arthritis, previous injuries, and other conditions. Smoking may also increase the risk. Anyone with any of these conditions — particularly obesity — should be especially careful about prevention.

7. CTD's can happen because of non-work activities. Hobbies, sports, driving, and even sleeping positions can contribute to them. Any attempts at treatment or prevention should include a look at off-the-job factors.
8. One of the most important preventive measures is 'variety.' In other words, change posture and activities often. If possible, take breaks before getting tired. Extremely short breaks can be very helpful of frequent enough. A "break" doesn't have to be a rest break — it can simply involve doing something else for awhile.
9. Don't follow CTD prevention rules without looking for consequences. Every fix has a drawback. Every ergonomic rule or gizmo has a downside, which can possibly make matters worse rather than better. The best way to evaluate ergonomic fixes is by considering all the ergonomic risk factors described above in #2. Example: a wrist rest may force a straighter wrist (vertically) but may put too much pressure on the underside of the wrist or make the individual bend the wrist sideways to reach side keys.
11. Total CTD prevention involves ergonomics (changing the environment), ergonomics education (changing work styles or habits), medical management (optimizing treatments and return-to-work procedures), and management (monitoring statistics to find the most hazardous jobs and working proactively). CTD's usually cannot be adequately dealt with without all four approaches happening together. Many obstacles to good ergonomics are not scientific, medical, or engineering reasons ... they are political in nature.

JOB STRESS

Job stress can be defined as the harmful physical and emotional responses that occur when the requirements of the job do not match the capabilities, resources, or needs of the worker. Job stress can lead to poor health and even injury. It results when there is Imbalance between the Demand of the job with the workers capability, need and resources.

Job stress results from the interaction of the worker and the conditions of work. Views differ on the importance of worker characteristics versus working conditions as the primary cause of job stress. There are many ways to prevent stress at work. According to one school of thought, differences in individual characteristics such as personality and coping skills are very important in predicting whether certain job conditions will result in stress. In other words, what is stressful for one person may not be a stressful or problem for someone else.

Causes for Job Stress

- *Nature of work.* Hectic and continuous long working hours, without rest and breaks.
- *Environment.* **Environment having sound and air pollution may also lead to stress.**

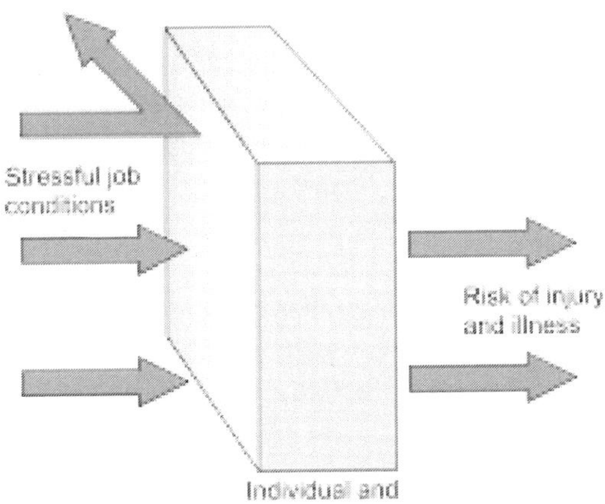

Fig. 7.3: Showing NIOSH model of Job Stress

- *Management Style.* Lack of participation by workers in decision-making, poor communication in the organization, lack of family-friendly policies.

- *Social Relationships.* Lack of support from the co-worker and senior administrative workers.
- *Job expectation.* Improper balance between Job Demand and Job expectation.
- *Job satisfaction.* **Worker feels that there is no job security,** slow growth and promotion in his career.

Early Warning Signs of Job Stress

- Depression
- Headache
- Insomnia
- Less concentration in work and other activities
- Loss of temperament
- Job dissatisfaction
- Anxiety
- Palpitations
- Mood swings
- High Blood Pressure
- Fatigue.

Nonetheless, there is some evidence that stress plays a role in the development of several types of chronic health problems—including cardiovascular disease, musculoskeletal disorders, and psychological disorders. These all problems may lead worker to have Injury, Illness, absenteeism and finally to leave the job.

Stress Management has a limited role in reducing organization stress because no effort is made to remove or reduce sources of stress at work. **Stress management has been identified as the best tool to eliminate the working stress. These can be achieves through many techniques. Few Examples are given below:**

Unhealthy strategy

- Drinking
- Smoking
- Overeating/Under eating
- Removing anger on family and friends
- Withdrawal from social activities

- Spending too much time in front of Television or Computer.
- Sleeping Pills.

Healthy strategy

- Exercise
- Relaxation Techniques
- Listening music
- Gardening
- Meditation/Yoga
- Power-nap
- Discussing problems with family and friends.
- Warm bath
- Laughter club

There are many way to combat stress and they may vary person to person, place to place.

Preventing and identifying the problem it may reduce majority of stress which also reduce chances that may lead to illness and injuries.

Preventive Organization Strategies

- Ensuring the worker can handle the workload efficiently.
- Giving opportunity to worker to show their skills and discussing new strategies that may improve work production.
- Defining workers' roles and responsibilities.
- Give workers opportunities to participate in decisions and actions affecting their jobs.
- Improving communications between supervisor, workers and co-workers.
- Making work place friendly.
- Managing work schedule, rest breaks properly.
- Combat workplace discrimination (based on race, gender, national origin, religion or language).

What Can Be Done About Job Stress?

The two methods are found to be more effective in combating Job stress:

1. Stress Management
2. Organizational Change.

No standardized approaches or simple "how to" manuals exist for developing a stress prevention program. Program design and appropriate solutions will be influenced by several factors—the size and complexity of the organization, available resources, and especially the unique types of stress problems faced by the organization.

Although it is not possible to give a universal prescription for preventing stress at work, it is possible to offer guidelines on the process of stress prevention in organizations. In all situations, the process for stress prevention programs involves three distinct steps: problem identification, intervention, and evaluation. For this process to succeed, organizations need to be adequately prepared. At a minimum, preparation for a stress prevention program should include the following:

- Building general awareness about job stress (causes, costs, and control)
- Securing top management commitment and support for the program
- Incorporating employee input and involvement in all phases of the program
- Establishing the technical capacity to conduct the program (e.g., specialized training for in-house staff or use of job stress consultants)

Steps Toward Prevention

Low morale, health and job complaints, and employee turnover often provide the first signs of job stress. But sometimes there are no clues, especially if employees are fearful of losing their jobs. Lack of obvious or widespread signs is not a good reason to dismiss concerns about job stress or minimize the importance of a prevention program.

Step 1 - Identify the Problem: The best method to explore the scope and source of a suspected stress problem in an organization depends partly on the size of the organization and the available resources. Group discussions among managers, labor representatives, and employees can provide rich sources of information. Such discussions may be all that is needed to track down and remedy stress problems in a small company. In a larger organization, such discussions can be used to help design formal surveys for gathering input about stressful job conditions from large numbers of employees.

Step 2 - Design and Implement Interventions: Once the sources of stress at work have been identified and the scope of the problem is understood, the stage is set for design and implementation of an intervention strategy.

Step 3 - Evaluate the Interventions: Evaluation is an essential step in the intervention process. Evaluation is necessary to determine whether the intervention is producing desired effects and whether changes in direction are needed.

The job stress prevention process does not end with evaluation. Rather, job stress prevention should be seen as a continuous process that uses evaluation data to refine or redirect the intervention strategy.

GUIDELINES: OCCUPATIONAL HEALTH PHYSIOTHERAPY: WORK CONDITIONING AND WORK HARDENING PROGRAMS

INTRODUCTION

Injured workers benefit from physiotherapist services from the onset of injury through their return to work. Early physiotherapy intervention consists of treatment for acute neuromusculoskeletal problems and other injuries. Many patient/clients who receive appropriate early care return to their job without additional rehabilitation services.

For those who are not able to return to work because of unresolved physical problems following acute care, the treatment focus changes to restoration of work-related function. Defined as *work conditioning*, these programs address the physical issues of flexibility, strength, endurance, coordination, and work-related function for the global outcome of return to work.

For the limited number of patient/clients with behavioral and vocational dysfunction, *work hardening* may be indicated. Work *hardening* programs are interdisciplinary and address the physical, functional, behavioral and vocational needs of the injured worker, with the global outcome of return to work. Physiotherapists provide the physical and functional components within both of these programs.

The following guidelines identify Work Conditioning and Work Hardening as separate and distinct programs for injured workers. These guidelines describe program elements that should be used to develop and guide practice.

The guidelines serve the following purposes:

- For Physiotherapists - to design, implement and evaluate structured programs for injured workers.
- For medical referral sources - to facilitate appropriate referral to structured programs.
- For insurance companies, and managed care organizations-to develop appropriate methods of program authorization, monitoring and payment.
- For Departments of Labor and Industry - to utilize as definitions and guidelines for worker compensation patients.
- For managed care organizations, regulators, and providers - to serve as a resource documents.

Guidelines

- Physiotherapy services for injured workers
- Physiotherapist professional education programs
- Professional development and staff education
- Peer review
- Education of legislators, employers, regulators and payers
- Marketing.

OPERATIONAL DEFINITIONS

Work Conditioning: an intensive, work-related, goal-oriented conditioning program designed specifically to restore systemic neuromusculoskeletal functions (e.g., joint integrity and mobility, muscle performance (including strength, power, and endurance),

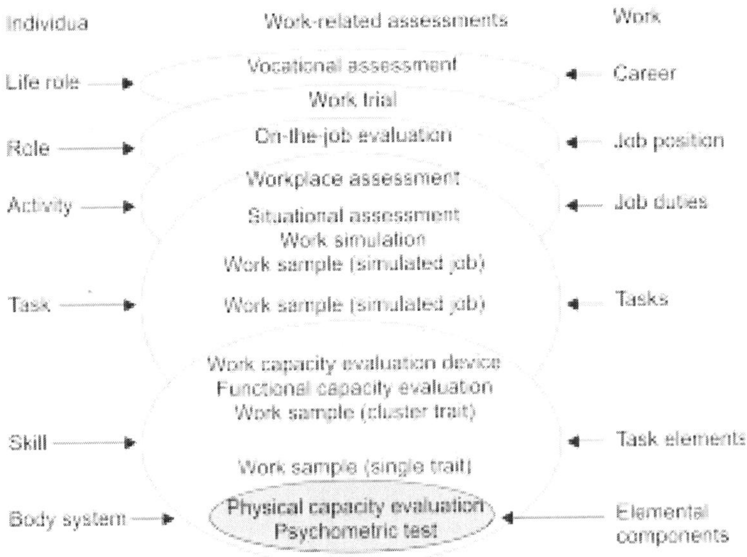

Fig 10.4: Need of Work Related Assessment

motor function (motor control and motor learning), range of motion (including muscle length), and cardiovascular/pulmonary functions (e.g. aerobic capacity/endurance, circulation, and ventilation and respiration/gas exchange). The objective of the work conditioning program is to restore physical capacity and function to enable the patient/client to return to work.

Work Conditioning Examination and Evaluation (see Fig. 10.4): Examination by history, systems review, and selected tests and measures required to identify the patient/client's individual work-related, systemic, neuromusculoskeletal restoration needs. Evaluation of examination data shall be used to identify eligibility, design a plan of care, monitor progress and plan for discharge and return to work.

Work Conditioning Provider: A Licensed Physiotherapist

Work Hardening: a highly structured, goal-oriented, individualized intervention program designed to return the patient/client to work. Work Hardening programs, which are multidisciplinary in nature, use real or simulated work activities designed to restore physical, behavioral, and vocational functions. Work Hardening addresses the issues of productivity, safety, physical tolerances, and worker behaviors.

Work Hardening Examination and Evaluation: multidisciplinary examination including history, systems review, and selected tests and measures required to identify the patient/client's individual restoration needs related to physical, functional, behavioral, and vocational status. The initial multidisciplinary evaluation of examination data is used to identify patient/client eligibility, design a plan of care, monitor progress, plan for discharge and return to work.

Work Hardening Providers: Work Hardening providers include the following professionals; physiotherapists, occupational therapists, psychologists, and vocational specialists.

Program Comparison

Table 10. 2

Work Conditioning	*Work Hardening*
Addresses physical and functional needs may be provided by one discipline (single discipline model)	Addresses physical, functional, behavioral, vocational needs within a multidisciplinary model.
Requires Work Conditioning examination and evaluation	Requires Work Hardening examination and evaluation.
Utilizes physical conditioning and functional activities related to work	Utilizes real or simulated work activities.
Provided in multi-hour sessions up to: • 4 hours/day • 5 days/week • 8 weeks	Provided in multi-hour sessions up to: • 8 hours/day • 5 days/week • 8 weeks

WORK CONDITIONING GUIDELINES

PATIENT/CLIENT ELIGIBILITY

To be eligible for Work Conditioning, a patient/client must:

- Have a job goal.
- Have stated or demonstrated willingness to participate.
- Have identified systemic neuromusculoskeletal physical and functional deficits that interfere with work.

Work conditioning generally follows acute medical care or may begin when the patient/client meets the eligibility criteria.

Work Conditioning should not begin after 365 days have elapsed following the injury without a comprehensive multidisciplinary examination and evaluation.

Provider Responsibility

The employer and/or carrier should be notified prior to initiation of the program.

The need for a program shall be established by a Work conditioning provider based on the results of a Work Conditioning examination and evaluation.

The program shall be provided by or under the direction and supervision of a Work conditioning provider.

The Work Conditioning provider shall document all examinations, evaluations, and services provided patient/client progress, and discharge plans. Information shall be available with appropriate authorization to the patient/client, employer, other providers, insurance carriers, and any referral source.

The Work Conditioning provider shall develop and utilize an outcome assessment system designed to evaluate, at a minimum, achievement of goals and outcomes, and program effectiveness and efficiency.

The Work Conditioning providers should be appropriately familiar with job expectations, work environments, and skills required of the patient/client through means such as site visitation, videotapes, and functional job descriptions.

Program Content

- Development of program goals in relation to job skills and job requirements.Interventions to improve strength, endurance, movement, flexibility, motor control and cardiovascular/ pulmonary capacity related to the performance of work tasks.
- Practice, modification, and instruction in work related activities.
- Education related to safe job performance and injury prevention.
- Promotion of patient/client responsibility and self-management.

Program Termination

The patient/client shall be discharged from the Work Conditioning program, when the goals and outcomes for the patient/client have been met.

Work Conditioning may be discontinued when any of the following occur:

- The patient/client is unable to continue to progress toward goals and outcomes because of medical or psychosocial complications or because financial/insurance resources have been expended.
- The patient/client declines to continue intervention
- The patient/client fails to comply with the requirements of participation.
- The physiotherapist determines that the patient/client will no longer benefit from physiotherapy.

When the patient/client is discharged or discontinued from the Work Conditioning program, the Work Conditioning provider shall notify the employer, insurance carrier and/or any referral source, and include the following information:

- Reasons for program termination
- Clinical and functional status
- Recommendations regarding return to work
- Recommendations for follow-up services.

WORK HARDENING GUIDELINES

PATIENT/CLIENT ELIGIBILITY

To be eligible for Work Hardening, a patient/client must:

- Have a targeted job or job plan for return to work at the time of discharge

- Have stated or demonstrated willingness to participate
- Have identified physical (systemic neuromusculoskeletal) functional, behavioral and vocational deficits that interfere with work
- Be at a point of resolution of the initial or principal injury such that participation in the Work Hardening program would not be prohibited.

  Work Hardening may begin only after the completion of the Work Hardening examination and evaluation.

Provider Responsibility

The employer and/or carrier should be notified prior to initiation of the program.

The need for a program shall be based on the results from a Work Hardening examination and evaluation performed by all of the Work Hardening providers.

The program components shall be provided by or under the direction and supervision of the appropriate Work Hardening providers.

The Work Hardening providers shall meet on a regular basis to discuss, coordinate and document program progress toward anticipated goals and expected outcomes.

The Work Hardening providers shall document all examination and evaluations, services provided, patient/client progress, and discharge plans. Information shall be available with appropriate authorization to the patient/client, employer, other professional providers, insurance carriers, and any referral source.

The Work Hardening providers shall develop and utilize an expected outcome assessment system designed to assess, at a minimum, patient/client care results, program effectiveness, and efficiency.

The Work Hardening providers should be familiar with job expectations, work environments, and skills required of the client through such means as site visitation, videotape, and functional job descriptions.

There should be an area that is designed, arranged and equipped for the specific purpose of providing Work Hardening programs.

Program Content

- Development of program goals and outcomes in relationship to specific job requirements.
- Interventions to develop joint integrity and mobility, motor function (motor control and motor learning), muscle performance (including strength, power, and endurance), range of motion, and cardiovascular/pulmonary capacity related to the performance of work tasks.
- Practice, modification, and instruction in simulated or real work activities.
- Education related to safe job performance and injury prevention.
- Provision of behavioral and vocational services as determined by the respective Work Hardening provider.
- Promotion of patient/client responsibility and self-management.

Assist the patient/client to obtain as appropriate:
- Counseling for substance abuse.
- Engineering and ergonomic services
- Medical services
- Nutrition and weight control services
- Smoking cessation counseling.

Program Termination

The patient/client shall be discharged from the Work Hardening program when, the goals and outcomes for the patient/client have been met.

Work Hardening may be discontinued when any of the following occur:
- The patient/client is unable to continue to progress toward goals and outcomes because of medical or psychosocial complications or because financial/insurance resources have been expended.
- The patient/client declines to continue intervention.
- The patient/client fails to comply with the requirements of participation.
- The physiotherapist determines that the patient/client will no longer benefit from physiotherapy services.

When the patient/client is discharged or discontinued from the

Work Hardening program, the Work Hardening provider(s) shall notify the employer, insurance carrier and/or any referral source, and include the following information:

- Reasons for program termination
- Clinical and functional status
- Recommendations regarding return to work
- Recommendations for follow-up services.

OUTCOME ASSESSMENT

Outcome assessment is a systematic data collection designed to assess, at a minimum, achievement of goals and outcomes, and program effectiveness and efficiency. Effectiveness is a measure of meeting established program goals and outcomes, including return to work. Efficiency reflects total cost and time utilized to achieve established goals and outcomes.

Elements

Identify services provided as either Work Conditioning or Work Hardening.

Demographic Data

- Age
- Gender
- Race and ethnicity

Occupational and Injury Data

- Primary and secondary medical diagnoses
- Diagnosis by physiotherapist
- Work status prior to injury
- History of other treatment for this injury prior to entering the Work Conditioning or Work Hardening program, identifying all disciplines involved
- Date of injury
- Same injury
- New injury

- Date Work Conditioning or Work Hardening program was initiated
- Current and future employability
- Time off work
- Length of the program
- Hours/day
- Days/week
- Total days

Discharge Data

- Total charges billed for the program
- Program status (terminated or discharged) regarding return to work
- Same employer or different employer
- Previous job or different job
- Full time or part time
- Patient/client status at time of program termination/discharge
- Referrals for additional services not available in the program
- Payment source
- Worker's compensation board
- Private insurance

EMPLOYEE FITNESS PROGRAMS: IDEAS FOR PROMOTING EXERCISE AT WORK

- Develop a safe walking path around your workplace (inside or outside) to encourage workers to take a 10-15 minute walk before, during or after work. Make sure to include maps, distances, steps, and durations of the routes selected. Place them in a location where all workers can access them either on a corporate site, newsletter, or regular fliers.
- Ask upper management to support environmental changes at the workplace. Recommend implementation of policies that include opportunities for workers to obtain exercise during their workday. An example of a policy might include fitness breaks (15-20) at least once per day for all workers.
- Implement a workplace stretching program before, during, or

after each shift. Even starting with one stretch break a day will make a big difference.

- Give or subsidize the cost of pedometers or step counters for all workers. This will help them keep track of how much exercise they accumulate each day. Help them locate their baseline and then provide regular challenges for them to enhance daily step activity.
- Educate workers about how much exercise they can accumulate by walking to a co-workers office or workstation rather than using the telephone or email. Post parking stall signs that encourage workers to park further away from the entrance.
- Encourage workers to take the stairs by hanging signs near elevators and stairs and educate them about how many steps they can accumulate by doing so.
- For workers that do want to join a health club provide reimbursements to workers based on usage of the facility. Many places will have the ability to give usage reports on a monthly or quarterly basis to help keep track of attendance.
- Encourage workers to host walking meetings when possible to enhance exercise while in the workplace.

Employee fitness programs should strive to enhance exercise at the workplace and outside the workplace. Think creatively and ask your wellness committee to help out in designing and maintaining your employee fitness programs.

RISK ASSESSMENT

There are good reasons for this. If the risk assessment process – the start of the health and safety management approach – is not done well or not done at all, the appropriate preventive measures are unlikely to be identified or put in place.

Significant Hazards and Risks

All hazards identified by risk assessment should be addressed. The type of hazard, the degree of risk it poses and the severity of harm that may result vary from workplace to workplace and sector to sector. The following are just some of the issues.

- **Work equipment and plant:**
  - Inadequate mechanical safeguards to prevent contact with dangerous objects lack of maintenance of work equipment and vehicles cuts and splinters from blades, corners, sheet metal, tools or edges electrical hazards.
- **Workplace:**
  - Poor housekeeping: order, cleanliness and control poor visibility in areas where vehicles and lifting equipment such as mobile cranes are working the mixing of people and vehicles, particularly at entrances and exits to garages, warehouses and depots.
- **Workplace transport:**
  - Uncontrolled movements of objects such as poorly secured barrels and other loads and containers in storage, transport, distribution or handling. People being struck or run over by moving vehicles, falling from vehicles, being struck by objects falling from vehicles or vehicles overturning.
- **Workforce:**
  - Lack of information, instruction, training, supervision and education.
- **Working at height:**
  - On scaffolding, ladders, staircases, mobile and ramps; also there is the risk of objects being dropped on people working below.
- **Burns:** thermal burns caused by working with hot surfaces, hot liquids, vapours, gases or heating systems chemical burns caused by corrosive substances, in particular by the strong acids and bases used in such as cleaning.
- **Fires and explosions**
  - Caused by the conjunction of three factors — fuel, oxygen and an ignition source.
- **Dangerous substances:**
  - Can be fatal when inhaled; for example, the 'silent killer' carbon monoxide generated by incomplete combustion such as exhaust fumes.
- **Asphyxiation:**
  - Some work involves exposure to the risk of asphyxiation, i.e.

to a lack of vital oxygen. This can be the case in confined spaces such as vats, tanks, reactors or tubes.

- **Psychosocial factors:**
  Stress can increase the risk of industrial accidents.

Purpose of Risk Assessment

Employers in each workplace have a general duty to ensure the safety and health of workers in every aspect related to their work. The purpose of carrying out a risk assessment is to enable the employer to take the measures necessary for the safety and health protection of workers.

These measures include:

- Prevention of occupational risks
- Providing information to workers
- Providing training to workers
- Providing the organisation and means to implement the necessary measures.

Whilst the purpose of risk assessment includes the prevention of occupational risks, and this should always be goal, it will not always be achievable in practice. Where elimination of risks is not possible, the risks should be reduced and the residual risk controlled. At a later stage, as part of a review programme, such residual risk will be reassessed and the possibility of elimination of the risk, perhaps in the light of new knowledge, can be reconsidered.

The risk assessment should be structured and applied so as to help employers to:

- Identify the hazards created at work and evaluate the risks associated with these hazards, to determine what measures they should take to protect the health and safety of their employees and other workers, having due regard to legislative requirements.
- Evaluate the risks in order to make the best informed selection of work equipment, chemical substances or preparations used, the fitting out of the workplace, and the organisation of work.
- Check whether the measures in place are adequate.
- Prioritise action if further measures are found to be necessary as a result of the assessment.

- Demonstrate to themselves, the competent authorities, workers and their representatives that all factors pertinent to the work have been considered, and that an informed valid judgment has been made about the risks and the measures necessary to safeguard health and safety;
- Ensure that the preventive measures and the working and production methods, which are considered to be necessary and implemented following a risk assessment, provide an improvement in the level of worker protection.

Common Workplace Hazard Groups

1. **Mechanical hazards include:**

By Type of Agent

- Impact force
  - Collisions
  - Falls from height
- Struck by objects
- Confined space
- Slips and trips
- Falling on a pointed object
- Compressed air/high pressure fluids (such as cutting fluid)
- Entanglement
- Equipment-related injury.

By Type of Damage

- Crushing
- Cutting
- Friction and abrasion
- Shearing
- Stabbing and puncture.

2. **Other physical hazards:**
   - Noise
   - Vibration
   - Lighting
   - Barotrauma (hypobaric/hyperbaric pressure)

- Ionizing radiation
- Electricity
- Asphyxiation
- Cold stress (hypothermia)
- Heat stress (hyperthermia)
- Dehydration (due to sweating).

3. **Biological hazards include:**
   - Bacteria
   - Virus
   - Fungi
     - Mold
   - Blood-borne pathogens
   - Tuberculosis.
4. **Chemical hazards include:**
   - Acids
   - Bases
   - Heavy metals
     - Lead
   - Solvents
     - Petroleum
   - Particulates
     - Asbestos and other fine dust/fibrous materials
     - Silica
   - Fumes (noxious gases/vapors)
   - Highly-reactive chemicals
   - Fire, conflagration and explosion hazards:
     - Explosion
     - Deflagration
     - Detonation
     - Conflagration.
5. **Psychosocial issues include:**
   - Work-related stress, whose causal factors include excessive working time and overwork
   - Violence from outside the organisation
   - Bullying, which may include emotional, verbal, and sexual harassment

- Mobbing
- Burnout
- Exposure to unhealthy elements during meetings with business associates, e.g. tobacco, uncontrolled alcohol.

6. **Musculoskeletal disorders**, avoided by the employment of good ergonomic design.

Risk Assessment Tools

There are many risk assessment tools and methodologies available to help enterprises and organisations assess their risks. The choice of method will depend on workplace conditions, for example the number of workers, the type of work activities and equipment, the particular features of the workplace and any specific risks.

The *most common risk assessment tools are checklists*, which are a useful tool to help identify hazards. Other kinds of risk assessment tools include: *guides, guidance documents, handbooks, brochures, questionnaires, and "interactive tools"* (free interactive software, including downloadable applications which are usually sector-specific).

Workplace Health Promotion

According to the definition of the World Health Organisation (WHO), health promotion includes all measures that enable individuals, groups or organisations to have increased control over the determinants of health. The objective of all measures is the improvements of the health of individuals, groups, organisations and communities.

Health Promotion can be described as a process that enables people to reach a higher level of self-determination about their health and to strengthen it. In this sense, health represents a resource for daily life that enables a person or a group to fulfil their expectations and has a highly positive influence on behavioural attitudes.

Workplace Health Promotion (WHP) is the combined efforts of employers, employees and society to improve the health and well-being of people at work. According to the Luxembourg Declaration on WHP in the European Union, this can be achieved through a combination of:

- Improving work organisation and the working environment
- Promoting active participation in the process of WHP
- Encouraging personal development.

Why WHP?

Society and enterprises are now more dependant than ever on well trained, highly qualified, highly motivated and contented employees. Health is more than the mere absence of disease and actively promoting employee health is a comprehensive task that goes beyond accident prevention and the avoidance of work-related illnesses.

Significantly, work satisfaction, a pleasant working environment, and intelligent work organisation are just as important as safety helmets and good ventilation systems for example.

Health promotion at work is beneficial for the employees, for "healthy" employees are a vital resource in the process of creating a truly "healthy" company. In reducing sickness-related costs and increasing productivity, health promotion at work also has a direct benefit for the company.

Research results based on a large number of Models of Good Practice in enterprises from different European regions show the common success factors for workplace health promotion. These general characteristics of successful workplace health practice are independent of enterprise size and economic sector. The success factors include:

- Workplace health action should be based on an analysis of the health requirements and needs of an enterprise
- Health actions should to involve all stakeholders in enterprises, especially the workers, and representatives of intermediary organisations (a participative approach)
- WHP actions should seek to improve the quality of working life and conditions as well as focusing on the behaviour of the individual worker
- Workplace health action should become an integral part of management practices and daily working life at all levels of an enterprise.

WHP and Work-Related Stress

WHP offers a way to reduce work-related stress. Its aim is to influence those factors that promote worker's health. It succeeds by improving the working conditions, by promoting the employee's participation and by strengthening personal competence. A major contribution of company health promotion is having a methodological approaches and procedures in place.

In order to analyse the initial position, both the work loads as well as the subjective disturbances of well-being are being identified using different methodological tools such as questionnaires, tools for health risk appraisal and health circles. Additionally, health circles offer the chance to have an immediate participation of the employees who are involved in the process of reducing stress as experts in their own affairs.

In order to preserve the employee's capability in the long term, those responsible must face the problem of stress at the workplace. Stress prevention, which primarily identifies the causes of stress, has to set off processes and at the same time to integrate the changes in ergonomic working conditions, work organisation and individual behaviour. The major prerequisite in order to reach this aim is that the employees will be enabled to improve their own working conditions.

By actively engaging with their work situation, employees can recognise sources of stress in their work, reconsider their personal methods of dealing with stress and tap into new resources (e.g. for changing their work situation). The way the individual experiences situations and his or her behaviour can also change in this way. The long-term aim of active stress management for employees consists in individually creating and maintaining a balance between the demands of work and their own capabilities, skills and needs.

An important precondition for this consists in diminishing the experience of stress by strengthening individual skills in dealing with stressors.

Within a process where each step is built up on the previous one it is particularly important in the group to:

- Actively perceive stress

- Recognise methods of dealing with stress which may be dangerous
- Mobilise one's own resources
- Recognise the possibilities and limits of individual stress management
- Deal with anger
- Improve self-assertion in discussions with superiors.

In connection with further measures for workplace health promotion, optimal stress management, depending on the particular requirements of the situation, can include the following:

- Improvement of knowledge and skills in order to be able to cope better with the situation
- Planning and organisation of work by the individual responsible for carrying it out
- Setting-up of a personal communication and co-operation network
- Re-evaluation of existing demands, change of attitude, change of behaviour
- Physical activity and healthy way of life.

WHP aims at identifying and improving organisational conditions for better health. This includes addressing the working conditions that are conducive to health (physical and psychosocial) and in particular all relevant issues around work organisation.

There is strong evidence that the quality of job and workplace design has an enormous impact on health and well-being of workers. In particular, job and task design constitute an important potential for strengthening worker's resources conducive to health. Other factors that have to be considered include:

- Leadership style
- Recruitment and appraisal procedures, and
- Recognition schemes.

At the centre of this level, WHP aims at influencing corporate policies that impact either directly or indirectly on health and well-being. The main objective is to support a development that leads to a health-promoting organisational culture. Relevant policy areas include human resource management, quality management, occupational health and safety, and environmental health.

Employer's Roles and Responsibilities

Employers should carefully prepare what they are going to do in order to meet their responsibilities to make a risk assessment, and put in place the measures necessary for the safety and health of workers. It is recommended that they do this through an action plan for the elimination or control of risks.

The action plan should include:

- Commissioning, organising and coordinating the assessment
- Appointing competent people to make the assessments
- The person carrying out the risk assessment can be:
  - The employers themselves
  - Employees designated by the employers
  - External assessors and service providers if there is a lack of competent personnel in the workplace.
- People can demonstrate their competence by showing that they have the following abilities:
  - An understanding of the general approach to risk assessment
  - The capacity to apply this understanding to the workplace
  - The ability to identify situations where they would be unable to adequately assess the risk without help, and be able to advise on the need for further assistance.
- Consulting worker's representatives on arrangements for the appointment of those who will make the assessments.
- Providing the necessary information, training, resources and support to assessors who are the employer's own employees.
- Ensuring adequate coordination between assessors (where relevant).
- Involving management and encouraging the participation of the workforce.
- Determining the arrangements to be made for reviewing and revising the risk assessment.
- Ensuring that the preventive and protective measures take account of the results of the assessment.
- Ensuring that the risk assessment is documented.
- Monitoring the protective and preventive measures to ensure that their effectiveness is maintained.

- Informing workers and/or their representatives of the results of the assessment and of the measures introduced (making the records available to them).

Worker's Roles and Responsibilities

It is important that workers participate in the risk assessment. They know the problems and the details of what really happens when, they perform their tasks or activities, so they should be involved in the assessment. Their practical knowledge or competence is also often needed to develop workable preventive measures.

Worker's participation is not only a right, it is fundamental to make the employer's occupational health and safety management effective and efficient.

Worker's and/or their representatives have the right/duty to:

- Be consulted on arrangements for the organisation of the risk assessment and for the appointment of those undertaking the task.
- Participate in the risk assessment
- Alert their supervisors or employers regarding perceived risks
- Report any changes in the workplace
- Be informed of the risks to their safety and health and of the measures necessary to eliminate or reduce these risks.
- Be involved in the process of deciding on the preventive and protective measures to be put in place.
- Ask the employer to put in place appropriate measures and to submit proposals to minimise hazards or to remove the danger at source.
- Cooperate to help the employer to ensure that the working environment is safe.
- Be trained/receive instructions on the measures to be put in place.
- Take care as far as possible of their safety and health and that of others persons affected by their acts in accordance with the training and the instructions given by the employer.

In addition, it is important workers representatives are trained so that they understand risk assessment and their role in it.

REFERENCES

1. Workers' Compensation Year Book. Elisburg D [1995]. Workplace stress: legal developments, economic pressures, and violence. In: Burton JF, ed. 1995 Workers' Compensation Year Book. Horsham, PA: LRP Publications, 1995; pp. I-217-I-222.
2. American Psychologist. Sauter SL, Murphy LR, Hurrell JJ. Prevention of work-related psychological disorders. American Psychologist Jr. 1990; 45(10):1146-1158.
3. Bureau of Labor Statistics. BLS [1996]. Bureau of Labor Statistics Homepage [http://stats.bls.gov/]. Tabular data, 1992-96: Number and percentage distribution of nonfatal occupational injuries and illnesses involving days away from work, by nature of injury or illness and number of days away from work.
4. Encyclopaedia of Occupational Health and Safety. Sauter S, Hurrell J, Murphy L, Levi L. Psychosocial and organizational factors. In: Stellman J, ed. Encyclopaedia of Occupational Health and Safety. Vol. 1. Geneva, Switzerland: International Labour Office, 1997; pp. 34.1-34.77.
5. Families and Work Institute. Bond JT, Galinsky E, Swanberg JE [1998]. The 1997 national study of the changing workforce. New York, NY: Families and Work Institute.
6. Journal of Applied Psychology. Jones JW, Barge BN, Steffy BD, Fay LM, Kuntz LK, Wuebker LJ. Stress and medical malpractice: organizational risk assessment and intervention. Journal of Applied Psychology. 1988;73(4):727-735.
7. Journal of Occupational and Environmental Medicine. Goetzel RZ, Anderson DR, Whitmer RW, Ozminkowski RJ, Dunn RL, Wasserman J, Health Enhancement Research Organization (HERO) Research Committee. The relationship between modifiable health risks and health care expenditures: an analysis of the multi-employer HERO health risk and cost database. Journal of Occupational and Environmental Medicine, 1998;40(10).
8. Northwestern National Life (now ReliaStar Financial Corporation) Northwestern National Life Insurance Company . Employee burnout: America's newest epidemic. Minneapolis, MN: Northwestern National Life Insurance Company. (Note: This reference is the source for the statistics cited, 1991; p 5.)
9. Northwestern National Life Insurance Company. Employee burnout: causes and cures. Minneapolis, MN: Northwestern National Life Insurance Company. (Note: This reference is the source for the information presented in the graph, 1992; on page 4.)

10. Princeton Survey Research Associates. Princeton Survey Research Associates [1997]. Labor day survey: state of workers. Princeton, NJ: Princeton Survey Research Associates. Barsade S, Wiesenfeld B, The Marlin Company. Attitudes in the American workplace III. New Haven, CT: Yale University School of Management, 1997.
11. Occupational Health Guidelines: Work Conditioning and Work Hardening Programs, Amended BOD 03-00-25-62; BOD 03-99-16-49; BOD 11-94-33-109; Initial BOD 11-92-29-134] [Guideline].

Eleven

Instrument to Measure Health and Fitness

PHYSICAL SELF MAINTENANCE SCALE (PSMS)

Self Rated version Extracted from the Multilevel Assessment Instrument (MAI)

Name ______________________________ Date ____________________

1. Do you eat
   a. Without any help, 3
   b. With some help (cutting food, identifying for blind, etc.) or 2
   c. Does someone feed you? 1
2. Do you dress and undress yourself
   a. Without any help (pick out clothes, dress and undress yourself) 3
   b. With some help (dressing or undressing) or 2
   c. Does someone dress and undress you? 1
3. Do you take care of your own appearance, things like combing your hair
   (FOR MEN: and shaving)
   a. Without help, 3
   b. With some help, or 2
   c. Does someone do all this for you? 1
4. Do you get around your (house/apartment/room)
   a. Without help of any kind (except for a cane) 3
   b. With some help (from a person or using a walker, crutches, chair), or 2
   c. Don't get around your home at all unless someone moves you? 1

5. Do you get in and out of bed
   a. Without any help or aid, 3
   b. Only with some help (from a person or a device), or 2
   c. Don't you get in and out of bed unless someone lifts you? 1
6. Do you bathe – that is, take a bath, shower or sponge bath
   a. Without any help, 3
   b. With some help (from a person or device), or 2
   c. Only when someone bathes you (lifts in and out or bathes) 1
7. Do you have trouble getting to the bathroom on time?
   a. Yes, 1
   b. No, 2
8. About how often do you wet or soil yourself during the day or night?
   a. Never, 4
   b. Less than once a week, 3
   c. Once or twice a week, 2
   d. Three times or more a week, 1

Brooke Grading Scale for Upper Extremity Function

Overview

Brooke et al developed a functional grading scale for the upper extremity. While developed for persons with muscular dystrophy, it can be applied to patients with other disorders of the upper extremity.

Level of Function	*Grade*
• Can raise the arm over the head, starting with the arm at the side and abducting the arm in a full arc until the hand is over the head	1
• Can raise the arm over the head only be flexing the elbow or using accessory muscles	2
• Can not raise the hands above the head AND can raise an 8 ounce glass of water to the mouth	3
• Can raise the hand to the mouth AND cannot lift an 8 ounce glass of water to the mouth	4
• Cannot raise hand to mouth AND has useful function in hand (can hold a pen, pick up coins off the table, etc.)	5

Contd...

Contd...

- Cannot raise hand to mouth AND has no useful function in hand — 6

where:

- The original wording of the functional descriptions describes both sides being affected, presumably to an equivalent degree.
- Flexing the elbow in Grade 2 reduces the circumference of movement and makes the task easier to do.
- Grades 1 to 4 might be subdivided into those with and without useful hand function.

REFERENCES

- Brooke MH, Griggs RC, et al. Clinical trial in Duchenne dystrophy: I. design of a protocol. Muscle Nerve. 1981; 4: 186-197
- Lord JP, Portwood MM, et al. Upper extremity functional rating for patients with Duchenne muscular dystrophy. Arch Phys Med Rehabil. 1987; 68: 151-154 (Table 1, page 152).

Clinical Mobility Scale

Overview

A clinical Mobility Scale can be used to assess a patient's degree of moblity over time.

Parameters (see Table 11.1)

1. Upright posture
2. Walking
3. Gait
4. Sitting
5. Stair climbint
6. Hand-held appliances
7. Wheelchair
8. Time usage

Table 12.1: Mobility Scale

Mobility Parameter	*Finding*	*Rating*
Upright posture (how patient functions with or without prosthesis)	does not stand	0
	stands only with personal assistance	1
	stands with the assistance of a hand-held appliance (crutch cane walker)	2
	stands without assistance	3
Waling (how patient functions with or without prosthesis)	does not walk	0
	walks only with personal assistance	1
	walks with the assistance of a hand-held appliance (crutch cane walker)	2
	walks without assistance	3
Gait (how patient functions with or without prosthesis)	walks slowly or not at all	0
	walks at a moderately slow space	1
	walks briskly	2
	can jog or run	3
Sitting (how patient functions with a without prosthesis)	sits only for short periods of time and prefers to lie down	0
	sits without discomfort for short periods of time (1 hour)	1
	sits without discomfort for longer periods of time (over 1 hour)	2
	sits without discomfort	3

Contd...

Contd...

Mobility Parameter	*Finding*	*Rating*
Stair climbing (how patient functions with or without prosthesis)	cannot climb stairs	0
stair climbing (how patient functions with or without prosthesis)	can not climb stairs	0
	climbs stairs with assistance of another person	1
	climbs stairs with assistance of hand rail and/or crutches	2
	climbs stairs unassisted	3
Handhheld appli-ances (crutches and canes)	cannot use crutches or cane	0
	must use crutches	1
	uses single crutch or cane or two crutches intermittenity	2
	use no hand-held appliance	3
Wheelchair	moves with the aid of wheelchair most of time	0
	moves with the aid of wheelchair only for long distances	1
	occasionally uses wheelchair	2
	never uses wheelchair	3
Time usage	spends most day in bed or on couch at home	0
	spends most of day in chair at home	1
	spends most of day ambulatory but confined to the hosue	
	spends most of day ambulatory	3

Mobi1ity assessment score = (points for upright posture) + (points for walking) + (points for gait) + (points for sitting) + (points for stair climbing) + (points for hand-held appliances) + (points for wheelchair) + (points for time usage)

Interpretation

- minimum score 0 = least mobile
- maximum score 24 = most mobile.

REFERENCES

1. Barofsky I Cohen S.J. Sugarbaker PH. Chapter 16: Selecting a quality of life assessment instrument. standardized tests clinical assessments or crustom-designed instruments. pages 239. IN.
2. Wenger NK Mattson ME et al. Assessment of Quality of Life in Clinical trials of Cardiovascular Therapies. Le Jacq Publishing inc. 1984.
3. Sugarbaker PH Barofsky I et al. Quality of life assessment of patients in extremity sarcoma clinical trials. Surgery. 1982;91:17-23.

EVALUATING WEIGHT GAIN IN A CHILD DURING REHABILITATION FOR SEVERE MALNUTRITION

Overview

The change in a child's weight during nutritional rehabilitation for severe malnutrition can help monitor the adequacy of the therapy. Parameters:

1. number of days in time interval.
2. body weight in kilograms at beginning of the interval.
3. body weight in kilograms at the end of the interval change in weight over time interval in grams.
   = (weight at end of interval in kilograms) - (weight at beginning of interval in kilograms)) * 1000
   average daily change in weight in grams per day over time interval
   = (change in weight over interval in grams) / (number of days in interval) weight gain in g per kg body weight per day
   = (change In weight in grams per day)/(average body weight in kilograms)

where:

- The method uses the "average body weight". This could either be based on the beginning and ending weights, or on the daily body weights, or on the child's preillness weight.

Contd...

Contd...

Gain	Interpretation
< 5 g/kg/day	poor
5 - 10 g/kg/day	moderate (fair)
> 10 g/kg/day	good

The therapeutic regimen should be reviewed if the weight gain is poor, both for calculations and compliance. For Bhan et al the endpoint is reaching a weight for height that is 90% of the national median (50th percentile).

REFERENCES

1. Bhan MK, Bhandari N, Bahl R. Management of the severely malnourished child: perspective from developing countries. BMJ. 2003; 326: 146-151.
2. World Health Organization. Management of the child with a severe infection or severe malnutrition. Guidelines for care at the first referral level in developing countries. Geneva. 2000. Chapter 7: Severe malnutrition, page 90. Appendix A4.2, page 149.

GERIATRIC FUNCTIONAL RATING SCALE (GFRS)

Overview:

The Geriatric Functional Rating Scale (GFRS) can be used to evaluate the functional capacity of an elderly patient. This can help identify those patients who are able to function alone or with some assistance from those WHO require institutionalization. The authors were from the McGill University and Royal Ottowa Hospital in Canada.

Measures:
1. Physical condition
2. Mental condition
3. Functional abilities
4. Support from the community
5. Living quarters
6. Relatives and friends
7. Financial situation

Physical Condition	*Finding*	*Points*
Eyesight	good (watches TV, reads, does needle work, etc.)	0
	distinguishes faces	-3
	sees light only (or totally blind)	-10

Contd...

Contd...

Physical Condition	*Finding*	*Points*
Hearing	good	0
	requires a loud voice	-3
	deaf	-5
Mobility	fully mobile (dresses, carries parcels, rides bus, etc.)	0
	uses cane or should use one, dependent on railings	-3
	requires cane and other support	-15
	wheelchair	-15
Pulmo-Cardiovascular Function	no restrictions	0
	1 flight of stairs	-3
	partly or totally bedridden	-20
Diet	no restrictions	0
	restricted	-3

where:

- Total blindness is not scored in the original table.

Mental Condition	*Finding*	*Points*
Disorientation	none	0
	to time	-3
	to person and/or place	-15
Delusions	none	0
	suspiciousness	-3
	overt	-10
Memory loss	none	0
	benign	-3
	malignant	-20
Energy and drive	normal	0
	hyperactive	-5
	hypoactive	-5
Judgmentint	act	0
	impaired	-5
Hallucinations	none	0
	auditory and/or visual	-10

Contd...

Contd...

Functional Abilities	*Finding*	*Points*
Reads and writes letters	yes	2
	no	0
Able to use telephone	yes	5
	no	0
Able to bank and shop	yes	5
	no	0
Able to prepare simple meals and bake	yes	7
	no	0
Washes, dresses and toilets self without assistanc	eyes	5
	no	0
Uses public transportation	yes	7
	no	0
Able or would be able to take own medication and follow diet	yes	10
	no	0
Support from the Community	*Finding*	*Points*
Ethnic compatibility	yes	2
	no	0
If living alone, can get support and help from a reliable relative, friend, neighbor or janitor	yes	10
	no	0
Able to shop at reliable grocer's who is willing to deliver when necessary	yes	5
	no	0
Club available who is geared to the aged	yes	2
	no	0
Church or synagogue available and supportive	yes	1
	no	0
Library available	yes	1
	no	0

Contd...

Contd...

Support from the Community	*Finding*	*Points*
Other facilities available and supportive (park, shopping center, restaurant, movie theaters, etc.)	yes	1
	no	0
Public health nurses available	yes	2
	no	0
Meals-on-wheels services available	yes	2
	no	0
Homemaker services available	yes	2
	no	0
Friendly visitors available	yes	2
	no	0
Hospital with emergency room and clinic facilities available	yes	2
	no	0
Public transportation	yes	2
	no	0

Other	*Finding*	*Points*
Living quarters	able to access (elevator, ground floor, etc.)	3
	difficult access	0
Relatives and friends	not married but lives with compatible and helpful relatives or friends	5
	lives with incompatible relative, friend or spouse	0
	lives with able and compatible spouse	10
Financial situation	totally independent	5
	dependent on helping relatives	3
	dependent on Social Security or other community resources	0

Geriatric functional rating scale
= SUM (points for all of the measures)

Interpretation:

- Minimum score: -118
- Maximum score: +101

Contd...

Contd...

Score	*Interpretation*
> 40	able to live in their own home setting; do not need to enter an institution 20 – 40requires some supportive care but does not need to enter an institution; may benefit from a day care program.
< 20	requires care in a suitable institution/

THE COPD SELF-EFFICACY SCALE OF WIGAL ET AL

Overview

Wigal et al developed the 34-item COPD Self-Efficacy Scale for evaluating a patient with chronic obstructive pulmonary disease (COPD). This can help determine how much (or little) confidence the patient has in being able to cope with the disease. The authors are from Ohio University in Athens, Ohio.

Statements - How I feel when

1. I become too tired.
2. There is humidity in the air.
3. I go into cold weather from a warm place.
4. I experience emotional stress or become upset.
5. I go up stairs too fast.
6. I try to deny that I have respiratory difficulties.

7. I am around cigarette smoke.
8. I become angry.
9. I exercise or physically exert myself.
10. I feel distressed about my life.
11. I feel sexually inadequate or impotent.
12. I am frustrated.
13. I lift heavy objects.
14. I begin to feel that someone is out to get me.
15. I yell or scream.
16. I am lying in bed.
17. During very hot or very cold weather.
18. I laugh a lot.
19. I do not follow a proper diet.
20. I feel helpless.
21. I drink alcoholic beverages.
22. I get an infection.
23. I feel detached from everyone and everything.
24. I experience anxiety.
25. I am around pollution.
26. I over eat.
27. I feel down or depressed.
28. I breathe improperly.
29. I exercise in a room that is poorly ventilated.
30. I am afraid.
31. I experience the loss of a valued object or a loved one.
32. There are problems in the home.
33. I feel incompetent.
34. I hurry or rush about.

Responses

- Very confident
- Pretty confident
- Somewhat confident
- Not very confident
- Not at all confident

Subgroups

1. Negative affect (12): 6, 11, 12, 16, 20, 21, 23, 24, 27, 31, 32, 33
2. Emotional arousal (8): 1, 4, 8, 10, 14, 15, 18, 30
3. Physical exertion (5): 5, 9, 13, 29, 34
4. Weather or environment (6): 2, 3, 7, 17, 22, 25
5. Behavioral (3): 19, 26, 28

NOTE: Some of the questions seem redundant. While this may be justified for a psychological test, a shorter scale might be more useful clinically. It may be possible to reduce the scale to 22 statements:

1. I become too tired
2. there is humidity in the air (29) I exercise in a room that is poorly ventilated
3. I go into cold weather from a warm place (17) during very hot or very cold weather
4. I experience emotional stress or become upset (32) there are problems in the home
5. I go up stairs too fast (34) I hurry or rush about
6. I try to deny that I have respiratory difficulties
7. I am around cigarette smoke (25) I am around pollution
8. I become angry (15) I yell or scream
9. I exercise or physically exert myself (13) I lift heavy objects
10. I feel distressed about my life (27) I feel down or depressed
11. I feel sexually inadequate or impotent (33) I feel incompetent
12. I am frustrated (20) I feel helpless
14. I begin to feel that someone is out to get me
16. I am lying in bed
18. I laugh a lot
19. I do not follow a proper diet (26) I overeat
21. I drink alcoholic beverages
22. I get an infection
23. I feel detached from everyone and everything
24. I experience anxiety (30) I am afraid
25. I breathe improperly
26. I experience the loss of a valued object or a loved one

REFERENCES

1. Wigal JK, Creer TL, Kotses H. The COPD self-efficacy scale. Chest. 1991; 99: 1193-1196 (Appendix, pages 1195-1196).

THE CUMULATIVE ILLNESS RATING SCALE FOR GERIATRIC PATIENTS CIRS(G) OF MILLER ET AL

Overview

The Cumulative Illness Rating Scale for Geriatrics CIRS(G) was developed by Miller et al based on the Cumulative Illness Rating Scale of Linn et al. This can be used to measure the burden of current and chronic illnesses in the older adult.

Body Systems Evaluated

1. Heart
2. Vascular
3. Hematopoietic
4. Respiratory
5. EENT (eyes, ears, nose, throat, larynx)
6. Upper GI tract
7. Lower GI tract
8. Liver
9. Renal
10. Genito-urinary (ureters, bladder, urethra, prostate, genitals)
11. Musculoskeletal/integument
12. Neurological
13. Psychiatric illness
14. Endocrine/metabolic

Differences from the Original CIRS

1. Addition of hematopoietic item
2. Addition of breast to endocrine/metabolic

Degree of Severity	Points
No problem	0
Mild current problem or past significant problem	1
Moderate disability or morbidity; requires "first line" therapy	2
Severe or constant significant disability; uncontrollable Chronic problem	3
Extremely severe (life threatening), end organ failure, Severe impairment in function	4

Total score = SUM(points for number of body systems evaluated)
Severity index = (total score) / (number of body systems evaluated)

Additional tabulations

1. Number of body systems with severity grade 3
2. Number of body systems with severity grade 4

Interpretation

- Minimum total score : 0
- Maximum total score : 56
- Minimum severity index : 0
- Maximum severity index : 4

Performance

- The scale showed good inter-rater reliability with intra class correlation coefficients in range 0.78 ro 0.88.
- The scale correlated with the physician's estimate of global disease burden. It also correlated with disability as measured with the Older Americans Activities of Daily Living Scale.

Limitations

- It may be difficult to accurately convey the burden of multiple conditions by using a single index.
- A person could have multiple problems within a single body system. One way to handle this would be to move to a higher score if, two or more conditions of similar magnitude are present.

REFERENCES

1. Guralnik JM. Assessing the impact of comorbidity in the older population. Ann Epidemiol. 1996; 6: 376-380.
2. Linn BS, Linn MW, Gurel L. Cumulative illness rating scale. J Am Geriatric Soc. 1968; 16: 622-626.
3. Miller MD, Paradis CF, et al. Rating chronic medical illness in burden in geropsychiatric practice and research: Application of the cumulative illness rating scale. Psychiatry Res. 1991; 41: 237-248. (Figure 1, page 240).

GENERALIZED SELF-EFFICACY SCALE (GSES) IN PATIENTS WITH ARTHRITIS

Overview

The Generalized Self-Efficacy Scale (GSES) can be used to assess a person's perceived coping ability when faced with a chronic condition. The scale is independent of age and health status. It is also available in at least 9 languages, permitting international comparisons.

Items in the scale

1. I always manage to solve difficult problems, if I try hard enough.
2. If someone opposes me, I can find ways and means to get, what I want.
3. It is easy for me to stick to my aims and accomplish my goals.
4. I am confident that I could deal efficiently with unexpected events.
5. Thanks to my resourcefulness, I know how to handle unforeseen situations.
6. I can solve most problems if I invest the necessary effort.
7. I remain calm when facing difficulties because, I rely on my coping abilities.
8. When I am confronted with a problem, I usually find several solutions.
9. If I am in trouble, I can usually think of something to do.
10. No matter what comes my way, I'm usually able to handle it.

Response	*Points*
Not at all true	1
Barely true	2
Moderately true	3
Exactly true	4

GSES = SUM(points for the 10 items)

Interpretation

- Minimum score : 10
- Maximum score : 40

The higher the score, the greater the self-perceived self-efficacy.

REFERENCES

1. Barlow JH, Williams B, Wright C. The Generalized Self-Efficacy Scale in people with arthritis. Arthritis Care and Research. 1996; 9: 189-196. (Table 2, page 191)

LIFE SATISFACTION INDEX A OF NEUGARTEN ET AL

Overview

Neurgarten et al developed two indices for measuring life satisfaction in older persons. These can help identify both those who are successfully aging and those who may be facing difficulties due to illness, loneliness or other factors. The study population was from Kansas City and the authors were associated with the University of Chicago.

Attitudes Found Associated with Life Satisfaction

1. Zest for life, as opposed to apathy
2. Resolution and fortitude, as opposed to resignation
3 Congruence between desired and achieved goals
4. High physical, psychological and social self-concept
5. Happy, optimistic mood tone

Instructions

Here are some statements about life in general that people feel differently about. Would you read each statement on the list, and if you agree with it, put a check mark in the space under "AGREE". If you do not agree with a statement, put a check mark in the space under "DISAGREE". If you are not sure one way or the other, put a check mark in the space under "?". PLEASE BE SURE TO ANSWER EVERY QUESTION ON THE LIST)

Questions/Statements

1. As I grow older, things seem better than I thought they would be.
2. I have gotten more of the breaks in life than most of the people I know.
3. This is the dreariest time of my life.
4. I am just as happy as when I was younger.
5. My life could be happier than it is now.
6. These are the best years of my life.
7. Most of the things I do are boring or monotonous.
8. I expect some interesting and pleasant things to happen to me in the future.
9. The things I do are as interesting to me as they ever were.
10. I feel old and somewhat tired.
11. I feel my age, but it does not bother me.
12. As I look back on my life, I am fairly well satisfied.
13. I would not change my past life even if I could.
14. Compared to other people my age, I have made a lot of foolish decisions in my life.
15. Compared to other people my age, I make a good appearance.
16. I have made plans for things I'll be doing a month or a year from now.
17. When I think back over my life, I did not get most of the important things I wanted.
18. Compared to other people, I get down in the dumps too often.
19. I've gotten pretty much what I expected out of life.
20. In spite of what people say, the lot of the average man is getting worse, not better.

Responses: agree, disagree, unsure ("?")

Scoring

- "Agree" scored 2 point: 1, 2, 4, 6, 8, 9, 11, 12, 13, 15, 16, 19
- "Disagree" scored 2 point: 3, 5, 7, 10, 14, 17, 18, 20
- "?" scored 1 point
- Otherwise 0 points
- In the initial version (Neugarten, 1961), (1) 1 point was used for all 2 point items above; everything else was 0; (2) scoring "?" as 0 points would tend to make the intermediate person look more dissatisfied than they really are.
  Life satisfaction index = SUM(points for the 20 statements)

Interpretation

- Minimum score : 0
- Maximum score : 40

The higher the score, the greater the life satisfaction.

REFERENCES

1. Adams DL. Analysis of a life satisfaction index. J Gerontology. 1969; 24: 470-474.
2. McDowell I, Newell C. Measuring Health. A Guide to Rating Scales and Questionnaires, Second Edition. Oxford University Press. 1996. pages 198-203.
3. Neugarten BI, Havighurst RJ, Tobin SS. The measurement of life satisfaction. J Gerontology. 1961; 16: 134-143 (page 141).
4. Wood V, Wylie ML, Sheafor B. An analysis of a short self-report measure of life satisfaction: Correlation with rater judgments. J Gerontology. 1969; 24: 465-469.

KARNOFSKY PERFORMANCE SCALE INDEX

Overview

The Karnofsky Performance Scale Index allows patients to be classified as to their functional impairment. This can be used to compare effectiveness of different therapies and to assess the prognosis in individual patients. The lower the Karnofsky score, the worse the survival for most serious illnesses. Other similar scales of performance status include the Zubrod , TNM and AJC-ECOG scales.

Contd...

Contd...

General Category	*Specific Criteria*	*Index*
Description Able to carry out normal activities; no special care required	normal; no evidence of disease and no physical complaints	100
	able to carry on normal activities but has minor signs or symptoms of disease	90
	normal activity with effort; some signs or symptoms of disease	80
Unable to work; able to live at home and care for most personal needs; varying amounts of assistance needed	unable to carry on normal activities or to work, but able to care for self	70
	requires occasional assistance from others but able to care for most needs	60
	requires considerable assistance from others and frequent medical care	50
Unable to care for self; requires institutional or hospital care or equivalent; disease may be rapidly progressing	disabled; requires special care and assistance	40
	severely disabled; death not imminent; stay in hospital indicated	30
	very sick; necessary to be in hospital; active supportive treatment necessary	20
	moribund	10
	dead	0

[after Table 1, page 386, O'Toole (1991)]

OVERT AGGRESSIVE SCALE (OAS)

Overview

Yudofsky et al developed the overt aggressive scale (OAS) to describe verbal and physical aggression by patients. It is easy to complete and provides a reliable rating of aggressive events. It can be used to monitor the type and severity of episodes shown by a patient over time. The authors are from Columbia University College of Physicians and Surgeons and the New York State Psychiatric Institute.

Each episode is treated as a separate event.

For each category, the most severe behavior observed and the most extreme intervention used were rated.

Aggressive behaviors

1. Verbal
2. Physical against self
3. Physical against objects
4. Physical against other people

Behavior	*Aggressive Action*	*Rating*
Verbal	none	0
	makes loud noises, shouts angrily	1
	yells mild personal insults	2
	curses viciously, uses foul language in anger, makes moderate threats	3
	makes clear threats of violence to self or others; requests help to commit self	4
Physical against self	none	0
	action with no or minor injury (picks or scratches self; pulls hair)	1
	hurts self without serious injury (bangs head, hits object with fist, throws self to the floor, throws self at something)	2
	small cuts or bruises, minor burns	3
	serious injury (mutilates self, deep cuts, bites that bleed, internal injury, fracture, loss of teeth, loss of consciousness)	4

contd...

contd...

Behavior	*Aggressive Action*	*Rating*
Physical against object	none	0
	slams door, scatters clothes, makes a mess	1
	throws objects down; kicks furniture without breaking it; marks the wall	2
	breaks objects, smashes windows	3
	sets fires, throws objects in a dangerous manner	4
Physical against others	none	0
	threatening gestures, swings at others, grabs at clothes	1
	action without injury (strikes, kicks, pushes, pulls hair)	2
	action with mild to moderate physical injury (bruise, sprain, welt, other)	3
	action with severe physical injury (broken bone, deep laceration, internal injury)	4

Interventions (one or more of the following)

1. None
2. Talking with patient
3. Places under closer observation
4. Holds patient
5. Immediate medication by mouth
6. Immediate medication by injection
7. Isolation without seclusion (time out)
8. Seclusion
9. Use of restraints
10. Injury requiring immediate medical attention
11. Injury to someone else requiring immediate medical attention

REFERENCES

1. Yudofsky SC, Silver JM, et al. The overt aggression scale for the objective rating of verbal and physical aggression. Am J Pyschiatry. 1986; 143: 35-39

PHYSICAL SELF-MAINTENANCE SCALE OF LAWTON

Overview

Lawton used the Physical Self-Maintenance Scale to evaluate the ability of a patient to live with complete independence. While developed for the elderly it can be used in other persons with disabilities. The author is from the Philadelphia Geriatric Center.

NOTE: The scale shows similarities to other scales in this section, such as the Katz Index of Independence in ADL.

Parameters

1. Use of toilet
2. Feeding
3. Dressing
4. Grooming (neatness, hair, nails, hands, face, clothing)
5. Physical ambulation
6. Bathing

Parameter	*Finding (Paraphrased from the Original Text)*	*Original points*	*Modified points*
Use of toilet	complete care for self on toilet and no incontinence	1	4
	needs to be reminded or help in cleaning self or has rare accidents	0	3
	soils or wets self while asleep more than once a week	0	2
	soils or wets self while awake more than once a week	0	1
	no control of bowel or bladder	0	0
Feeding	prepares meals, eats and cleans up without assistance	1	4
	requires minor assistance	0	3
	requires moderate assistance and is untidy	0	2
	requires extensive assistance for all meals	0	1
	does not feed self at all and resists efforts of other to feed	0	0

Contd...

Contd...

Parameter	*Finding (Paraphrased from the Original Text)*	*Original points*	*Modified points*
Dressing	does completely on own	1	4
	sses and undresses self with minor assistance	0	3
	needs moderate assistance	0	2
	needs major assistance and cooperates with others	0	1
	completely unable to do and resists efforts of others to help	0	0
Grooming	always neatly dressed and groomed without assistance	1	4
	grooms self adequately but needs help occasionally with some activities	0	3
	needs moderate and regular assistance or supervision	0	2
	needs total grooming care but can remain well-groomed	0	1
	actively works against any effort to groom	0	0
Ambulation	completely independent ambulates about residence or for up to a block outside	1	4
	ambulates with assistance of a person or mobility device (cane, walker, wheelchair, etc.)	0	2
	sits unsupported in chair or wheelchair but cannot propel self without help	0	1
	bedridden most of the time	0	0
Bathing	bathes self without help	1	4
	bathes self but needs help getting in and out of tub	0	3
	washes face and hands but needs help elsewhere	0	2
	does not wash self but cooperates with efforts to clean	0	1
	does not wash self and resists efforts of others to wash	0	0

Contd...

Contd...

where :

- The original scale awards points only to full independence.
- Something not seen in many scales is the description of the patient working against attempts to dress, feed, groom or bathe.
- Use of toilet could be broken up into 2 parameters - use of toilet and incontinence. These could then be combined into a single result.

Total score in original scale = SUM(points for all 6 items)

Total score in modified scale = SUM(points for all 6 items)

Number of items at a given level in modified scale = SUM (number of parameters at given level)

Interpretation

- Minimum score in original or modified scale: 0
- Maximum score in original scale: 6
- Maximum score in modified scale: 24
- The higher the score the greater the independence.

Twelve

Role of International Organizations in Health Sector

- WHO
- ICRC
- DPI
- SPI
- SIDA
- CARE
- UNICEF

NGO

Non-governmental organization (NGO) is a term that has become widely accepted as referring to a legally constituted, non-*governmental* organization created by natural or legal persons with no participation or representation of any government. In the cases in which NGOs are funded totally or partially by governments, the NGO maintains its non-governmental status and excludes government representatives from membership in the organization.

The number of *internationally operating NGOs* is estimated at 40,000. National numbers are even higher: *Russia* has 277,000 NGOs. *India* is estimated to have between 1 million and 2 million NGOs.

Apart from "NGO", often alternative terms are used as for example: independent sector, volunteer sector, civil society, grassroots organizations, transnational social movement organizations, private voluntary organizations, self-help organizations and non-state actors (NSA's).

Non-governmental organizations are a heterogeneous group. A long list of acronyms has developed around the term "NGO".

World Health Organization

World Health Organization (WHO) (http://www.who.int/en/)

The **World Health Organization** (**WHO**) is a specialized agency of the *United Nations* (UN) that acts as a coordinating authority on international *public health*. Established on 7 April 1948, and headquartered in *Geneva, Switzerland*, the agency inherited the mandate and resources of its predecessor, the Health Organization, which had been an agency of the *League of Nations*.

WHO operates through three principal organs: the World Health Assembly, which meets annually as the general policy-making body; an Executive Board of health specialists elected for three-year terms by the assembly; and a Secretariat, which has regional offices and field staff throughout the world. The organization is financed primarily from annual contributions made by member governments on the basis of relative ability to pay. In addition, after 1951, WHO was allocated substantial resources from the expanded technical-assistance program of the UN.

The work of WHO may be divided into three categories:

Health Information: WHO provides a central clear inghouse and research services. It established a codified set of international sanitary regulations, for example, designed to standardize quarantine measures without interfering unnecessarily with trade and air travel across national boundaries. The central WHO Secretariat also keeps member countries informed of the latest developments in the use of vaccines, cancer research, nutritional discoveries, control of drug addiction, and health hazards of nuclear radiation.

Disease Control: WHO sponsors measures for the control of epidemic and endemic disease by promoting mass campaigns involving nationwide vaccination programs, instruction in the use of antibiotics and insecticides, the improvement of laboratory and clinical facilities for early diagnosis and prevention, assistance in providing pure-water supplies and sanitation systems, and health education for people living in rural communities. These campaigns have had some success against tuberculosis, malaria, and venereal disease. There has also been considerable progress against cholera, trachoma, yellow fever, and yaws. In May 1980 smallpox was globally eradicated, a feat due largely to the efforts of WHO.

Consultation and Education: WHO encourages efforts to strengthen and expand the public health administrations of member nations. The organization, on request, provides technical advice to governments in the preparation of long-term national health plans, sends out international teams of experts to conduct field surveys and demonstration projects, helps set up local health centres, and offers aid in the development of national training institutions for medical and nursing personnel. It also makes teachers available for on-the-spot training, and it grants traveling-fellowship awards to doctors, public-health administrators, nurses, sanitary inspectors, and laboratory technicians.

In 2003 WHO came under the searchlight of the global media with its role in coordinating the international efforts designed to deal with the epidemic of severe acute respiratory syndrome (SARS). In this context it was again clear that WHO is indispensable to health on this earth.

www.nrcissi.org

The Spastics Society of India is India's most noted *non-profit* and a *Non-governmental organization* (NGO), working for Neuro-Muscular and Developmental Disabilities. Started in 1972, to provide education and treatment services for the *spastics* (children suffering from *cerebral palsy*).

Role of International Organizations in Health Sector

Today it has broadened its scope to include programs on teacher training, vocational training of young adults with Cerebral Palsy, Autism, Mental Retardation, Multiple Disabilities and Learning Disabilities. It also works in the field of advocacy and awareness and offers support to parents and other professionals. It has led to the formation of independent Spastic societies in 16 states in India. In 1999, it established the 'National Resource Centre for Inclusion (NRCI), in *Mumbai*, to include disabled children from special schools into normal schools.

State wise Spastics Societies in India

- Spastic Society of Eastern India, *Kolkata* now known as Indian Institute of Cerebral palsy IICP. (www.IICPindia.com)
- The Spastics Society of *Karnataka* (SSK), *Bangalore*
- The Spastics Society of Northern India, *New Delhi*
- The Spastics Society of Sikkim
- The Spastics Society of Tamil Nadu (SPASTN), *Chennai.*

www.dpi.org

Disabled People's International (DPI) is an *international non-governmental organization* (INGO) headquartered in Canada, with regional offices in Asia Pacific, Middle East, Europe, Africa, Latin America and the Caribbean. DPI is a network of national organizations or assemblies of people with disabilities, established in 1981 to promote the *human rights* of people with disabilities through full participation, equalization of opportunity and development.

DPI assists organizations in over 120 nations with the day to day discrimination and lack of equal opportunity faced by people with disabilities. The Goals of DPI are to:

- Promote the human rights of people with disabilities

- Promote economic and social integration of people with disabilities
- Develop and support organizations of people with disabilities.

DPI holds special consultative status with the United Nations and collaborates with many international organizations and Governments of the world.

ICRC

www.icrc.org

The **International Committee of the Red Cross (ICRC)** is a private *humanitarian* institution based in *Geneva, Switzerland*. States parties (signatories) to the four Geneva Conventions of 1949 and their Additional Protocols of 1977 and 2005 have given the ICRC a mandate to protect the victims of international and internal *armed conflicts*. Such victims include war wounded, *prisoners, refugees,civilians*, and other *non-combatants*.

The ICRC is part of the *International Red Cross and Red Crescent Movement* along with the *International Federation* and 186 *National Societies*. It is the oldest and most honoured organization within the movement and one of the most widely recognized *organizations* in the world, having won three *Nobel Peace Prizes* in 1917, 1944, and 1963.

The official mission statement says that: "The International Committee of the Red Cross (ICRC) is an impartial, neutral, and independent organization whose exclusively humanitarian mission is to protect the lives and dignity of victims of war and internal violence and to provide them with assistance." It also directs and coordinates international *relief* and works to promote and strengthen *humanitarian law* and universal humanitarian principles. The core tasks of the Committee, which are derived from the Geneva Conventions and its own statutes, are the following:

- To monitor compliance of warring parties with the Geneva Conventions
- To organize nursing and care for those who are wounded on the battlefield
- To supervise the treatment of prisoners of war and make confidential interventions with detaining authorities
- To help with the search for missing persons in an armed conflict (tracing service)
- To organize protection and care for civil populations
- To act as a neutral intermediary between warring parties

The ICRC drew up seven fundamental principles in 1965 that were adopted by the entire Red Cross Movement. They are humanity, impartiality, neutrality, independence, volunteerism, unity, and universality.

care

http://www.care-international.org/About-Care/

CARE is one of the largest international development and *humanitarian organizations* in the world, with programmes in over 70 countries. The CARE International Secretariat is located in Geneva, Switzerland.

Worldwide staffing exceeds 14,000, most of who come from the nation in which they work.

CARE (originally "Cooperative for American Remittances to Europe", and later "Cooperative for Assistance and Relief Everywhere"), was a co-founded in 1945 by *Arthur Ringland* who had the idea and the perseverance to secure financial backing for overseas food relief packages, Lincoln Clark who focused on practical administration and Wallace Campbell who limited its scope to include voluntary agencies. The relief came in *"CARE Packages"*. Each CARE Package cost $10 and was guaranteed to reach its addressee within four months.

CARE's mission has evolved over the decades. CARE continues to provide emergency relief during and after disasters, but the organization today focuses on addressing underlying causes of poverty. In areas such as health, HIV/AIDS, natural resources, education and economic development, CARE works to empower women, because experience has shown those women's gains yield dramatic benefits for families and communities. CARE also advocates for policies that defend human rights and promote the eradication of poverty.

Today CARE International is an international confederation composed of twelve national members. Each member is an autonomous non-governmental organisation in its own right, registered and governed according to national law as a charitable body.

CARE's Campaigns in the Fight Against Global Poverty Include

- **The World Hunger Campaign** – Donations to CARE sponsor feeding programs, education, microcredit loans, sustainable agriculture and other projects designed to reduce world hunger and poverty.
- **Education** – CARE partners with governments, communities and organizations to improve the quality and accessibility of basic education.
- **HIV/AIDS** – CARE provides educational programs and supports grassroots efforts to reduce the spread of the disease and to aid those affected by HIV/AIDS.
- **Victories Over Poverty** - CARE works with communities to provide emergency relief, and long-term solutions to poverty.
- **CARE for the Child** - Supporters may automatically contribute funds via the CARE for the Child monthly giving program.

CARE supplies and equipment, including food, water, repair water systems and sanitation kits to pediatric hospitals, health centers, and vulnerable families.

http://www.unicef.org

The **United Nations Children's Fund** (or **unicef**) was created by the *United Nations General Assembly* on December 11, 1946, to provide emergency food and healthcare to children in countries that had been devastated by *World War II*. In 1953, UNICEF became a permanent part of the *United Nations System* and its name was shortened from the original **United Nations International Children's Emergency Fund** but it has continued to be known by the popular *acronym* based on this old name. Headquartered in *New York City*, UNICEF provides long-term *humanitarian* and developmental assistance to *children* and *mothers* in *developing countries*.

UNICEF relies on contributions from governments and private donors and UNICEF's total income for 2006 was $2,781,000,000. Governments contribute two thirds of the organization's resources; private groups and some 6 million individuals contribute the rest through the National Committees. UNICEF's programs emphasize developing community-level services to promote the health and well-being of children. UNICEF was awarded the *Nobel Peace Prize* in 1965 and the *Prince of Asturias Award* of Concord in 2006.

Sida

www.sida.org

Sida is the Swedish Governmental agency providing technical assistance and funding throughout the world. Sida is a government agency of the country of Sweden with over 650 employees. Sida channels its resources through NGOs, multilateral cooperation, and the EU, among others and is interested in promoting the idea of "international development cooperation" to replace the one-sided giving indicated by the term "assistance." Supporting over 2,000 projects in over 100 countries (over 20 of them are specially designated as target countries), Sida seeks to create partnerships with companies, popular movements, organizations, universities, and government agencies for its development projects. Sida's geographic focus is on countries in Africa, Asia, Latin America, and Central and Eastern Europe.

Goals

1. **Economic growth:** To help increase the production of goods and services.
2. **Economic and social equality:** To help reduce differences between rich and poor and ensure that everyone's basic needs are met.
3. **Economic and political independence:** To help to ensure that countries can make their own decisions on their economies and policies and create the conditions necessary for national self-determination.
4. **Democratic development:** To help to ensure that people are given greater opportunities to influence developments locally, regionally and nationally.
5. **Environmental protection**: To promote the sustainable use of natural resources and protection of the environment.
6. **Gender equality:** To promote equality between men and women.

Table 12.1: International Days

Date	Days
January 24	National girl child day of India, recognized by India
February 4	World Cancer Day
February 20	World Day of Social Justice, recognized by the UN
March 8	International Women's Day , recognized by the UN
March 15	World Consumer Rights Day

Contd...

Contd...

Date	Days
March 20	International Day of the Francophonie (site (French))
March 20	World Day of Theatre for Children and Young People
March 24	International Day for Achievers, World Tuberculosis Day, recognized by the UN
April 2	World Autism Awareness Day, recognized by the UN
April 7	World Health Day, recognized by the World Federation of Hemophilia
April 17	World Hemophilia Day, recognized by the UN
April 25	World Malaria Day, recognized by the WHO
May 8	World Red Cross & Red Crescent Day
May 10	International Mothers Day
May 12	International Nurses Day
May 19	World Hepatitis Day
May 31	World No Tobacco Day, recognized by the UN
1st Tuesday of May	World Asthma Day
June 5	World Environment Day, recognized by the UN
June 8	World Brain Tumour Day
June 19	World Sickle Cell Anaemia Awareness Day
July 11	World Population Day, recognized by the UN
August 12	International Youth Day, recognized by the UN
September 11	World First Aid Day
September 21	World Alzheimer's Day
September 28	World Rabies Day
October 1	International Day of Older Persons, recognized by the UN
October 2	International Day of Non-Violence, recognized by the UN, observed on M.K. Gandhi's birthday
October 10	World Mental Health Day, recognized by the UN
October 15	International Day of Rural Women, recognized by the UN
October 16	World Food Day, recognized by the UN
October 17	International Day for the Eradication of Poverty, recognized by the UN

Contd...

Contd...

Date	Days
October 24	United Nations Day, recognized by the UN
November 14	World Diabetes Day, recognized by the UN
December 1	World AIDS Day, recognized by the UN
December 3	International Day of Persons with Disabilities, recognized by the UN
December 10	Human Rights Day, recognized by the UN.

REFERENCES

WHO

1. Constitution of the World Health Organization (PDF). World Health Organization. Retrieved 2007-07-18. – For an easier to read version see "Constitution of the World Health Organization (English only version)"(PDF). World Health Organization. Retrieved 2008-02-11.
2. Chronicle of the World Health Organization, April 1948 (PDF). World Health Organization. pp. 54. Retrieved 2007-07-18.
3. Chronicle of the World Health Organization, 1947 (PDF). Retrieved 2007-07-18.
4. United Nations General Assembly Resolution 61 session 1 Establishment of the World Health Organization on 14 December 1946
5. Iriye, Akira (2002). Global Community: The Role of International Organizations in the Making of the Contemporary World. Berkeley: University of California Press. ISBN 052023179.
6. ^ Collin N, de Radiguès X; the World Health Organization H1N1 Vaccine Task Force. Vaccine production capacity for seasonal and pandemic (H1N1) 2009 influenza. Vaccine. 2009 Jun 27. [Epub ahead of print]PMID: 19563891
7. Hayden FG, Howard WA, Palkonyay L, Kieny MP. Report of the 5th meeting on the evaluation of pandemic influenza prototype vaccines in clinical trials: World Health Organization, Geneva, Switzerland, 12–13 February 2009. Vaccine. 2009 Jun 24;27(31):4079–89. Epub 2009 May 9. PMID: 19406184
8. Xinhua - English
9. WHO | WHO reports some promising results on avian influenza vaccines
10. Sugar industry threatens to scupper WHO | Society | The Guardian
11. Diet, nutrition and the prevention of chronic diseases. Report of the joint WHO/FAO expert consultation. World Health Organization and Food and Agriculture Organization of the United Nations, Geneva, 2003. See section 1.3 A summary of population nutrient intake goals

of Chapter 5, Population nutrient intake goals for preventing diet-related chronic diseases
12. World Health Organization. Workers' health: global plan of action. Sixtieth World Health Assembly, May 23, 2007. Retrieved September 15, 2008.
13. WHO Collaborating Centres. World Health Organization. Accessed September 14, 2009.
14. http://ftp.who.int/gb/pdf_files/EB105/ee17a1.pdf
15. WHO liaison and other offices
16. http://www.who.int/fctc/en/index.html
17. Vatican: condoms don't stop Aids
18. New York Times, February 16, 2008 Gates Foundation's Influence Criticized By DONALD G. McNEIL Jr.

Spastic Society of India

1. Encyclopaedia of Social Work in India, by India Ministry of Welfare. Publications Division, Ministry of Information and Broadcasting (India), 1987. Page 197.
2. Spastics Society, Bandra, Mumbai - Profile Tata, www.tatainternational.com.
3. The Spastics Society of India Profiles of Nonprofit organizations. www.karmayog.com.
4. Focus on education for disabled children The Hindu, Jan 28, 2003.
5. Social Entrepreneurs provide examples of Leadership and Vision...: Mithu Alur, NRCI & Spastics Society of India
6. History www.nrcissi.org.
7. Touch of Herosim - Forming The Spastics Society Of India Godrej, www.change.godrej.com.
8. Indian Institute of Cerebral palsy
9. Indian Institute of Cerebral palsy Profile
10. Spastics Society ties-up with PACER Center, IBM India The Economic Times, Oct 24, 2007.
11. The Spastics Society of Karnataka Official website.
12. Major Activities of the Spastics Society Official website of Sikkim state.
13. Spastics Society of Tamil Nadu (SPASTN), Official website.
14. Spastics Society celebrates 24th anniversary The Hindu, Feb 05, 2005.
15. The Spastics Society of India, Chennai www.ngosindia.com.
16. Before the match, Pakistani players visited the spastics society in Madras BBC News, January 28, 1999.

ICRC

1. ICRC. 2008. ICRC 2007 Annual Report (Headquarters section). 35.

2. ICRC. 2008. ICRC 2007 Annual Report (Headquarters section). 32.
3. Discover the ICRC. 2007. Retrieved 2009-05-12. p.6.
4. Nobel Laureates Facts - Organizations". Nobel Foundation. Retrieved 2009-10-13.
5. Favez, Jean-Claude (1999). The Red Cross and the Holocaust. Cambridge: Cambridge University Press. ISBN 9780521415873.p. 75.
6. Mégevand-Roggo, Béatrice. Srebrenica – remembering the missing. 5 July 2005.
7. Red Cross Condemns Burman 'Abuses'" BBC News. 29 Jun 2007. *http://news.bbc.co.uk/2/hi/asia-pacific/6252024.stm*
8. ICRC in WW II: the Holocaust". Retrieved 2007-10-19..
9. Buignion, François (2002-11-05). "Dialogue with the past: the ICRC and the Nazi death camps". Retrieved 2007-10-19..
10. ICRC: Official Statement (2005-01-27). "Commemorating the liberation of Auschwitz". Retrieved 2007-10-19..
11. Reports: 'Disastrous' Iraqi humanitarian crisis. CNN. 2008-03-17. Retrieved 2008-03-17..
12. ICRC. The Mission.. 7 May 2006.
13. David P Forsythe, The Humanitarians: The International Committee of the Red Cross, (Cambridge, NY:Cambridge University Press, 2005), 161.
14. ICRC. The Fundamental Principles, 1 Jan 1995.
15. Forsythe, The Humanitarians, 233.
16. Forsythe, The Humanitarians, 225.
17. Forsythe, The Humanitarians, 203-6.
18. Forsythe, The Humanitarians, 208.
19. Bugnion, La Protection, 1138-41.
20. ICRC. New ICRC vice-president, 9 Dec 2005.
21. ICRC. ICRC presidency, 1 Jan 2006.
22. Forsythe, The Humanitarians, 211.
23. Forsythe, The Humanitarians, 219.
24. Philippe Ryfman, La question humanitaire (Paris:Ellipses, 1999), 38.
25. Ryfman, La question humanitaire, 129.
26. Georges Willemin and Roger Heacock, The International Committee of the Red Cross, (Dordrecht: Martinus Nijhoff Publishers, 1984).
27. Le CICR manqué de bras. LM, 20 July 2002, 15.
28. Forsythe, The Humanitarians, 231.
29. Andre Durand, History of the International Committee of the Red Cross: From Sarajevo to Hiroshima, (Geneva:ICRC, 1984), 147.
30. Forsythe, The Humanitarians, 52.
31. Forsythe, The Humanitarians, 37.
32. ^ Merson MH, Black RE, Mills AJ, eds.,International Public Health: Diseases, Programs, Systems, and Policies, 2nd ed, (Boston: Jones and Barlett, 2006), 497.

33. ^ David P. Forsythe, "Choices More Ethical Than Legal: The International Committee of the Red Cross and Human Rights," Ethics and International Affairs, 7 (1993): 139-140.
34. ^ Nelson Mandela, Speech before the British Red Cross, London, 10 July 2003. [1].
35. Fiona Terry, Condemned to Repeat? The Paradox of Humanitarian Action, (London: Cornell University Press, 2002), 45.
36. Nelson Mandela, Interview on Larry King Live, 16 May 2000. [2].
37. Nelson Mandela, Long Walk to Freedom (London: Little, Brown, 1994), 396.

CARE

1. http://www.care-international.org/About-Care/
2. CARE Campaigns", [www.care.org], Accessed December 7, 2007.
3. CARE readies humanitarian deliveries from Jordan to Iraq. Relief Web", April 18, 2003. Accessed December 8, 2007.
4. Director of CARE Iraq Abducted in Baghdad." "Fox News." October 20, 2004. Accessed December 8, 2007.
5. CARE profoundly saddened by the apparent death of Mrs. Margaret Hasan, [CARE.org], November 14, 2004. Accessed December 8, 2007.

UNICEF

1. UNICEF, Dictionary.com Unabridged, retrieved, 2009-06-04
2. US Fund for UNICEF
3. http://www.irishtimes.com/newspaper/ireland/2009/0725/1224251305112.html
4. http://www.independent.ie/business/irish/tesco-in-clash-with-unicef-1841427.html
5. UNICEF Team Canada
6. Newstrack India "International Tent Pegging", January 14, 2008
7. UNICEF, Hammarby strikes partnership (In Swedish)
8. Art in All of Us
9. NGO Monitor Analysis, (Vol. 1 No. 5), 11 March 2003
10. The Truth About UNICEF
11. UNICEF, WHO Want ' Alliance' with Church but Promote Abortion
12. Guatemala's baby business
13. The Guatemala 5000 Initiative
14. Innocenti Research Centre